Health & Social Care

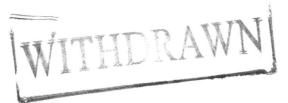

www.harcourt.co.uk

✓ Free online support
✓ Useful weblinks
✓ 24 hour online ordering

01865 888118

Series editor: **Beryl Stretch**

Heinemann, Halley Court, Jordan Hill, Oxford OX2 8EJ
Heinemann is the registered trademark of Harcourt Education Ltd

© Harcourt Education Ltd

First published 2007

12 11 10 09 08 07
10 9 8 7 6 5 4 3 2 1

British Library Cataloguing in Publication Data is available
from the British Library on request.

10-digit ISBN: 0 435 46425 6
13-digit ISBN: 978 0 43546425 7

Designed by Carolyn Gibson and Wooden Ark
Layout by Tower Design
Printed by CPI Bath Press
Illustrated by Calow2Craddock, HL Studios and Tower Design

Cover design by Wooden Ark
Cover photo: © Getty Images/Steve Krongard

Websites

Please note that the examples of websites suggested in this book were up to
date at the time of writing. We have made all links available on the Heinemann
website at www.heinemann.co.uk/hotlinks. When you access the site, the
express code is 4256P.

CONTENTS

Acknowledgements

Harcourt Education Ltd and the authors would like to thank the following people:

- Angela Clark and the CPA for permission to reproduce the extract on page 54.
- Jane Hancock and CMI for permission to use the '5 a day' logo on page 144.
- Ted Grossbart for permission to reproduce an extract of his article 'Is your itch medical or psychological?' on page 162.

'Summary of recommendations – a check list, Nos 148–157' in CPA *Home Life: A Code of Practice for Residential Care* ©1984 Centre for Policy on Ageing, London. Reproduced on page 54 with permission.

The definitions of addiction and substance abuse on pages 158 and 159 are taken from Sarafino, E.P. (1998) *Health Psychology – Biophysical Interactions*. (3rd ed.). Reprinted with permission of John Wiley & Sons, Inc.

The extract on page 186 is taken from *Advisory Committee on Dangerous Pathogens – Infection at work: controlling the risks*. Crown copyright and reproduced with permission of the Controller of HMSO and the Queen's Printer for Scotland.

Dee Spencer-Perkins would like to acknowledge the support given by Gail Lincoln and Neil Moonie who were both very generous both with time and resources.

Photos

AJ Photo/Hop Americain/Science Photo Library, p116; A. Parada/Alamy, p35 (right); Ashley Cooper/Alamy, p159; Blackburn North Healthy Living Centre, p260; Brenda Prince/Photofusion Picture Library, p21; Bubbles, p230; Charles Thatcher/Stone/Getty Images, p1; Chris Steele-Perkins/Magnum, p215; Comesa GesmbH, p157; Daemmrich Bob/Sygma/Corbis UK Ltd, p136; David M. Martin/Science Photo Library, p97; Deep Light Productions/Science Photo Library, p99; Digital Vision/Rob Van Petten, p16; Gareth Boden/Harcourt Education, p2; George Blonsky/Alamy, p182; Getty Images/PhotoDisc, p105, p265; Ghislain and Marie David de Lossy/Photographer's Choice/Getty Images, p133; Gianni Muratore/Alamy, p41; ImageState/Alamy, p269; Jack Sullivan/Alamy, p262; Jacky Chapman/Photofusion Picture Library, p207; Janine Wiedel Photolibrary/Alamy, p40; Jim Varney/Science Photo Library, p170; Jim West/Alamy, p13; John Powel/Rex Features, p35 (left); Mark Lloyd/Handout/Reuters/Corbis UK Ltd, p33; Mary Evans Picture Library, p211; Mauro Fermariello/Science Photo Library, p267; Medical-on-Line/Alamy, p195; Medisana AG, p151; Megapress/Alamy, p148; Mike Goldwater/Alamy, p43; Noah Clayton/The Image Bank/Getty Images, p65; Paul Doyle/Photofusion Picture Library, p249; Paula Solloway/Photofusion Picture Library, p222; PhotoDisc/PhotoLink, p35 (middle); Photofusion Picture Library, p29, p212; Photofusion Picture Library/Alamy, p258; Princess Margaret Rose Orthopaedic Hospital/Science Photo Library, p123; Rex Interstock/Rex Features, p253; Richard Smith/Harcourt Education, p56; Robert Brook/Photofusion Picture Library, p181; Scimat/Science Photo Library, p81; Tim De Waele/Corbis UK Ltd, p138; Voisin/Phanie/Rex Features, p165; Zooid Pictures, p159.

INTRODUCTION

Core Themes in Health and Social Care will support anyone undertaking a health and social care related course or pursuing a career in a health and social care setting. This book will be a valuable reference source if, for example, you are:

- a Level 3 student wishing to read around a subject and relate it to real-life practice
- a student on an OCR or BTEC course who needs up to date materials to refer to
- a student completing an Access to Nursing or Health Studies course and need a good textbook to use whilst studying.

Written by an experienced and respected team of authors, you can be sure that whatever health and social care course you are completing, you will find the information within this book relevant, up to date and thought provoking. Each chapter and its content has been carefully written to ensure coverage of the major themes and issues that form an integral part of health and social care studies. From anatomical and physiological information, basics of common disorders, the fundamentals of psychology and the influence of the mind on health and illness, to principles of first aid, health and safety issues and research methodology – if it's relevant to health and social care, you will find it in *Core Themes in Health and Social Care*.

How to use this book

This book incorporates many features that have been designed to make it user-friendly and actively encourage your learning and reflection on health and social care topics.

The first page of each chapter lists the key points that will be covered. Reading this list before you proceed with the chapter will give you a brief overview of the chapter and allow you to identify topics of interest. These key points should also be used to ensure that, after you have read the chapter, you take away with you the main messages of the chapter.

All chapters begin with a brief introduction to the main topic area. The various themes and issues explored within the chapter utilise the following features:

Scenario

The real-life examples from the health and social care environment in Scenario features enable you to put theory into practice and learn about situations you may or may not already be familiar with.

Did you know?

Did you know? features reveal a fact or statistic relating to the topic being explored.

Over to you

Activities and tasks suggested for you to carry out in Over to you features will develop your first-hand knowledge and understanding of the issues you have read about. Many Over to you features will ask you to collect data or try new experiences relating to health and social care work. These activities can often be used as starting points for assignments or can be further developed into research projects if desired.

It's my story

It's my story features give you a personal account from service users and individuals working in health and social care settings. By reading them you will gain valuable insight into the thoughts and feelings of those on both sides. You may be able to relate to some of the stories, whilst others may open up a new understanding of health and social care issues.

Reflection

Reflection features ask you questions relating to information you have recently read within a chapter or relating to your own experiences and knowledge of the health and social care environment, both as a service user and an employee.

Key concept

Key concept features highlight fundamental and integral concepts relating to learning about health and social care issues.

View Point

The world of health and social care is one of many different voices, views and opinions. Viewpoint features offer up two or more often opposing views on aspects of health and social care theory or practice. Use them to challenge your own views and beliefs and to start discussions with colleagues.

Working in health and social care environments exposes you to a host of often unfamiliar words, terminology and phrases. Definition features explain in clear terms what is meant by a word **emboldened** in the text, allowing you to fully understand the topic under discussion. Those words defined in Definition features can also be found in the glossary at the back of the book (see pages 300–302). A great quick reference tool.

Test yourself

Test yourself features appear at the end of chapters and at the end of some large topic areas within chapters. Answer the questions to check your knowledge and understanding of what you have read and identify any areas you may wish to read again or explore in more depth.

Working in health and social care is both challenging and rewarding. *Core Themes in Health and Social Care* has been written to help prepare you for both the theoretical and practical issues you will encounter every day and the core themes that will be a feature of your career.

Beryl Stretch
Series Editor

CHAPTER 1

Interpersonal skills in health and social care

Key points

- Working with people involves encounters of an emotional and social nature as well as the communication of information.

- The social and emotional outcomes of a conversation can often be more important than the communication of information.

- Observable interpersonal skills can be categorised as verbal, non-verbal and process skills.

- Successful interpersonal interaction requires the ability to understand other people's thoughts and emotions.

- Working within the system of care values involves demonstrating respect and value for others; essential to this is the ability to listen to and develop an understanding of other people.

- An essential starting point for providing emotional support to others is the ability to reflect on and question your own understanding of and assumptions about people.

- Reflective thinking skills provide a basis for the development of effective listening and support skills, and may be central to the delivery of interpersonal care.

Introduction

Interpersonal skills are the techniques people use in order to communicate and maintain effective social relationships.

> **Interpersonal** means 'between people'.

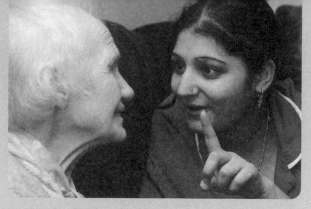

Interpersonal skills enable people to maintain effective social relationships

Tola

I work with older people. I can't imagine anyone coping with the role if they didn't enjoy working with other people. In my job, the things you say and the tone of your voice can really affect individuals.

One of the people I work with has dementia and she often says that she has to leave in order to go home and get dinner for her children. I guess she is imagining her life fifty years ago. I think if anyone tried to stop her or argue with her she would become very distressed. Confronting any person with the fact that they don't know where they are or how old they are must be incredibly painful. But on the other hand, if you ignore the person and let him or her walk out the door, then he or she is going to be at risk and will become distressed anyway – so you can't do that either. I approach this situation by engaging the individual in a friendly conversation. For example, the other day when she said that she had to 'go home now', I replied, 'Well, it's cold outside. You will need your coat – do you know where your coat is?' She immediately said, 'It's in my room'. So I suggested we went to her room to get it. As we walked to her room I talked to her about her daughter and grandchildren who visited last Sunday. When we got to her room, where there is a photograph of her daughter's wedding, I encouraged her to talk about her grown-up children. After a couple of minutes I asked if she'd like to go downstairs for a cup of tea. She thought that would be nice. I suppose she had forgotten about 'going home'.

Tola is able to prevent emotional distress because of her highly skilled caring behaviour. Tola's skills include:

- *Communication* skills – Tola is good at engaging individuals in conversation. Communication skills are analysed in detail in this chapter.
- *Understanding* – Tola has learned a little about the individual's past life. By imagining how she might feel in the individual's situation, Tola can also anticipate some of the feelings and emotions that the individual experiences.
- *Supportive skills* – Tola combines the skills of communication and understanding in order to make the individual feel respected and valued. Tola is able to create a conversational situation where the individual chooses to go downstairs for a cup of tea. Tola has made the person feel safe and has perhaps met her emotional need for company and purpose. Tola has used a basic approach which is similar to the way a counsellor might work.

Reflection

1   What might have happened if Tola had just communicated information to the individual without involving her in a supportive conversation?

2   Tola knew about the individual's past life – why was this so important?

3   Tola's interpersonal approach can be described as showing respect and value for the individual. Can you describe the interpersonal behaviour that shows this respect and value?

Communication skills

Verbal skills: formal and informal speech

We often use informal communication when we know people well, such as friends and family. This may include terms that other people would not understand or particular ways of speaking, for example, 'How's it going?' is an informal way of saying 'How are you today?' Because different groups of people use different informal language, it can be difficult to understand the informal communication of people from diverse social groups.

Health and social care work often involves the need for formal communication. For example, you might expect a hospital receptionist to say something like: 'Good morning. How can I help you?' This formal communication will be understood by a wide range of people. Formal communication also shows respect for others. It is possible that some people might prefer an informal greeting, since this could put them at ease. However, in many situations an informal greeting can cause people to feel that they are not being respected.

The degree of formality or informality of language is called the **language register**, and it establishes a context. For example, at a hospital reception you are unlikely to want to spend time making friends with the receptionist; you may be seeking urgent help. Your expectations of the situation might be that you want to be taken seriously and put in touch with professional services as soon as possible. You might see the situation as a very formal encounter. If you are treated informally, you may interpret this as not being taken seriously, or 'not being respected'.

> **Language register** — the degree of formality or informality of language.

Speech communities

Informal speech is very likely to identify a specific **speech community**. Different localities, ethnic groups, professions and work cultures each have their own special words, phrases and speech patterns. For example, an elderly middle-class woman is unlikely to start a conversation with the words 'Alright mate'. Some individuals may feel threatened or excluded by the kind of language they encounter. However, simply using formal language will not necessarily solve this problem. Technical terminology (often called **jargon**) may also create barriers for people who are not part of a speech community.

> **Speech community**
>
> A speech community might be based on people who live in a geographical area, a specific ethnic group, or different professions and work cultures. Speech communities are evidenced by their own special words, phrases and speech patterns.

> **Jargon** — terminology that people in a specific social or occupational speech community use.

Non-verbal communication

When people communicate, they generally use two language systems: a verbal or spoken language and non-verbal or body language. Within a few seconds of meeting an individual, even before the person speaks, you will usually be able to tell whether he or she is tired, happy, angry, sad or frightened. We can deduce what people are feeling by their non-verbal communication.

Non-verbal communication is the messages that people send without putting them into words. These messages are communicated through the eyes, the tone of voice, facial expressions, the hands and arms, gestures, the angle of the head, the way a person sits or stands (known as body posture) and the tension in the muscles. For example, when a person is sad, he or she may signal this emotion by looking downwards and avoiding eye contact. There may be tension in the person's face and neck, and the mouth may be firmly closed. In comparison, a happy person will smile, with 'wide eyes' that make contact with you. If excited, a person may show this by animatedly moving his or her arms and hands.

Understanding body language

To communicate effectively, care workers need to understand the non-verbal behaviour of the individuals they work with. They also need to understand their own body language and what this communicates to others. This is because non-verbal messages can be sent without deliberately meaning to communicate such messages.

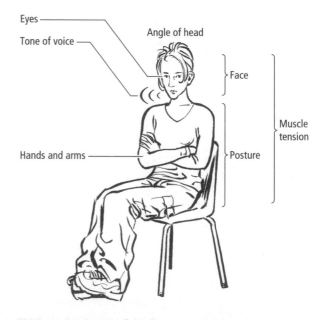

Figure 1.01 Areas of the body used in communication

The eyes

It is possible to guess a person's feelings and thoughts by looking in his or her eyes. One poet called the eyes 'the window of the soul'. The eyes get wider when a person is excited and attracted to or interested in someone else. A fixed stare may send the message that someone is angry. In European culture, looking away is often interpreted as being bored or disinterested.

The face

The face can send very complex messages which can be read relatively easily, even in diagram form. The face often indicates a person's emotional state.

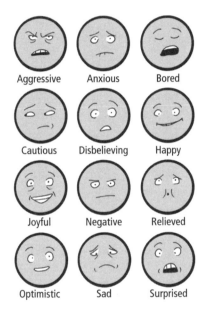

Aggressive   Anxious   Bored

Cautious   Disbelieving   Happy

Joyful   Negative   Relieved

Optimistic   Sad   Surprised

Figure 1.02 The face expresses emotion

Voice tone

It's not just what we say, but the way that we say it. If we talk quickly in a loud voice with a fixed tone, people may see us as angry. A calm, slow voice with varying tone may send a message of being friendly.

Body movement

The way a person walks, moves their head, sits, crosses their legs and so on, sends messages about whether he or she is tired, happy, sad or bored.

Posture

How we sit or stand can also send messages. Sitting with crossed arms can mean 'I'm not taking any notice' or 'I'm feeling defensive'. Leaning can send the message that a person is relaxed or bored. Leaning forward can show interest.

Muscular tension

Muscular tension in the feet, hands and fingers can indicate how relaxed or tense a person is. If an individual is stressed, tension will appear in the facial muscles and shoulders, and the person might sit or stand rigidly. A tense face is shown by a firmly closed mouth with lips and jaws clenched tight. A tense person might breathe quickly and become hot.

Figure 1.03 Communicating through body posture

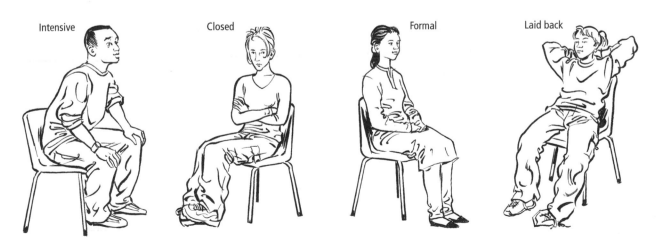

Intensive   Closed   Formal   Laid back

Gestures

Gestures are hand and arm movements that help to communicate what a person is saying. Some gestures carry a meaning of their own.

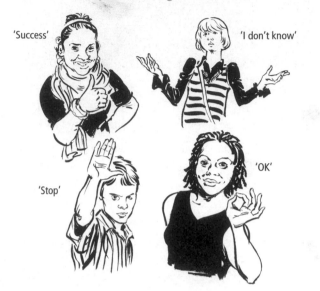

Figure 1.04 Some gestures common in the UK

Touch

Touching another person can send messages of care, affection, power or sexual interest. The social setting and person's body language usually help others to understand what touch might mean. Care workers should be careful not make assumptions about touch – holding someone's hand might be seen as an attempt to dominate.

Proximity

The space between people can sometimes show how friendly or 'intimate' the conversation is. Different cultures have different behaviours with respect to the appropriate space between people. In the UK, the expectation is that when talking to a stranger, people remain at arm's-length apart. The ritual of shaking hands indicates that you have been introduced, so the people may move closer together. When you are friendly with someone, you may accept him or her being in close proximity to you. Relatives and partners may not be restricted in how close they can come.

Proximity is a very important issue in health and social care work. Many individuals have a sense of personal space and it is important that this is treated with respect. A care worker who assumes it is fine to enter an individual's personal space without asking or explaining may come across as domineering or aggressive.

Face-to-face positions (orientation)

Standing or sitting eye-to-eye can send a message of being formal or being angry. A slight angle can create a more relaxed and friendly feeling.

Silence

One definition of friends is 'people who can sit together and feel comfortable in silence'. Sometimes a pause in conversation can make people feel embarrassed or uncomfortable. A silent pause can mean 'let's think' or 'I need time to think'. Silent pauses are fine as long as non-verbal messages which show respect and interest are given. Silence doesn't always stop the conversation – some care workers use pauses in a conversation to show that they are listening and thinking about what the client has said.

Barriers to effective communication

Communication can become blocked if individual differences are not understood. There are three main ways in which this happens:

- a person cannot see, hear or receive the message
- a person cannot make sense of the message
- a person misunderstands the message.

Examples of the first kind of block include visual disabilities, hearing disabilities, speaking from too far away and environmental problems such as poor lighting and background noise.

Barriers to communication
Barriers can exist at a physical and sensory level, when making sense of a message, and when misunderstanding arises within a particular cultural and social context. Effective communication depends on identifying the barriers that may block understanding.

Examples of situations in which people may not be able to make sense of a message include:

- the use of different languages, including signed languages
- the use of different terms in language, such as jargon (technical language), **dialect** or **slang**
- physical and intellectual disabilities, such as dysphasia (difficulty with language expression or understanding), aphasia (an absence of language ability), illness, memory loss or learning difficulty.

Dialect – words and the pronunciation of words that is specific to a geographical community. For example, people who live in the north-east of England generally use a different dialect to those who live in the south-west of England.

Slang – informal words and phrases that are not found in standard dictionaries but are used within specific social groups and communities.

Reasons for misunderstanding a message include:

- cultural influences – different cultures interpret non-verbal and verbal messages and humour in different ways
- assumptions about race, gender, disability and other social groupings
- the labelling or **stereotyping** of others
- the social context – statements and behaviour that are understood by friends and family may not be understood by strangers
- emotional barriers – a care worker's own emotional needs may stop him or her from wanting to know about others
- time pressures can mean that staff withdraw from wanting to know about others
- emotional differences – these can sometimes be interpreted as personality clashes or differences. Very angry, very happy or very shy people may misinterpret communication from others.

Stereotype – a fixed way of thinking involving generalisations and expectations about an issue or a group of people.

Strategies to overcome communication barriers

In order to minimise communication barriers, it is important to learn as much as possible about others. Individuals may have preferred forms of interaction. These may include a reliance on non-verbal messages, sign language, lip-reading, use of description, slang phrases, choice of room or location for a conversation, and so on. Everyone has communication needs of some kind. Table 1.01 details a range of strategies for overcoming communication barriers.

Barriers	Strategies for overcoming communication barriers
Visual disability	• Use language to describe things. • Assist people to touch things (e.g. touch your face to recognise you). • Explain details that sighted people might take for granted. • Check what people can see (many registered blind people can see shapes or tell light from dark). • Explore technological aids such as information technology that can expand visual images. • Check glasses, other aids and equipment.
Hearing disability	• Do not shout; speak clearly and normally; ensure your face is visible for people who can lip-read. • Display pictures or write messages. • Learn to sign (for people who use signed languages). • Ask for help from, or employ, a communicator or interpreter for signed languages. • Check that technological aids such as hearing aids are working.
Environmental barriers	• Check and improve lighting. • Reduce noise. • Move to a quieter or better-lit room. • Move to smaller groups. • Check seating arrangements.
Language differences	• Communicate using pictures, diagrams and non-verbal signs. • Use translators or interpreters. • Be careful not to make assumptions or to stereotype people. • Increase your knowledge of jargon, slang and dialects. • Re-word your messages: find different ways of saying things appropriate to the individual's speech community. • Check the formality of your language; speak in short, clear sentences if appropriate.
Intellectual disabilities	• Increase your knowledge of disabilities. • Use pictures and signs as well as clear, simple speech. • Be calm and patient. • Set up group meetings where people can share interests, experiences or reminiscences. • Check that people do not become isolated. • Use advocates – independent people who can spend time building an understanding of the needs of specific individuals, to assist with communication work.
Preventing misunderstandings based on cultural differences	• Try to increase your knowledge of different cultures and speech communities. • Watch out for different cultural interpretations. • Avoid making assumptions about or discriminating against people. • Use active listening techniques to check that your understanding is correct. • Stay calm and try to create a calm atmosphere. • Be sensitive to different social settings and the form of communication that would be most appropriate in different contexts. • Check your work with advocates who will try to represent the best interests of the people that you are working with.

Table 1.01 Minimising barriers to communication

Emotional barriers to communication

Individuals may have serious emotional needs; for example, they are afraid or depressed because of the stresses they are experiencing. Sometimes individuals may lack self-awareness or appear to be shy or aggressive. Listening involves learning about frightening and depressing situations. Care workers sometimes shun listening to avoid unpleasant emotional feelings.

Emotion can create barriers because care workers:

- are tired (listening fully requires mental energy)
- believe they do not have sufficient time to communicate properly
- are emotionally stressed by the needs of individuals
- react with negative emotions towards the culture of others
- make assumptions about, label or stereotype others.

Over to you

Complete the grid in Table 1.02 below to help you reflect on an interpersonal interaction that you have witnessed within a care setting. Use the following rating scale:

1. Good – there is no barrier.
2. Quite good – a few barriers.
3. Not possible to decide / not applicable.
4. Poor – barriers identified.
5. Very poor – major barriers to communication.

Table 1.02 Barriers to communication grid

In the environment					
Lighting	1	2	3	4	5
Noise levels	1	2	3	4	5
Opportunity to communicate	1	2	3	4	5
Language differences					
Appropriate use of language (terminology and level of formality)	1	2	3	4	5
Care worker's skills with different languages	1	2	3	4	5
Care worker's skills with non-verbal communication	1	2	3	4	5
Availability of translators or interpreters	1	2	3	4	5
Assumptions and/or stereotypes	1	2	3	4	5
Emotional barriers					
Stress levels and tiredness	1	2	3	4	5
Care workers stressed by emotional needs of others	1	2	3	4	5
Cultural barriers					
Inappropriate assumptions made about others	1	2	3	4	5
The labelling or stereotyping of others	1	2	3	4	5
Interpersonal skills					
Degree of supportive non-verbal behaviour	1	2	3	4	5
Degree of supportive verbal behaviour	1	2	3	4	5
Appropriate use of listening skills	1	2	3	4	5
Appropriate use of assertive skills	1	2	3	4	5
Appropriate maintenance of confidentiality	1	2	3	4	5

Communication skills for developing understanding

You can recognise other people's emotions just by watching their non-verbal communication, but you can't easily learn about other people's thoughts without good listening skills.

Listening skills

Listening is not the same as hearing the sounds that people make when they talk. Listening involves paying attention to another person's words and then thinking about what he or she means and what to say in response. Sometimes this process is called **active listening**; it is also called **reflective listening**. As well as thinking carefully about and remembering what a person says, good listeners make sure that their non-verbal behaviour shows interest. Good listening can feel like really hard work – instead of just being around when people speak, you have to build an understanding of them.

Active listening
Active listening involves being able to demonstrate what you have understood when you listen to another person.

Reflective listening
The word 'reflective' is used because the person's conversation is reflected back (like the reflection in a mirror) in order to check understanding.

Skilled listening involves:
- being interested in what the other person has to say
- hearing what is said
- remembering what is said
- checking understanding with the other person.

Checking understanding

Good listening involves thinking about what you hear the other person say and checking your understanding as the conversation goes along. This is an active process in which you both hear and reflect on the other person's ideas. Checking understanding in this way can involve listening to what the other person says and then asking questions about it. It may also involve putting what a person says into your own words then saying this back to him or her.

Did you know?
When you listen to complicated details of other people's lives, you often begin to form mental pictures based on what they say. Listening involves checking these mental pictures with the person who is speaking.

Reflection
Shona is very worried about the clinical health checks she must have. She says to you: 'But supposing they find that there is something wrong with me?'

How can you respond to Shona in a supportive way? Consider some of the possibilities in Table 1.03.

Possible response	Considerations
Try to be reassuring, e.g. 'I'm sure you'll be all right.'	Unless you are an expert with detailed knowledge of the person's condition, any attempt at reassurance is likely to sound false.
Offer advice, e.g. 'Try not to worry about it.'	Receiving unwanted advice can be very irritating. Many people will find advice such as 'don't worry' very unhelpful (and even patronising). They may perceive the advice as you trying to avoid the issue, i.e. the message you are communicating is 'please don't talk to me about health checks'.
Repeating what was said, e.g. 'Supposing they find that there is something wrong?'	Parroting phrases back to a person can come across as though you are behaving in a mechanical way. The person might respond: 'That's what I just said – didn't you hear me?'
Repeating the other person's message, e.g. 'You feel worried about the health checks.'	This response shows that you have listened and is an invitation to keep talking. The person's experience of being actively listened to may leave him or her feeling supported.

Table 1.03 Responding to an individual's concerns

Over to you

Take a piece of paper and divide it into four areas; for example:

- *where I live*
- *an important thing that happened in the past*
- *something I am looking forward to*
- *where I work or study.*

You can choose any four areas, as long as you can talk in detail about each one. Think through what you can tell another person about yourself. Then get together with a colleague who has planned his or her speech and explain the four areas to each other. This should take at least 10 minutes. Finally, see what you can remember about the other person and how detailed and accurate it is! How good are you at understanding and remembering?

Variation between cultures

Skilled care workers will be sensitive to variations in culture. Culture is the history, customs and ways that people learn as they grow up. The expressions that people use and the meanings that non-verbal signs have vary from one culture to another. For example, white middle-class people often expect others to 'look them in the eye' while talking; if a person looks down or away a lot, this is considered a sign that he or she is dishonest, sad or depressed. In other cultures, looking down or away while talking is a sign of respect.

Cultural variation
Communication is always influenced by cultural systems of meaning. Different cultures interpret verbal and non-verbal behaviours in different ways.

It would be impossible to learn every cultural variation of a non-verbal message, but it is possible to learn about the non-verbal messages that the individuals you work with are using. You can do this by first noticing and then remembering what others do – that is, which non-verbal messages are they sending? The next step is to interpret the non-verbal message. Finally, check your understanding with the person. This process involves active listening skills and thinking carefully about the person's responses.

Care workers have to be mindful not to assume that phrases, words and signs always have the same meaning, because these vary with culture, race, class and geographical location. Consequently, there are a vast range of meanings that can be given to any type of eye contact, facial expression, posture or gesture. Every culture develops its own special meanings. Care workers have to respect these differences and remember that it is impossible to learn all the possible variations of meaning.

SOLER principles

SOLER is an acronym formed from the words Squarely, Open posture, Lean, Eye contact and Relaxed. These words are drawn from a theory of non-verbal supportive behaviour identified by Gerard Egan (1986) (see Table 1.04). Egan states that the SOLER principles should not be used rigidly and that individual and cultural differences might require some modification of the principles.

Table 1.04 Egan's SOLER principles

Principle	Explanation
S: [Face] Squarely	Egan (1986) states: 'In North American culture, facing another person squarely is often considered a basic posture of involvement… what is important is that the bodily orientation you adopt conveys the message that you are involved with the client. If, for any reason, facing a person squarely is too threatening, then an angled position may be called for. The point is the quality of your attention'. The key issue is that you have to face other people in a way that shows that you feel involved.
O: [Keep an] Open Posture	Egan (1986) says: 'In North American culture, an open posture is generally seen as non-defensive'. Crossed arms or legs might send a message that you do not feel involved with the person you are talking to. An open posture involves not crossing the arms or legs.
L: Lean	Egan (1986) states: 'In North American culture a slight inclination towards a person is often interpreted as saying, "I'm with you; I'm interested in you and what you have to say" '. A degree of movement may help to convey interest in another person.
E: [Use good] Eye Contact	Egan (1986) argues that 'Maintaining a good eye contact with a client is another way of saying "I'm with you" '. Steady but varied eye contact is associated with deep conversation within a North American cultural context.
R: [Be] Relaxed	Egan argues that it is important not to fidget, and to feel comfortable and relaxed with your own non-verbal behaviour.

Egan's SOLER principles are open to debate, however. In a multi-cultural society, different communities may interpret specific non-verbal behaviours in different ways. In some situations (for instance, a middle-class social worker interviewing a working-class individual), sitting or standing squarely, maintaining an open posture and fixing the individual with steady eye contact might be perceived as a non-verbal attempt to dominate that person. Some individuals might, therefore, interpret SOLER behaviour as overly formal, officious or even patronising.

View point

It is possible to identify specific non-verbal skills that communicate a caring approach.

Viewpoint 1

Gerard Egan (1986) argues that there are some basic 'micro skills' that can help to create a sense of involvement when working with individuals. These should be enacted within all social and cultural contexts.

Viewpoint 2

Non-verbal behaviour can only be interpreted in relation to its specific social and cultural context. Care workers should, therefore, monitor how their behaviour appears to be received and adapt it through a process of self-reflection.

Reflection

How far do you believe that the five SOLER principles are likely to be effective in conveying care and involvement within social groups that you belong to?

Providing emotional support

Some communication between people is simply about sharing or 'transmitting' information. For example, a person may want to know what number bus to catch or may ask for a drink of water. A great deal of communication in the health and social care sector involves building an understanding of the individual and providing emotional support within a caring relationship.

Burnard and Morrison (1997) argue that caring and communicating are inseparably linked: care workers need to care about the people they work with in order to communicate effectively with them.

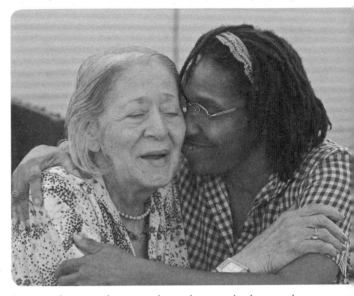

Care workers need to care about the people they work with in order to communicate effectively with them

Most individuals will have emotional needs that will not be satisfied by the simple provision of information. Consider the following three situations:

- *Situation 1* – a woman with a terminal illness is receiving care in a hospital setting. She says to her care worker: 'Please stay with me. I want someone to be with me. I don't want to be alone.'
- *Situation 2* – a young man with a learning difficulty comes to his care worker in tears and says, 'Nobody likes me. Will you be my friend?'
- *Situation 3* – a mother is experiencing intense grief following the death of her son. She explains, 'I just don't know how I can go on living. I feel like I have lost my insides – you can't begin to imagine how it feels.'

The examples above illustrate a range of situations where a caring response or caring interpersonal interaction is required. The first person wants someone simply to listen or provide a 'caring presence'; the second person is looking for an emotional response which suggests he is valued socially; the third person may experience some emotional support if she believes that others respect and understand something of her experience. These three people are expressing emotional needs and an appropriate response will have to address these needs; providing answers or information, or offering to undertake practical tasks, will not meet the individuals' requirements.

Interpersonal interaction and the need for 'someone to be there'

To some extent, everybody has an emotional need for someone to 'be there for them'. This 'being there' is not necessarily about personal attachments or relationships, but rather that many people cannot function effectively in isolation. If you experience threat, rejection or grief, you may need someone to provide support simply by being present. One way of explaining this need is to note that people develop an understanding of themselves and the world that they live in within a framework of social assumptions. Contact with other people may provide an increased feeling of security – a feeling of being 'connected' to others.

Finnegan (2004) uses the concept of interconnectedness to explain social interaction. He argues that effective communication depends on a sort of social inclusion where people can understand and share common assumptions. For example, interaction between people involves a wide range of social and emotional assumptions, and speech only conveys meaning within a framework of social and linguistic conventions.

Perhaps some people need to feel the presence of others in order to function. Just being with someone – touching a person's shoulder or holding his or her hand – may help to maintain a sense of interconnectedness. If you undergo an emotional crisis, your experience may be less traumatic if you do not feel socially isolated. In this sense, some communication may serve the purpose of establishing a common sense of 'interconnectedness' rather than the transmission of information.

Teresa Thompson (1986), writing about health work, argues that communication is important for two major reasons: firstly, it enables people to share information; secondly, it enables relationships between people. She states that 'communication is the relationship', and that speaking or signing is central to establishing relationships between people. Care workers, therefore, must have highly developed social skills in order to work with the wide range of emotional needs that individuals have.

Caring presence

Engebretson (2004) uses the idea of a caring presence to emphasise the importance of building an understanding within health or social care work of the feelings that individuals may be experiencing. A caring presence involves being open to the experience of another person through a two-way encounter with that person, and might develop from reflective listening. If an individual believes that a care worker understands his or her needs and is concerned about him or her, then just knowing that the care worker is nearby may help the individual to feel supported.

Empathy

Care work sometimes involves developing a sense of empathy with an individual. Empathy involves a caring attitude where an individual person can see beyond his or her own assumptions about the world, and can imagine the thoughts and feelings of the other person.

Empathy

Egan (1986) defines empathy as 'the ability to enter into and understand the world of another person and communicate this understanding to him or her'.

At a basic level, empathy develops from communicating that you have understood not only the thoughts but also the feelings of another person. A health and social care professional will, therefore, be able to imagine the emotions that an individual is experiencing, including physical pain and grief. A person who is supported by a caring and empathetic listener will feel that he or she can explore his or her situation with someone who understands. Individuals may become more relaxed, communicative and appreciative of a conversation that involves an attempt to understand their thoughts and feelings.

View point

Is empathy a learnt skill, the outcome of personal development, and can it be understood at different levels?

Viewpoint 1

At a basic level, empathy is an interpersonal skill. Good listeners tend to show respect and value for the thoughts and feelings of others. Listening and showing respect and value are practical skills that can be developed by reflecting on experience. You can be trained to develop caring, empathetic skills.

Viewpoint 2

Carl Rogers (1975) argued that empathy could be regarded as 'a state of being', not a communication skill. Empathy involves a particular way of experiencing self and others, and is not a tool or technique that can simply be picked up and used when you think it might be useful. You have either developed yourself to the point where you can experience the thoughts and feelings of others or you haven't.

Viewpoint 3

Egan (1986) suggests that there are different levels of empathy. He states, 'at its deepest it is a way of being', but it is also 'a communication skill that can be learned'. McLeod (2003) agrees: 'Empathy is like

a state of being. But in so far as this understanding must be offered back to the client, it is also a communication skill'. It may be that people can begin to develop empathy through developing listening skills. At an advanced level, perhaps empathy becomes something that 'you are' rather than a technique you have learned.

Reflection

To what extent is being good at caring a matter of using the right skills? To what extent is it the result of how you understand yourself and others?

When should care workers try to understand the thoughts and feelings of individuals?

Sometimes care workers can be stressed by the emotional needs of individuals. Listening to others might involve learning about frightening and depressing situations, and care workers sometimes avoid listening to avoid experiencing unpleasant emotional feelings. A lack of time, tiredness or a desire to avoid emotional stress can also create barriers to providing caring communication. It is important, therefore, that health and social care workers can identify whether a situation simply requires a practical response, such as the sharing of information, or whether a more sensitive, empathetic approach is needed.

The importance of emotional needs

Care workers often support vulnerable people who are likely to have a range of communication needs. Individuals may have experienced abuse, feel afraid, not understand their situation or feel threatened by what they are experiencing. In the past it was sometimes assumed that physical needs should take priority over social and cultural needs. Today, however, codes of practice (such as the General Social Care Council code) make it essential to address the social and emotional needs of individuals.

One way of understanding human needs is through the work of Abraham Maslow (1908–70). His hierarchy of needs is often set out as a pyramid, as shown in Figure 1.05; the role of interpersonal communication in meeting human needs is described to the right of the hierarchy.

Consequences of individuals' emotional needs not being met

Listening skills may provide a basis for establishing emotional safety and thereby reduce the threat that individuals might feel. If a person does not feel that he or she has been listened to, he or she may feel disrespected. A lack of respect can create feelings of low self-esteem and emotional vulnerability. Furthermore, the individual may feel that he or she is physically at risk because his or her needs have not been understood. Effective communication is, therefore, vital to professional relationships and in creating a sense of safety and belonging for people in your care.

Using interpersonal skills to support others

Muscle tone, facial expression, eye contact and posture can send messages of friendliness. When meeting a person it is usually appropriate to smile, express interest through eye contact and maintain a relaxed posture free of muscle tension; together, these indicate a readiness to talk and to listen.

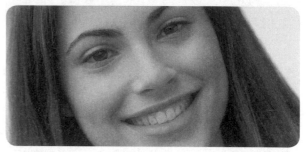

Smiling and eye contact indicate a readiness to talk and to listen

It is difficult to define a simple set of rules for supportive body language because each individual will have his or her own expectations about what is appropriate and normal. The most important thing about supportive body language is to learn to monitor the effects that your behaviour is having on the individual. One indication of providing effective support is the other person reflecting your behaviour; in other words, the individual may become relaxed and friendly if you are relaxed and friendly.

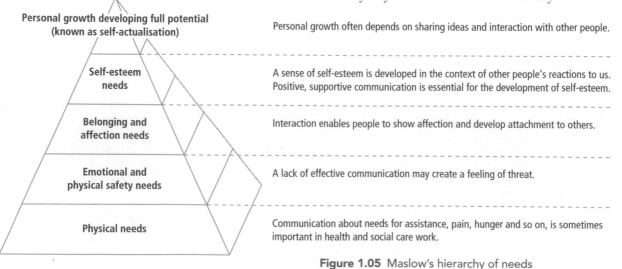

Personal growth developing full potential (known as self-actualisation) — Personal growth often depends on sharing ideas and interaction with other people.

Self-esteem needs — A sense of self-esteem is developed in the context of other people's reactions to us. Positive, supportive communication is essential for the development of self-esteem.

Belonging and affection needs — Interaction enables people to show affection and develop attachment to others.

Emotional and physical safety needs — A lack of effective communication may create a feeling of threat.

Physical needs — Communication about needs for assistance, pain, hunger and so on, is sometimes important in health and social care work.

Figure 1.05 Maslow's hierarchy of needs

Supportive skills

Carl Rogers (1902–87) identified six 'core conditions' that would create a successful helping relationship within a counselling context. As Murgatroyd (1985) proposed, it is possible to simplify these core conditions and to suggest that, within a helping or supportive relationship, the care worker needs to communicate three basic qualities:

- warmth (showing respect and value; not making assumptions about others)
- understanding (or basic empathy)
- sincerity (not putting on an act; not imposing own needs on others).

Warmth

In order for individuals to view you as a warm and accepting person, you will need to demonstrate that you do not stereotype, label or judge others. This is sometimes referred to as having a non-judgemental attitude.

To convey warmth, it is also necessary that you actively listen to others. That is, you give your attention to the person when he or she talks and remember what the person has said. You can then reflect the individual's words back again (see Figure 1.06).

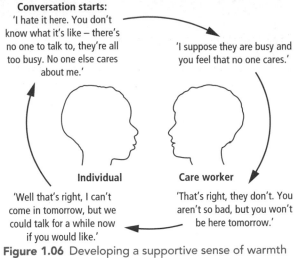

Conversation starts:

'I hate it here. You don't know what it's like – there's no one to talk to, they're all too busy. No one else cares about me.'

'I suppose they are busy and you feel that no one cares.'

Individual   **Care worker**

'Well that's right, I can't come in tomorrow, but we could talk for a while now if you would like.'

'That's right, they don't. You aren't so bad, but you won't be here tomorrow.'

Figure 1.06 Developing a supportive sense of warmth involves being non-judgemental

As Figure 1.06 illustrates, the care worker is able to show the individual that she is listening by repeating some of the things that the individual has said. The repetition is not 'parrot fashion'; the care worker uses her own words. The care worker has also avoided being judgemental. For example, when the individual says that no one cares, the care worker does not argue with him. The care worker might have felt like saying, 'How can you say that? Don't you know how hard we work for you? There are plenty of people here who don't complain'. However, such a statement does not value the other person and fails to convey warmth. If the care worker had said these things to the individual, it would have blocked the conversation. Warmth makes it safe for the individual to express his feelings. Warmth means that, although the care worker may disagree with what an individual has said, the individual can trust that he will not be put down.

In developing the skill of showing warmth, it is important not to judge. Care workers should accept that people have the right to be the way they are and to make their own choices. While you may disapprove of a person's behaviour, you must show that you do not dislike him or her as an individual. This is particularly important when working with people with difficult behaviour. It is essential that individuals know it is the behaviour which is disliked, not them as a person.

Understanding

Understanding means learning about the identity and beliefs of another person. Carl Rogers saw understanding or empathy as the ability to experience another person's world as if it were your own. The key part here is the 'as if': it is important to try to really understand the thoughts and feelings of others.

Active listening provides a useful tool to enable care workers to learn about people. If the care worker is warm and non-judgemental, it becomes safe for an individual to talk about his or her life. If an individual is listened to, he or she will feel understood and valued, and this may encourage him or her to talk further. The more the person talks, the more the care worker has a chance to learn about him or her.

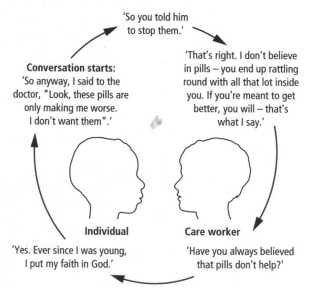

'So you told him to stop them.'

Conversation starts: 'So anyway, I said to the doctor, "Look, these pills are only making me worse. I don't want them".'

'That's right. I don't believe in pills – you end up rattling round with all that lot inside you. If you're meant to get better, you will – that's what I say.'

Individual

Care worker

'Yes. Ever since I was young, I put my faith in God.'

'Have you always believed that pills don't help?'

Figure 1.07 Developing a supportive sense of understanding involves active listening

As the example in Figure 1.07 shows, through listening and conveying warmth the care worker is given the privilege of learning about the individual's religious views. In this way, shared understanding and a sense of trust has developed from a conversation in which the care worker conveys value for the individual.

Sincerity

Being sincere means being open. It also means not acting and not using set phrases or professional styles which are not really you. In some ways, being sincere means being honest and real. (Though remember, being real also has to involve being non-judgemental – understanding people rather than disagreeing with them or giving them advice.)

When you engage with other people, be sure to speak as you do normally. Sometimes it is necessary to share your thoughts to keep a conversation going. It might be useful for you to think about how you might describe yourself and occasionally share details of your own life with the people you are supporting. Sharing personal information in this way may help to convey sincerity in some situations.

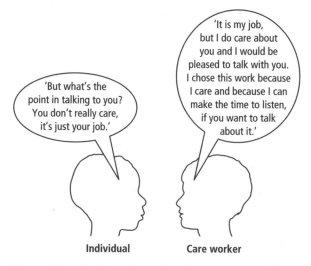

'But what's the point in talking to you? You don't really care, it's just your job.'

'It is my job, but I do care about you and I would be pleased to talk with you. I chose this work because I care and because I can make the time to listen, if you want to talk about it.'

Individual

Care worker

Figure 1.08 Sharing information about your own life may help to convey sincerity

The supportive skills of warmth, understanding and sincerity have to be combined in order to provide a safe and caring setting. These three qualities all belong together in any person-centred approach that creates emotional safety for others.

Values

Social care professionals must work within the standards established by the General Social Care

Council (GSCC) Code of Practice and to National Minimum Standards established for different types of service. These standards require that interpersonal interaction should:

- promote independence and choice for individuals
- show respect for the dignity and privacy of individuals
- respect diversity and different cultures and values.

These principles are sometimes described as care values (see Table 1.05).

Care values
Occupational standards and codes of practice identify a framework of values and moral rights of individuals that can be referred to as care values. These values include promoting equality and diversity, maintaining confidentiality, and promoting individual rights and beliefs.

Care workers should value the dignity, privacy, independence and diversity of others. Skilled listening provides a basis for developing an understanding of other people and may also help to develop empathy. If care workers can develop an understanding of an individual's needs then it is likely that this will provide a basis for valuing and respecting that person.

Sometimes, listening involves 'switching into' a store of knowledge and understanding. For some people this is a conscious process: you 'switch on' by remembering details of another person, perhaps recalling when you last spoke with him or her and what was said. If you get to know each person as an individual and you make it clear that you can remember his or her personal details, this will convey respect and value for that person. In this way you will be working within appropriate care values. Showing respect for differences may depend on being able to remember these important details, for example:

- greeting another person using a word of welcome in his or her own first language
- remembering a recent event in that person's life, such as a visit from grandchildren
- discussing an interest that you know an individual has previously expressed.

Table 1.05 Some key ideas for communicating care values

Communicating care values through...	Key ideas
Awareness of needs	It is very important to understand the self-development, self-esteem and belonging needs of individuals and not be limited to understanding only their basic physical needs.
Supportive skills	Use the supportive skills of understanding, warmth and sincerity in order to create emotional safety for individuals.
Understanding the individual	Learning about others is a key way to show that you value them. Formal techniques for understanding an individual's life history include: life story work with children and adults; life review and reminiscence work with older people.
Respect for difference	Do not treat everybody the same – this is not what is meant by equal opportunity. Alter your verbal and non-verbal behaviour to show respect for each individual.
Maintaining personal dignity	Physical care such as washing, dressing, feeding and cleaning should focus on making the individual feel that he or she is respected. Feeding someone should not be just about putting food in his or her mouth; it should also involve interaction that meets emotional and social needs.
Providing choice	Always offer choices when individuals cannot do things for themselves; a person can still be offered a choice of how he or she would like you to do things. For example, how does a person like to be fed; when would he or she like to eat; what would he or she like to eat?
Encouraging independence	A sense of self grows out of the choices and decisions that people make. For instance, learning to travel, learning independent living skills and learning to operate a computer helps to create a sense of self-esteem. Care work often focuses on helping people to be independent rather than dependent on others.

Sarah

I am a home care worker for older people in their own homes. When I first meet a person I try to learn as much as possible about him or her. So, while carrying out my practical tasks, I adopt a friendly manner and chat to the person about his or her life – the work the person used to do, his or her family and interests, and so on. I can imagine that some older people find it very threatening to have a stranger come into their home and take over, so I always try to 'go carefully'.

I remember one woman I worked with asked me to clean the kitchen but told me not to look in the fridge. She probably had lots of out-of-date food in there and she didn't want me to discover it. I suppose for her it was an issue of dignity and pride: she always used to look after the fridge and she didn't want me taking over. However, there might be a food safety issue, so it was important for me to earn her trust; that way, she would trust me not to make her feel stupid. So I tried to build up trust by talking a little about my family and listening a lot about her family. We were able to have a laugh and we seemed to get on. In the end the fridge stopped being an issue – she was happy to let me clean it because she trusted me not to criticise her.

It's really important not to come over 'all official' and start quoting regulations and so on. Sometimes you think a person is going to be difficult, but once you get to know him or her there usually isn't a problem. I think if you give people respect you often get respect back. Also, if you do care work you have to be prepared to make the first move – you have to show respect for the individual's wishes and then the person relaxes a bit and says what a wonderful person you are!

1 Can you identify some interpersonal skills that Sarah uses in order to meet the self-esteem needs of others?

2 What care values may guide the way in which Sarah works?

3 Sarah uses effective interpersonal skills in order to support individuals. How would Sarah know that she is providing effective support to others?

Reflective thinking skills

How do people develop effective interpersonal skills? The obvious answer is that people copy the behaviours of others: they learn to imitate interpersonal skills that appear to be successful. However, although people learn many practical and life skills by imitating others, they also need to think about, or reflect on, their actions in order to fine tune them and develop advanced skills. Many people need to be able to 'think things through' before they can feel confident in their performance.

Reflective thinking

The term 'reflective thinking' is used to identify the way in which people develop their own personal knowledge of interpersonal skills.

Reflective thinking can help people to:

- discover new ideas or insights
- feel confident in their own abilities
- understand their own interpersonal skills.

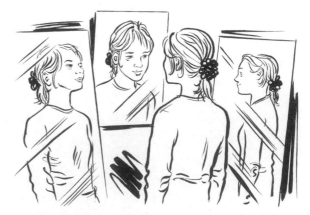

Figure 1.09 Reflective thinking involves bouncing ideas around in your mind in the same way that an image bounces between mirrors

Nathaniel

Nathaniel works with older people and has worked with Alf for some time. Alf has been diagnosed as having dementia and can become disorientated and frustrated. The following interaction took place one morning. Alf had become very aggressive and was threatening to attack Nathaniel with a walking stick.

Alf: Who do you think you are? You get out of it or I'll knock your head off.

Nathaniel: Alf – I'm Nathaniel – you remember me? We talked about your daughter Janice yesterday. Janice said she would be coming to visit you – do you remember?

Alf: [looking puzzled] You don't know Janice – you're having me on!

Nathaniel: Yes, Janice spent some time talking to me when she last came to visit. She told me about your career as a boxer – you won lots of trophies for boxing.

Alf: Well, help me get these people out of the room – they shouldn't be here, you know.

Nathaniel: Perhaps we could sort that out later. It would be nice to talk about your daughter's visit. Have you got the time to talk to me? We could go down to the office and talk there.

Alf: What and leave all these people here?

Nathaniel: Yes, just for the moment – they're not doing any harm. Perhaps we could talk about it over a cup of tea and a biscuit. What do you think?

Alf: Alright, but I'm not having it you know – not all these people.

Nathaniel: No, we'll sort it out later.

Alf became much calmer and was prepared to walk down the corridor with Nathaniel.

Later, Nathaniel discusses the incident in an interview.

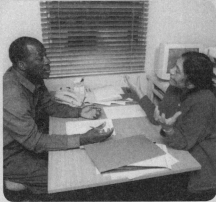

Interviewer: You handled that really effectively; you prevented any aggression and you treated Alf with respect and dignity. You seemed so calm and confident, and you knew exactly what to do.

Nathaniel: Well, inside I was scared. Alf may be old but he is still very strong. I think he could have injured me if I had handled it badly.

Interviewer: Did you put yourself at risk then?

Nathaniel: No – I know Alf and thought I could talk him round. But there's always that little doubt.

Interviewer: But if you were not certain then you were putting yourself at risk.

Nathaniel: Well, I did sort of assess the risk in my head. You see, I do understand Alf – he has a heart of gold. I only had to get him to remember me and think about his daughter and I knew it would work out. It wasn't as if I had a written plan or anything – it just all came together in my mind as Alf started to threaten me. I did feel tense inside, but I also knew that it would work out – so I would say that I didn't put myself at risk.

Interviewer: How do you learn to think like that? How can you work it all out with just a few seconds before things turn bad?

Nathaniel: I think it comes from knowing the people I work with and having confidence in my 'people skills'. I think it's also something that comes with experience – I imagine how things might happen and anticipate what I would do in these situations, and sometimes I find that these events do occur. In this way, I think a good imagination helps me to cope with these difficult situations.

1 What skills might Nathaniel have used in order to build an understanding of Alf's behaviour?

2 What are good 'people skills'? How might Nathaniel have developed these?

3 Nathaniel says you have to have a good imagination. Analyse what this 'good imagination' may involve and explain how it might be developed.

Reflection and imagination

In the story on page 21, Nathaniel explains that he uses his imagination to improve his interpersonal skills. Nathaniel is not simply recalling past experiences; nor is he 'daydreaming' or indulging in fantasy. Instead, he is trying to predict how the individuals in his care might react in future situations based on his memories and understanding of them. Nathaniel is actively developing his ability to react to difficult situations at work using the thought process of reflection. Reflection involves imagination and thinking, but it is a specific kind of focused thinking that may help you to understand the situations you experience.

Kolb's theory of reflective practice

David Kolb (1984) argues that effective learning results from a four-stage learning cycle, which is summarised in the diagram below.

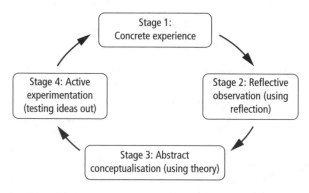

Figure 1.10 Kolb's four-stage learning cycle of reflective practice

Kolb states that learning may start from practical experience but it is then important to reflect on and understand more about the experience. He argues that, in order to make sense of your experience, it might be important to use knowledge and theory to explain what has happened. Once you can explain events that have happened, you can then test out your ideas (active experimentation).

Consider the scenario below and then read through the analysis using Kolb's four-stage process.

> ## Concrete experience
>
> Imagine that you are working with a man with a learning difficulty. It is the first time you have met him and you are offering him a drink at lunchtime. You offer him a glass of orange squash by placing it in front of him. He immediately pushes the glass away with a facial expression that you take to express disgust. But why has the individual reacted this way?

Using reflection

Using the above scenario, you might reflect on some possible reasons for the person's behaviour. (This process is often one of 'bouncing' ideas around.)

- Perhaps the individual doesn't like orange squash?
- Is there a cultural or religious reason (such as Ramadan)?
- Perhaps he doesn't like the way the drink was put in front of him?
- Does he not like to take a drink with his meal?
- Is there an issue to do with status; for example, could a cold drink symbolise childhood status for this individual; does he see adult status as defined by having a hot drink?

Reflection on the non-verbal behaviour of the individual may provide a range of starting points for interpreting his actions.

Using theory

The more you know about human psychology, the better your analysis of his reaction. You need to choose the most likely explanation for the individual's behaviour using everything you know about people. Given the different cultural interpretations of non-verbal behaviour, perhaps the way you placed the drink in front of the person has been seen as an attempt to control or dominate him. This message would not have been intentional, but the individual may have interpreted your behaviour as unpleasant.

Testing ideas out

Finally, you can try to identify any assumptions you have made. You might attempt to modify your non-verbal behaviour to look supportive. For example, you might show the individual a china cup and saucer to indicate the question 'Is this what you would like?' If the individual responds with a positive non-verbal response then you would have solved the problem in a way which values his individuality.

Kolb's theory in practice

In real life, health and social care workers might not always find a fixed four-stage cycle to be practical. Making sense of day-to-day experiences is often a chaotic and unstructured process, and linking past knowledge to reflective thinking may be an automatic process with no deliberate effort to analyse theory. Sometimes it may be difficult to identify a stage of 'testing ideas', especially if you are involved in a fast-moving conversation.

Making links

Whilst the idea of a learning cycle may not always explain how personal learning develops, Kolb's theory does identify some key processes involved in developing the personal knowledge necessary for effective interpersonal interaction. It may be more useful to understand learning about others' needs as a complex interaction of the components that Kolb identified in his theory (see Figure 1.11). Reflective thinking may involve making links between any or all of the four areas described in Table 1.06.

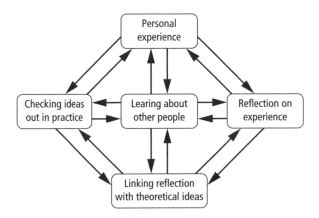

Figure 1.11 The development of personal and professional learning may involve making links between many different kinds of knowledge

Table 1.06 Different kinds of knowledge used in reflective thinking

Knowledge	Different types of knowledge include: • knowledge of theory and the ability to use theory to explain experiences • knowledge of codes of practice, legislation, organisational policies and procedures • knowledge gained by reading books, attending courses or studying • knowledge gained informally from other people.
Personal experience	Memories of events previously experienced including: • experiences of interaction with other people • general social experiences • experiences in employment, care placements or through voluntary work.
Skills and 'know-how'	This is sometimes called tacit knowledge – knowledge which is not easily put into words. It may include: • interpersonal skills • the ability to understand and get on with others • the ability to solve problems • the ability to organise yourself.
Care values	Life experience results in the development of a range of attitudes and beliefs that influence the way in which you value others. You will, therefore, make assumptions when you interpret the behaviour of others. Health and social care work requires you to explore your personal beliefs and the way in which you value vulnerable people. You will need to be familiar with the GSCC Code of Practice and refer to its principles when evaluating your own assumptions about individuals.

Levels of reflection

Jennifer Moon (1999) reviewed a great deal of research and theory on the nature of reflective thinking. Her work makes it clear that the term 'reflection' can mean different things to different authors. 'Reflection' can mean just making memories or it can imply the restructuring of the way in which a person thinks. Moon (1999) suggests that it is possible to identify five different levels of reflective thinking – five different 'depths' of thinking and learning (see Table 1.07).

Reflection provides an alternative to labelling

Consider the following scenario.

A difficult resident

Every morning a resident who lives in a supported housing complex comes to the office to complain. The complaints might be about anything: sinks that don't empty quickly enough, cars that park too close to a wall, light bulbs that need changing even though they still work! Naturally this behaviour is annoying for the people who work in the office.

When care workers are stressed, they may believe that they do not have time to reflect on individual need. If staff do not think about why a person complains, they may simply label the individual using terms such as 'difficult', 'attention-seeking' or 'suffering from mental health difficulties'. These labels classify the person and may appear to provide some sort of explanation. However, labelling in this way might mean that care workers never really understand a person's situation and needs. If care workers are too stressed to build an understanding of the people they work with, they may be perceived as not showing respect and value for individuals and may fail to provide appropriate caring responses or care services.

Reflection offers an alternative thought process to classifying or labelling individuals. Using Jennifer Moon's analysis, it may be possible to identify different levels of reflection that a care worker might achieve.

Just noticing what happens

Perhaps the interaction in the scenario always follows a pattern. For example, the person waits for a short period then launches into a verbal outburst about what is wrong. During this outburst the resident is unresponsive to the reactions of others. Having completed the outburst the resident will look for a reaction and then storm off.

Just noticing this detail – and thinking long enough to create a memory – might provide a start to the reflective process. It is easy to label an individual as 'difficult' or 'challenging' then use the label to block further thinking. Just noticing the detail of what happens may help to avoid labelling.

Reflection in order to make sense of a situation

What does the resident's pattern of behaviour mean? Perhaps this confrontational exchange

Level	Description	Explanation
1	Noticing	Recalling experiences, remembering
2	Making sense	Making links between memories and other theories and ideas in your understanding
3	Making meaning	Developing an understanding that you can use in other situations
4	Working with meaning	Developing and reorganising the way you think
5	Transformative learning	Restructuring assumptions about important issues; powerful learning experiences may be accompanied by strong emotional reactions

Table 1.07 Moon's five levels of reflective thinking

represents a release of tension; perhaps the resident does not have the social and emotional skills needed to engage in more sociable conversations; perhaps the resident is trying to create a sense of belonging within the housing complex. Confrontation might be chosen because the person is trying to communicate. Reflection may not give the correct answer but trying to make sense of a situation helps open it up to new ideas.

Going deeper – imagining yourself in another person's situation

What does the resident feel like when she comes to complain? Perhaps she feels a little isolated or insecure and is thinking, 'If I don't feel good then someone else is to blame!' Perhaps these emotions become focused on trivia such as light bulbs. Imagining how another person might experience a situation can help to generate extra ideas about what could be happening.

Reflecting on wider issues

A care worker reflecting on why the woman always complains might consider the significance of some ideas. For example, many people search for others to blame whenever anything is perceived to be less than perfect. This might manifest as saying that 'they' should do something about climate change, house prices or AIDS, for instance. Perhaps it is a basic human reaction to retreat into a childlike state and expect a kind parent to make the world comfortable and ideal. In this sense, the individual who complains is tapping into the same way of thinking that most people adopt from time to time.

Reflection that takes a wider view can involve new thoughts that could, for example, help you to understand yourself better. Perhaps the difference between the individual's behaviour and your own is that you are more skilled at knowing how, when and where it is acceptable to complain.

Reflection that results in new ways of thinking

To what extent do you take responsibility for your own emotions? Do you assume that your emotions are caused by outside events, or do you believe that your own thinking can directly influence your feelings? Many of the assumptions people make about life are hard to change. Abandoning the belief 'they should make my life better' and deciding 'I am responsible for my life' could represent a huge shift in thinking.

Reflection on your own life assumptions is not something that can happen on a daily basis. This kind of reflection involves an extreme shift in thinking.

Over to you

What positive benefits for care workers might arise from practising reflective thinking?

Labelling other people can create a simple and comfortable way of coping with difficult behaviour. Reflection requires time and mental energy, especially for 'deeper' reflective thinking. How deeply does reflective thinking need to go? As long as you reflect enough to get beyond the labelling stage, you are on the right path. Learning to notice and remember detail may help to prevent labelling. The ability to make sense of behaviour by thinking of different possibilities may enable care workers to use experience effectively.

Using reflection to develop interpersonal skills

The idea of different levels of reflective thinking may be useful if you explore the development of interpersonal skills within the context of professional development. Reflection might start with just noticing your own performance. For example, you might record your behaviour in a one-to-one or group discussion. This could identify the degree to which you have used appropriate language, non-verbal, listening and supportive skills.

At a more advanced level, it will be possible to reflect on how you are coming across to another person during an interaction. Donald Schön (1983) argued that professional people were those who had learned to reflect on their own actions whilst engaged in interactions with others. Schön referred to this ability as 'reflection in action'. The ability to check that you are keeping an open mind and to reflect on the effectiveness of your skills may be an important component of effective interpersonal interaction. Active listening and the development of 'basic empathy' will involve some degree of reflection on your performance and awareness of the impact your behaviour is having on others.

Test yourself

1 What does non-verbal communication mean?

2 Why is eye contact important during communication?

3 What is the difference between active listening and just hearing what someone has said?

4 How could you try to communicate with people who have difficulty in hearing?

5 What is meant by a 'speech community'?

6 What is meant by 'empathy'?

7 Effective interpersonal interaction in health and social care work involves more than the clear transmission of information to individuals. What other issues are likely to be important when working with individuals?

8 How are active listening skills or the ability to convey warmth, understanding and sincerity associated with care values?

9 What is meant by reflective thinking?

10 How can you develop your understanding of interpersonal skills using reflective thinking?

References and further reading

- Burnard, P. (1996) *Acquiring Interpersonal Skills*. (2nd ed.) London: Chapman & Hall
- Egan, G. (1986) *The Skilled Helper*. Monterey California: Brooks/Cole Publishing Company
- Engebretson, J. (2004) 'Caring presence: a case study' in *Communication, Relationships and Care*. Robb, M., Barrett, S., Komaromy, C. and Rogers, A. (Eds) London & New York: OU & Routledge
- Finnegan, R. (2004) 'Communicating humans but what does that mean?' in *Communication, Relationships and Care*. Robb, M., Barrett, S., Komaromy, C. and Rogers, A. (Eds) London & New York: OU & Routledge
- Kolb, D. (1984) *Experiential Learning: Experience as the Source of Learning and Development*. New Jersey: Prentice Hall
- McLeod, J. (2003) *An Introduction to Counselling*. (3rd ed.) Maidenhead: Open University Press
- Moon, J.A. (1999) *Reflection in Learning and Professional Development*. London: Kogan Page Ltd
- Moonie, N., Bates, A. and Spencer-Perkins, D. (2004) *Diversity and Rights in Care*. Oxford: Heinemann
- Morrison, P. and Burnard, P. (1997) *Caring and Communicating*. Basingstoke and London: Macmillan Press
- Murgatroyd, S. (1985) *Counselling and Helping*. London and New York: Methuen
- Rogers, C.R. (1975) Empathy: An unappreciated way of being. *Counselling Psychologist* 21: 95–103
- Schön, D. (1983) *The Reflective Practitioner*. San Francisco: Jossey-Bass
- Thompson, T. L. (1986) *Communication for Health Professionals*. New York: Harper & Row

CHAPTER 2

Promoting equality of opportunity within health and social care settings

Key points

- Equality of opportunity in health and social care is underpinned by valuing each individual as a unique person with his or her own abilities, needs, wants and desires.

- The health and social care needs of each individual are unique to him or her, and services should be provided based on these.

- Inequalities and unfair treatment of individuals can thrive simply through a lack of knowledge and understanding.

- Learning about diversity, equality of opportunity and the care value base is central to work routines and qualifications within health and social care.

- Gaining knowledge and confidence about people from cultures other than your own will enable you to provide high quality and acceptable services to all.

- Understanding the wide range of legislation that supports the rights of individuals is key to promoting equality of opportunity within health and social care settings.

- Promoting the rights of others or challenging inequalities wherever they are found requires sound knowledge and confidence in the subject.

Introduction

This chapter is designed to enable all health and social care learners to recognise the importance of equality, diversity and rights within the caring process. Recognising diversity and the richness of experience and culture that every individual brings with him or her is central to the role of a health and social care worker. Treating people equally and fairly is a way of demonstrating respect for diversity and the individual. Treating people differently due to their race, religion or anything else is not acceptable and would not be tolerated under any circumstances. Some of the information and the knowledge covered in this chapter might make you feel uneasy, but think of this in a positive way – it never hurts to challenge your assumptions.

In light of this, a sound knowledge of policy and practice and an understanding and recognition of the importance of equality, diversity and rights underpins all your future studies in health and social care and any development you may undertake in the workplace.

Understand concepts of equality, diversity and rights in relation to health and social care

A good starting point for your studies in equality, diversity and rights is the terminology (words or jargon) used to describe issues involved within the subject. For example, you need to understand the meaning applied to such words as equality, diversity and empowerment in the context of equality, diversity and rights. Without this understanding, you would be unable to participate appropriately in the provision of good practice in the workplace and wider community. Therefore, this chapter commences with an exploration of the key terms that you need to be able to understand and use comfortably.

Key terms

Equality

> **Equality**
> The meaning behind the word equality can be best summarised as 'treating all people fairly'.

The word equality is often linked to 'opportunity', creating the term 'equal opportunity'. By law, all workplaces should have an equal opportunities policy. This should aim to create a fair working environment and to ensure that all people are treated equally in relation to:

- access to work
- pay and conditions of work.

Equal opportunities policies also cover access to services and organisations. The UK healthcare system is based on 'need' rather than the ability to pay, and in any health and social care setting, everybody should have access to the treatment and care that they need. It is the responsibility of services and organisations to ensure that their actions or lack of them do not **discriminate** against any individuals requiring treatment and care.

> **Discriminate** – to treat a person differently (unfairly) because of prejudices (bias) about his or her sex, race, religion, etc.

Communication difficulties

Mabel Sziler has been living and working in London since 2001. She is from the Ukraine and is still struggling a little with her English. She is able to get by from day to day, can access banking services and is able to carry out her work as a leisure centre attendant without too much difficulty.

Mabel has recently been to a Well Woman Clinic held at her local GP centre and has been given information on blood pressure, cholesterol, weight and urine. She could not understand the points the nurse raised with her but felt too embarrassed to ask for clarification. She has been given two leaflets on blood pressure and cholesterol and cannot understand the contents. However, Mabel has decided not to worry about it, since she thinks it won't matter in the long run.

1 Has Mabel been able to gain access to this service?
2 What could the organisation do to improve the service to Mabel?
3 How could equal opportunities be better met in this case?

Equity

The dictionary would tell you that equity is a term describing fairness. However, in health and social care, equity is also about ensuring that all people have fair and equal access to services, such as doctors, treatment and medication. It also highlights the need to all individuals that they can and should expect fair and equal treatment from medical practitioners no matter where they live in the UK.

Diversity

> **Diversity**
> Diversity means recognising, acknowledging, accepting and valuing difference between all individuals. Diversity is about respect for people.

It is expected that all health and social care workers recognise that there are key differences between people that could affect their health and healthcare in a variety of ways. For example, gender has the potential to affect how long people live (in general, women live longer than men); religion can affect the food choices made by individuals; ethnic origin can affect a person's experience of ill health. However, it is important to recognise that none of these differences should be allowed to act as a barrier to equal access to services and all that life has to offer.

> **Over to you**
>
> *Create your own glossary of terms as you go through this section. Write any key words you don't understand in a notebook then find out the definition for each one.*

Rights

Rights are often linked with responsibilities: every individual has the right to live his or her life in the way he or she chooses as long as this does not affect anyone else in a negative way. In other words, everyone has access to basic human rights and in turn has a responsibility to ensure other people's basic human rights.

In the UK, sixteen human rights are incorporated into the legal system by the Human Rights Act 2000 (see also page 52). The rights are taken from the European Convention on Human Rights and, as you might expect from reading them, affect every aspect of human life (see Table 2.01 overleaf). They are central to the way individuals are cared for in the UK health and social care system.

1	The right to life.
2	The right to freedom from torture and inhuman or degrading treatment or punishment.
3	The right to freedom from slavery, servitude and forced or compulsory labour.
4	The right to liberty and security of person.
5	The right to a fair and public trial within a reasonable time.
6	The right to freedom from retrospective criminal law and no punishment without law.
7	The right to respect for private and family life, home and correspondence.
8	The right to freedom of thought, conscience and religion.
9	The right to freedom of expression.
10	The right to freedom of assembly and association.
11	The right to marry and found a family.
12	The prohibition of discrimination in the enjoyment of convention rights.
13	The right to peaceful enjoyment of possessions and protection of property.
14	The right of access to an education.
15	The right of free elections.
16	The right not to be subjected to the death penalty.

Table 2.01 The sixteen human rights enshrined in UK law

The right of access to an education

Read the following newspaper article.

Ruth Kelly: 'Tensions between different ethnic groups and faiths must be tackled'

In August 2004, Communities Secretary Ruth Kelly launched a Commission on Integration and Cohesion, a body which will look at how communities in the UK tackle tensions and extremism. Ms Kelly says the commission will create a 'new and honest' debate on diversity, but will not look at whether faith schools are a good thing, insisting that parents should have a choice. In fact, the government plans to have more faith schools, even though critics say that they increase segregation between people of different faiths.

Ms Kelly was quoted as saying: 'The fact that Britain is open to people of all faiths and none has been a huge strength of this country. But what we have to do is recognise that while there have been huge benefits, there are also tensions created. The point of the commission... is to try and examine how these tensions arise and what local communities can do on the ground practically to tackle those and make a difference.'

Speaking about faith schools, Ms Kelly said that Church of England schools were among the most 'diverse' in the country. She also said that Muslim parents should have the same opportunity as Christians and Jews to send their children to faith schools. However, Ms Kelly did suggest that faith schools should be encouraged to interact with one another, suggesting that they play sports matches against each other or perhaps twinned themselves with schools of another faith.

1 How could the right of access to an education affect the health and well-being of an individual?
2 Investigate initiatives in your local community to bring together people of different cultural and ethnic backgrounds.

Opportunity

Every individual should have the same opportunities open to him or her as every other person. These opportunities range from access to jobs through to becoming transplant patients or having access to life-saving medicines.

Postcode lottery

Manjeet and Kevin both have cancer. Each wants to be treated with a new drug that has been shown to improve the life chances of individuals with cancer. Manjeet lives in the south-west of England and her health authority has approved the decision to treat her with the new drug. Kevin lives in the north-east of England and his health authority has refused his treatment with the new drug.

1 How has 'opportunity' been affected in this situation? Should this be allowed to happen?
2 What might be the reasons behind a refusal?

Difference

The concept of 'difference' is linked to diversity. Each individual is different; even conjoined twins have their own talents, aspirations, needs and wants. There are some obvious differences between people which will affect their health and social care provision; these include age, gender, physical ability and disability. As a care worker, it is important to recognise that all individuals must be respected and valued for their differences.

Hilary Lister

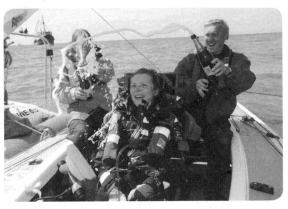

In 2005, Hilary Lister became the first quadriplegic (a person who is paralysed in both arms and both legs) to sail solo across the English Channel. Hilary is only able to move her head, eyes and mouth, and navigated a specially-adapted eight-metre boat by sucking and blowing through straws. She was quoted as saying 'I want to get able-bodied people to rethink their views about disabled people...We do not need wrapping up in cotton wool and can go out and do silly or dangerous things if that's what we want to do.'

Reflection

Before reading about Hilary's success, would you have thought it possible for someone who is a quadriplegic to have achieved what she did? Have your assumptions about what disabled people can do been challenged? What other assumptions might you hold about disabled people?

Discrimination

Discrimination

Discrimination can be defined as treating an individual less favourably than another because of his or her age, gender, religion, sexual orientation, nationality or colour, etc. Discrimination can be classed as direct or indirect (see below).

Discrimination is illegal in the UK and as such there is wide-ranging legislation to support any individual who feels unfairly discriminated against. Discrimination can take place for a variety of reasons; three common causes of awards being made to individuals in discrimination cases are sex discrimination, race discrimination and disability discrimination.

Overt and covert discrimination

Discrimination can be **overt** or **covert** – also known as direct or indirect discrimination. An example of overt, or direct, discrimination is paying a man more money than a woman for doing the same job. An example of covert, or indirect, discrimination might be a short-listing panel for a job vacancy deciding not to call someone for interview based on his or her name or the area in which he or she lives.

> **Overt** – open to view; not concealed.
> **Covert** – hidden, concealed.

Gina

I am an Irish traveller. I have lived in caravans all my life and thoroughly enjoy travelling from one place to another.

The other day, I arranged to visit a 'drop-in' GP surgery to have my diabetes checked. When I arrived the receptionist told me to come back at the end of surgery, when all the local people had been seen first. It was obvious to me that I should have been second on the appointment schedule. But I thought if I argued with the receptionist, I would never get in to see the doctor, so I just did what she said.

1 How is this covert discrimination?
2 What forms of health-related overt discrimination could you envisage taking place for someone similar to Gina?

Stephen

I am 45 years old and have had multiple sclerosis (MS) for two years. I work in a small company as a computer programmer. I am able to work most of the time but I have started to experience weakness in my hands, blurred vision and fatigue. The effects and progress of MS vary greatly from person to person but tend to be slowly progressive. I am unable to work when these relapses take place. The relapses are starting to increase in frequency and I will be taking a couple of days a month off as sick leave. My employer has told me if this time off increases, I will need to leave the company. She says that a small company cannot afford to have a key member of staff absent on regular sick leave.

1 MS means 'many scars'. What is being scarred and how can this affect the individual?
2 Are Stephen's employer's actions an example of prejudice or discrimination? Explain why.
3 How are the employer's actions likely to affect Stephen's self-image?
4 What medium- to long-term effects could this situation have on Stephen?

Institutional discrimination

Discrimination can also take place at an institutional level. This is when the rules of an organisation or the laws of a country discriminate against individuals and groups, thereby preventing them from enjoying the same rights and opportunities as others. Before the establishment of the 1995 Disability Discrimination Act, the rights of disabled people were not protected by UK law. Another example of institutional discrimination was against homosexuals: by 1994, the age of consent for heterosexuals was 16 years but for homosexuals it was 21 years; however, in 1994 the age limit for consenting to homosexual sex was reduced to 18 years. This then led to another three years of campaigning to have the age limit reduced to 16 years. It is interesting to note that the consenting age for sex amongst homosexual men in Ireland is 17 years and not 16 years.

Stereotyping

To 'stereotype' a person is to characterise or categorise him or her too simplistically. Stereotypes are based on the belief that all people are the same in certain circumstances, for example:

- all football fans are hooligans
- teenagers who wear hooded tops are violent
- overweight people are unhappy with their body image
- all drug users are burglars.

It is highly likely that you will have experience of many stereotypes as stereotypical attitudes are developed as part of the socialisation (growing-up) process. However, stereotyping individuals is a dangerous practice. The end result can be discrimination against individuals based on false assumptions.

What stereotypes do you hold about people? What labels do you apply to them?

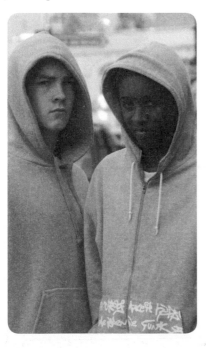
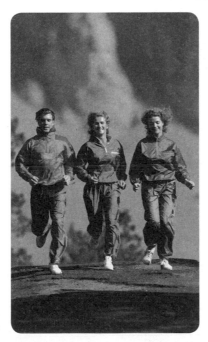
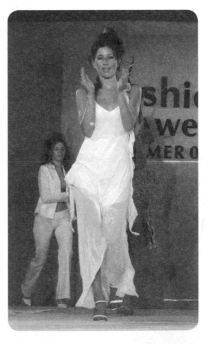

Labelling

A label is a word or term applied to an individual that is considered to 'sum up' him or her. Labelling is another form of discrimination. Unfortunately, most people often do this without even realising. Examples of frequently used labels are:

- thick
- aggressive
- lazy
- weak.

Labelling an individual takes away his or her identity. The danger is that people lose their dignity and are treated differently (discriminated against) as a result.

A 'difficult' person

Lizzie has been labelled 'difficult' by the residential care home that has organised her admittance into hospital. Consequently, all the ward nurses have been warned about Lizzie.

- How might Lizzie's treatment be affected by the label that has been applied to her?

Prejudice

Prejudice

Attitudes and opinions that are biased and pre-judge individuals and groups.

Prejudice is usually demonstrated by individuals who show a negative attitude towards some groups of the population. The term is often used to describe the way people can judge others without knowing them (the word 'prejudice' is based on the term 'pre-judgement'). Such judgements are based on labels and stereotypes and not the individual in question.

Acting on a prejudice is a form of discrimination. For example, believing that disabled people are not capable of working is a prejudiced view; not employing disabled people because of this view is an example of discrimination.

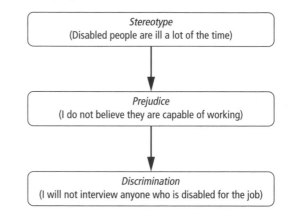

Figure 2.01 Stereotypical thinking leads to prejudice and discrimination

Again, the danger of prejudice is that people will be treated disadvantageously because of someone else's lack of knowledge about them. In other words, discrimination results from prejudice.

Self-image

The way other people 'see' you can affect your self-image. Their view of you can produce a 'looking glass' effect (Cooley, 1902). In other words, what is mirrored or reflected back to you from others can become part of what you believe about yourself.

Disadvantage

In health and social care, people often use the term 'disadvantage' to refer to a person's experience of life chances as being lower than average. In other words, individuals and families from poorer economic areas can (and usually do) experience poorer health. In addition:

- services available for healthcare may be of a lower quality
- access to education may be more limited
- housing is often of a poorer quality
- parks and play areas may be unavailable in the immediate areas.

As you might imagine, this list is not exhaustive; there are many other aspects of life, including employment and income, that have the potential to 'disadvantage' whole families and their communities.

Beliefs and values

A person's beliefs are those things that he or she regards as true. For example, the belief that there is or is not a God; the belief that it is always wrong to harm another living being or the belief that violence is justified under some circumstances. Beliefs reflect the way a person sees the world and the opinions he or she holds about what is happening in that world. For instance, how you feel about marriage reflects part of your belief system. Beliefs are formed over many years and are very powerful in terms of the way they influence a person's behaviour towards other people and towards his or her own self.

An individual's values reflect those things that he or she recognises as being good or having intrinsic worth. Values are developed through a person's experiences and can be strongly influenced by other people (often family and friends). A person's 'value system' – the totality of the values he or she holds – will be based upon a diverse range of things. For example, some people value ambition over loyalty; others value friendship over personal gain. The decision to be vegetarian or vegan could be based on religious values, an abhorrence for cruelty to animals (ethical or moral values), or a preferred diet. Some people value expensive cars as symbols of status, wealth and power; those who value the environment may view cars as dangerously polluting.

Today, people with many different beliefs and values live in the UK; some happily accept these differences while others do not. Tolerating different beliefs and values can be challenging, particularly if there is a perception that those with different views to us are dangerous, misguided or wrong. For example, if a person believes that it is okay to eat a high-fat diet, he or she will be more likely to develop heart or circulatory disease in the future.

Over to you

Beliefs and values are two very powerful influences on your life. Complete Table 2.02 by describing two beliefs and two values that you feel strongly about, then discuss your answers in a group.

Table 2.02 Key beliefs and values

	Belief 1	Belief 2
One thing that I strongly believe…		
Where this belief comes from		
How this belief might affect my work in health and social care		
	Value 1	**Value 2**
One thing that I strongly value…		
Where this value comes from		
How this value might affect my work in health and social care		

Vulnerability

This term is used to describe people who are potentially at risk from something or someone else. For example, older people who are frail and sick may be vulnerable to colds in winter; hence, flu vaccinations are provided for some groups of the population. Individuals with Alzheimer's disease may be more vulnerable to abuse because of challenging behaviour patterns and an inability to protect themselves.

Abuse

The term abuse is applied to a wide range of negative behaviours which have the potential to harm or damage individuals. Abuse is often categorised into four types, as follows:

- *Physical abuse* – causing physical harm to a person, e.g. by hitting, biting or scalding.
- *Emotional or psychological abuse* – the persistent ill-treatment of an individual, e.g. conveying to a person that he or she is worthless or inadequate; causing a person to feel humiliated, afraid or exploited.
- *Neglect* – the failure to meet a person's basic living needs, i.e. failing to feed or clothe a person adequately; failing to provide access to appropriate medical treatment, care and social opportunities.
- *Sexual abuse* – forcing or enticing a person to participate in sexual activities whether or not that person is aware of what is happening. These activities may involve inappropriate physical contact or may be non-physical acts such as inappropriate comments or displays.

Individuals can be subject to more than one type of abuse at once, for example, neglect alongside sexual abuse.

Empowerment

The term empowerment generally means: to enable an individual (or group of people) to take control of his or her life (or in some cases, specific tasks and actions) rather than relying on other people.

There are a variety of different ways in which empowerment can be considered. For example, on a macro (whole population) level, some people argue that the NHS is too paternalistic, i.e. telling people what to do and when, and should be empowering individuals to take responsibility for their own health. At an individual level (micro), a person who is given access to his medical records may be empowered to take more responsibility for his health and to question the health professionals involved in his care.

Reflection

How might an older person living in residential care be empowered to take control of her medication regime? What information would she need and who should supply it?

Independence

This word is often linked to 'empowerment'. In its simplest sense, independence is about enabling individuals to live life to the full without having to rely on others to fulfil tasks for themselves or tell them how and when to do something. All health professionals strive to have client independence at the centre of a healthcare regime. A good health professional will always endeavour to carry out caring and health tasks *with* (never *to*) the individual.

Interdependence

Interdependence means to depend on one another. A good way to see this term in action is through the work of a multi-disciplinary healthcare team. Each member of the team has a key role to play in improving the health of an individual and no one role is more important than another.

Racism

The term racism refers to a whole range of negative behaviours and unfair treatment patterns towards other people based on their **ethnicity** or **race**.

> **Ethnicity** – the customs of a particular cultural or racial group.
> **Race** – group of people of common descent and with a common set of characteristics.

Sexism

The term sexism refers to a whole range of negative behaviours and unfair treatment patterns towards other people based on their **sexuality** or **gender**.

> **Sexuality** – a person's sexual orientation, i.e. heterosexual, homosexual, bisexual.
> **Gender** – indicating differences in biological sex, i.e. whether a person is male, female, transgender, etc.

Homophobia

Homophobia means aversion to homosexuals. The term homophobia is not used very often today, but where it is used the meaning often refers to those people who discriminate against an individual on the basis of his or her sexual orientation. Whilst attitudes in the UK towards sexuality have changed significantly in recent decades, there remains a minority of people who are homophobic.

The benefits of diversity

The benefits of diversity are numerous. The wide range of cultures, skills and expertise inherent within a multicultural society increases opportunities to access learning and new experiences, all of which will ultimately contribute to an improvement in health and social care experiences, systems and structures.

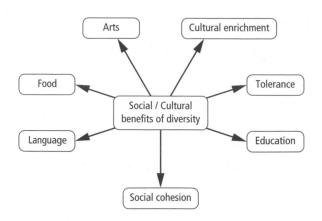

Figure 2.02 The social and cultural benefits of diversity

Economic

The economic benefits of diversity can be clearly seen through the contributions made to society by those people living and working in the community. These include, for example, opportunities for employment. These can arise when an individual is entrepreneurial and starts a new business, and when companies from abroad relocate to the UK.

Expertise

There are many doctors and nurses from other countries working in the UK. This enriches the UK's health services with new levels of expertise and knowledge. There is a wide range of medical advancements that have originated abroad and are now being used to improve medication and treatment services in this country.

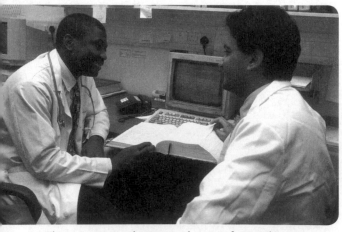

There are many doctors and nurses from other countries working in the UK

Did you know?

Almost 30 per cent of doctors and 43 per cent of nurses currently working in the UK were born in another country.

Education

Education has benefited from cultural diversity in many ways. These include, for example:

- The subjects studied in schools and colleges now incorporate the observances of a wide range of religious groups, whereas many years ago religious studies were generally confined to Christian traditions. Today, the celebration of different traditions and cultures is a feature of all syllabuses.
- Teachers and managers from diverse cultural backgrounds often bring new perspectives to their roles, thereby helping to break down traditional ways of working. This can benefit all those who study and work within the educational system.

Learning new languages

The opportunity to live and work with people from other countries and cultural backgrounds offers the chance to learn something new and exciting; language is just one example of this. Colleges of further education and schools provide the opportunity to study modern foreign languages at every level, which greatly supports people who wish to travel and work abroad. The teachers of this provision are most often from the corresponding cultural background.

View point

Viewpoint 1

Modern languages have dropped down the popularity polls in schools. That's fine – everyone speaks English anyway.

Viewpoint 2

I think it's great to learn different languages. Why should people in Spain be expected to speak to me in English?

The Arts

One of the benefits of living in a socially diverse society is the easy access people have to a range of different traditions and art forms from around the world. For example, Bollywood films and circus troops from Russia and China.

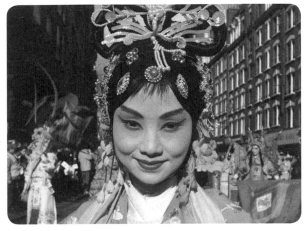

Different art forms enrich our lives

Food

A clear benefit of living in a multicultural society is the wide variety of foods that become available. The choice of fresh foods in supermarkets and markets that are grown in other countries has never been so good. In addition, restaurants serving traditional meals from around the world are available in most towns and cities throughout the UK.

Cultural enrichment

If the benefits of diversity explored above, for example, an increased range of food types and greater access to new languages, are available and accessed by all people in the UK, then the population will be culturally enriched. This means that people living in the UK have more experiences and opportunities available to them, to enable a wider perspective on people and life in general.

Promoting equal opportunity in health and social care settings

The key concepts described so far in this chapter apply to many health and social care settings. A good understanding of these concepts is, therefore, central to any job role within health and social care. However, in addition to understanding the terminology, it is important to recognise the wide variety of settings in which healthcare takes place.

Types of health and social care setting

Residential care settings

As the name suggests, residential care involves an individual leaving his or her home and moving into a setting that will allow the individual to live in a safe and secure environment and which caters for his or her social care needs. The individual shares the accommodation with other people who are usually in need of the same type of care and attention.

Moving into residential care

Shirley is moving into the Happy Mount Residential Care Home for older people. She is a bit apprehensive about the move but has been to visit and found that she can have her own room and even take some of her furniture with her. Since she fell and broke her hip, Shirley has lacked confidence in her own ability to 'get about', especially during the night. She is glad to know that someone will always be there if she needs them, and that she will still have her own doctor, solicitor and bank manager.

- What might be the benefits to Shirley of living in residential care?

Day care settings

Day care serves a variety of purposes and is provided in a range of ways by different day care providers. In the main, day care is used to support care that takes place mainly in the home.

Another form of day care is that attached to hospitals. In this instance, individuals may be collected by ambulance from home and taken to the centre. Once there, they have the opportunity to be treated by healthcare professionals, for example, physiotherapists and occupational therapists.

Nursing care settings

The care provided in this type of setting is by trained nursing staff. The service they provide goes beyond social care and often involves assessments, routine treatment and medication. However, when discussing nursing care, it is important to remember that there are several different types of trained nursing staff. These include:

- Practice Nurse
- Health Visitor
- Ward Nurse
- School Nurse
- Occupational Health Nurse
- Midwife
- Mental Health Nurse
- Paediatric Nurse.

Each of the nursing jobs specialises in a particular kind of care and works in a range of different settings with specific client groups. For example, school nurses are often based in schools and health centres, and mental health nurses are generally based in hospitals, GP practices or the local community.

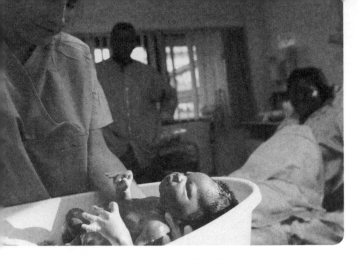

Midwives work in hospitals, health centres and the community

Over to you

1 Select two of the nursing jobs listed on page 42 and research:

 - the settings where the jobs are carried out
 - the qualifications needed to do the job
 - what the job role involves.

 Identify ways in which both nursing posts can work towards the empowerment of their client groups. Prepare a presentation to share your findings with others.

2 Health Care Assistants work in a wide variety of settings including hospitals, GP practices, care settings and the local community. Their role is to support and work alongside qualified nursing staff to assist in the care and/or treatment of individuals.

 - Use the Internet to find out more about the training and work roles of these new health posts.

Domiciliary settings

The phrase 'domiciliary setting' means that all the health and social care work pertaining to an individual is carried out in his or her own home. The kind of service provided in the home can vary from something relatively simple, such as preparing and cooking meals, through to the medical care required for a person who is terminally ill. Clearly, a wide range of health professionals could be involved in a domiciliary setting, depending on the needs of the individual.

Promoting equality and individual rights

A clear role and responsibility for people working in health and social care is to ensure that they take positive action to promote equality and individual rights in their work settings. It is often expected, by the public at large, that health professionals will continue to actively promote diversity in their personal as well as their professional lives.

Tolerance

Tolerance means acceptance of someone or something. With regard to diversity, tolerance is about accepting the differences that diversity brings; for example, the differences in political and religious beliefs, and in cultural ways and values. Tolerance requires that we are non-judgemental of others – that is, open to the differences rather than forming stereotypes or labels because of them. Tolerance does not mean that, in the workplace, you should be friends with everyone, but it does mean that you should behave at all times in a professional and caring manner to those whom you care for and your colleagues.

Social cohesion

Social cohesion can perhaps be best explained by the use of the word 'community' instead of social. A cohesive community is one where there is a common sense of belonging for all individuals living in that place. A community area could be a school, workplace, neighbourhood, town or country. For people to feel that they belong in their community there is a need for:

 - everyone's circumstances and background to be valued
 - positive relationships between people from different backgrounds.

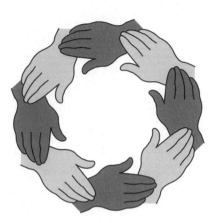

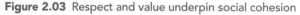

Figure 2.03 Respect and value underpin social cohesion

Treating people equally

All people deserve to be treated equally by health professionals and by the employing organisations that are providing healthcare for them. This means not discriminating against individuals because of their age, gender, sexual orientation, religion or anything else. However, actually carrying this out can be difficult in some situations.

Over to you

Fred, who is aged 63 years old with two adult children, needs to have a heart bypass operation if he is to live a full and active life for his remaining years. His heart surgeon has told him he must stop smoking if the operation is to be a success.

Myra, who is aged 47 years old with two children under 13 years of age, also needs a heart bypass operation if she is to live a full and active life. She smokes 20 cigarettes a day but is trying hard to quit.

- *Unfortunately there is only enough money to pay for one operation. Who should have it and why?*

It is fortunate that we do not often have to make decisions such as the one about Fred and Myra. Care workers are expected to provide equal care for all individuals no matter what their circumstances. If we fail to do this we can be accused of discrimination.

However, research has demonstrated that there are inequalities in health experiences and healthcare. These take various forms, for example, people from low income groups tend to suffer more illness and die at an earlier age than those from high earning groups. In many cases, these people and the areas where they live tend to face more barriers to effective healthcare than other areas. As a health professional, it is important to recognise that everyone should be treated according to their needs rather than treated according to the resources available.

Reflection

How realistic is it to treat everyone according to their needs rather than treating them according to the resources available?

Confidentiality

Confidentiality

Confidentiality means not passing an individual's private information to anyone unless there is a legitimate reason to do so. Maintaining confidentiality is a central part of the care value base.

Care value base

Occupational standards and the General Social Care Council (GSCC) code of practice identify a framework of values and moral rights of individuals that can be referred to as care values or a value base for care. This underpinning philosophy guides the work, beliefs and values of all health and social care workers. It can perhaps best be described as a series of features that put the individual at the centre of the caring process. The features are:

- promoting anti discriminatory practice
- providing individualised (personalised) care
- maintaining confidentiality

- promoting and supporting individual rights
- acknowledging and respecting diversity
- protecting individuals from abuse
- promoting effective communication and relationships.

Key words that align with the care value base are: respect, privacy, safety, dignity, choice and fulfilment.

Respecting confidentiality is an important part of the active promotion of individual rights. However, there may be occasions when confidentiality cannot and should not be maintained. For example, if an individual confides in you about an abusive situation, this must be passed on to a line manager or supervisor. The individual needs to be told (preferably before the disclosure, if possible) that this kind of information cannot be kept secret. In addition, anything that puts the life of another individual in danger must be disclosed.

Over to you

Using the Internet or other research methods, find out why disclosures about abusive situations cannot and should not be kept secret.

Practice implications of confidentiality

The Data Protection Act 1998 provides clear guidelines about the use of personal information (see also page 53). These state that care workers must ensure that only relevant information is collected about individuals and that personal information is stored in a secure place. It is also the responsibility of all care workers to maintain individual confidentiality at all times. Consequently, individuals have the right to expect that any information disclosed to a care worker will be kept safe and secure. This means that a care worker should never:

- gossip about individuals
- seek out information that he or she does not need to know
- discuss information about individuals in the hearing of other people

- leave notes lying around for others to read
- move individual records from one place to another without a valid reason
- disclose information to a third party without permission.

Over to you

The Data Protection Act 1998 states that individuals must be allowed access to any personal information relating to them upon their request.

1 What might be the implications of this legislation for healthcare practice?
2 How might a nurse be affected by this law?
3 How might an individual be affected by this right?

All records must be kept safe and secure, and each workplace must have a confidentiality policy or guidelines for staff to follow (see page 58). Whenever you are handling information, it is important to ensure that you respect the individual's wishes, follow the guidance and procedures of your organisation, and comply with the requirements of the Data Protection Act. Bringing these three key aspects together will help ensure that you provide an equitable and high quality service to all individuals.

Over to you

Obtain a copy of your setting's confidentiality policy. Make notes of the contents and their purpose in promoting access and individual rights.

Communication

Communicating with people is not as simple as just talking. Communication involves a whole range of different aspects. These include:

- active listening
- verbal communication
- non-verbal communication
- language
- level and pace
- aids to communication.

Communication is an entire subject in its own right and can only be touched upon here. (You may wish to research this interesting aspect of healthcare.) For the present, the focus is on the way you use communication to help or hinder equality and individual rights.

Communication barriers

Almira is having a baby. She is seven months pregnant and speaks limited English. She can understand if people speak slowly and use gestures to support their words. Her midwife is from Scotland and has a strong Glaswegian accent. Almira is pleased that her midwife is a woman but is worried because she cannot understand what she is saying, no matter how slowly she speaks.

The midwife is desperate to find a solution to their communication barrier as she wants Almira to have a positive birth experience.

- What action might the midwife take to improve the communication between her and Almira?

When using communication to actively promote individual rights and equality of access, as a health professional you will need to:

- use appropriate language
- actively listen to the responses given
- avoid the use of jargon or technical language
- use more than one method to communicate, i.e. verbal and written
- use interpreters when necessary
- check understanding by **paraphrasing** or asking questions.

Paraphrase – to express something a person has said but in your own words.

Tensions and contradictions

There are always difficult decisions to be taken in the provision of healthcare to others. You have already considered the examples of the need to pass on confidential information about individuals in certain circumstances, and the need to allocate tight resources and how this affects which individual receives which care. Imagine also: one ambulance and two heart attack victims living at opposite ends of a town. Where does the ambulance go first? Who decides?

Fortunately, no one health professional need carry the burden for such difficult decisions. Team work is an essential part of healthcare and when this is used alongside guidance, quality standards and evidence-based practice, decisions become easier and fairer.

The effects of sickness

Hilda has leg ulcers and cannot move around easily. She is waiting in her own home for the district nurse to arrive and dress her leg, which is extremely inflamed and painful. The dressing has to be changed everyday. Unfortunately, what Hilda does not know is that her nurse is off work today with a broken arm and her case load is being covered by another district nurse who has her own individuals to see. It is beginning to look like Hilda may not get a visit today.

1 What are the tensions and contradictions being shown in this scenario?
2 What action could the district nurse take to help improve the situation?
3 What other examples can you think of that demonstrate tensions and contradictions in the health service?

Staff development and training

Undertaking staff development and training are key ways in which health professionals can increase their knowledge about individual rights and equality of opportunity. Finding out about key legislation can help to keep care workers up-to-date and provide a sound basis from which to work.

Training and development does not just consist of attending college or completing qualifications. Whilst these are important for career development, the knowledge required to provide sound, high quality individual care can be derived from a variety of sources.

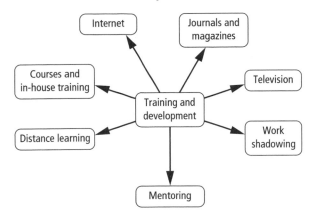

Figure 2.04 Training and development needs can be met from a variety of sources

Individual rights

Human rights were briefly outlined at the beginning of the chapter (pages 31–32). In this section, you will explore the following rights in detail:

- the right to be treated with respect
- the right to be treated equally and not discriminated against
- the right to be treated as an individual
- the right to be treated in a dignified way
- the right to privacy
- the right to protection from danger and harm
- the right to access information held about oneself
- the right to use preferred methods of communication and languages
- the right to be cared for in a way that meets the individual's needs, accounts for his or her choices and protects him or her.

The right to be treated with respect

All individuals have the right to be treated with respect, irrespective of age or circumstance. It is the responsibility of all healthcare professionals to communicate this respect through the way they approach and treat the individuals in their care.

Bed bath

Albert has had a stroke and cannot move the right side of his body. He has been in hospital for four days and is on a ward with twelve other men. He needs to have a bed bath and Nurse Baker has been asked to carry out this procedure. Nurse Baker is feeling very harassed, with a huge workload, but he goes off to prepare.

Version 1
Nurse Baker then approaches Albert, pulls off the bed clothes and removes Albert's pyjamas without once speaking to him. The curtains remain open while Nurse Baker gets on with his task, so that he can keep an eye on Harry who keeps getting out of bed and wandering off.

1 Consider the implications of this scenario for Albert.

2 How could respect for Albert be demonstrated?

Version 2
Nurse Baker asks a Health Care Assistant to monitor Harry while he baths Albert. He approaches Albert and gently touches his hand, saying 'Good morning' and asking whether he would like a bath to help him feel more comfortable. The curtains are closed whilst Nurse Baker removes the bed clothes and then takes off Albert's pyjama jacket, explaining everything to him as he goes along. Once his arms and chest are washed and dried, the nurse puts Albert's jacket back on and then removes his pyjama bottoms. He uses a towel to cover Albert as he washes each section of his lower body so he does not feel exposed. Once Nurse Baker is finished, he makes sure that Albert is comfortable and dry before re-covering him with the bedclothes and opening the curtains.

3 How does this scenario demonstrate respect for Albert?

Over to you

Develop your own scenario to show how respect could be demonstrated in other situations. Make notes of the key points in your reflective diary.

Respect for others is a core responsibility of a care worker. This means respecting an individual's:

- dignity
- beliefs and wishes
- need for privacy
- right to choose the kind of healthcare he or she receives.

Each individual's beliefs, wishes, needs and choices must be respected, even when these clash with your own.

The right to be treated equally and not discriminated against

All individuals have the right to be treated equally and not discriminated against. Healthcare professionals must take especial care to ensure that they do not discriminate against any person during the course of their work. In this respect, it is helpful to be aware that some actions which come naturally to us may in fact be discriminatory. For example, in many care settings, health professionals working with groups of people tend to spend more time with individuals whose company they prefer.

A discriminatory attitude

Maria does not want to help Marco to eat his evening meal again, as she finds his foreign accent difficult to understand, particularly since his stroke. Maria struggled to understand and respond to Marco's conversation yesterday. 'Someone else can take him on today', she thinks to herself.

1 Why can Maria's actions and thoughts be classed as discriminatory?

2 What could Maria do differently to aid both Marco and herself in this situation?

The right to be treated as an individual

Treating each person as an individual is central to the care value base. To do this, it is necessary to recognise and value difference. Abraham Maslow (1908–70) demonstrated some key similarities in the needs of all human beings, for example, the need for warmth, shelter and food, love, self-esteem and personal growth (see also page 16).

Whilst it is important to recognise that all people share these basic needs, it is also important to recognise that people also have individual needs based on difference. Treating everyone the same regardless of these differences is failing to respect diversity.

The right to be treated in a dignified way

All individuals deserve to be treated in a manner that preserves their dignity and self-worth. The second scenario about Albert on page 47 demonstrates how simple the maintenance of dignity can be. All care workers should be sensitive to and aware of the needs of the individuals in their care, especially at times when the body and its functions could be exposed.

The right to privacy

All human beings have the right to expect that their treatment and care will be kept private. This means that:

- information about the individual will be passed only to those people who need to access it (for more on confidentiality, see pages 58–59)
- the individual's dignity and privacy will be maintained throughout any procedures.

Reflection

Discuss with others how you would want your privacy to be maintained if you had to undergo an operation for a bowel disorder. Think about procedures during an initial consultation and then the treatment that might be required in a large ward setting.

The right to protection from danger and harm

All individuals have the right to expect their care workers to keep them safe from danger and harm. To this end, all hospitals and nursing homes must have a policy that describes the necessary actions to be taken, and rules and regulations to be followed, to ensure the health and safety of staff and individuals. In many hospitals the health and safety policy includes a 'locked door' policy, especially on children's wards and wards caring for vulnerable adults.

The right to access information held about oneself

As described on page 53, by the terms of the Data Protection Act 1998, individuals are entitled to access their records and any information held about them. In addition, the Freedom of Information Act 2005 requires that all healthcare professionals (as well as those from other sectors and industries) must respond to any written request for information within twenty working days. This means that healthcare professionals must:

- keep their records in order
- be able to find information quickly and easily
- enable colleagues to find information quickly and easily in their absence.

Reflection

What skills will be required from healthcare workers to ensure they can respond to the Freedom of Information Act effectively? Make notes for yourself.

The right to use preferred methods of communication and languages

All individuals have a preferred method of communication and language. This will vary, which means that enabling good communication in health and social care can be challenging for the healthcare workers involved. However, it is important to work to overcome any difficulties because, without good communication between an individual and his or her care worker, the treatment and recovery process are likely to be slower than usual.

Offering individuals the opportunity to communicate in their preferred language can mean:

- having staff who communicate in the same language as the individual
- using the skills of interpreters and translators
- having the information in a variety of formats, for example, leaflets, pictures, tapes, etc.
- asking an individual's family members to be involved in the communication process.

View point

Viewpoint 1
Asking family members to interpret on behalf of the individual is a good way to improve communication between two people who speak different languages.

Viewpoint 2
Family members should never be asked to interpret health information for family members.

The right to be cared for in a way that meets the individual's needs, accounts for his or her choices and protects him or her

Essentially, this is about individuals having their rights protected. For example, caring for individuals in a way that ensures their:

- privacy
- freedom to follow their own beliefs and values
- equality and fair treatment
- safe access to medication and treatment
- safety at all times.

Meeting the individual's needs

Meeting an individual's needs is not always easy. There are often limited resources available (as illustrated by the examples on page 44) and competing pressures on staff caring for the individual. However, as a health professional it is essential that you do all you can to ensure that each person's individual needs are met. For example, if you refer to Maslow's hierarchy of needs (see also page 16), it is essential that the individual's basic health needs are met before addressing his or her spiritual needs.

Taking account of choices

People should always be given a choice: it is the act of choosing that gives them a sense of control over their lives. When illness strikes, many individuals feel disempowered; at such times, making even simple choices becomes vital to restoring feelings of control. These 'simple' choices could include choosing from a menu, deciding which clothes to wear or when to have a bath or shower.

> **Did you know?**
>
> *Many hospitals and hospices now put pain control into the hands of the individual following an operation, as this has been shown to reduce distress and the experience of pain.*

Protecting individuals in your care

When people are frail and sick they become vulnerable and reliant on others. All healthcare workers have a duty to protect the people they care for. Not only should individuals be protected from harm, they should also be kept safe from exploitation by others. The Health and Safety at Work Act 1974 is a key piece of legislation that promotes the protection of both individuals and healthcare workers (see also Chapter 5 page 193).

> ### Keeping the individual safe from harm
>
> Jim is recovering from major brain surgery, and needs to be sedated and kept safe. He is in a high dependency bed with nurses who are monitoring his condition at all times. His heart, blood pressure, pulse and breathing are monitored by equipment that alerts the nurse to any fluctuations. His bed has high sides that can be lowered when the bedding needs to be changed. The ward is locked and entry is by permission only.
>
> **1** Working with another person, note the different ways Jim is being kept safe from harm.
>
> **2** Consider how Jim's dignity could be maintained in this situation.

Understand discriminatory practice in health and social care

Discriminatory practice does occur within health and social care settings. It could be assumed that, where it does happen, it is through ignorance and lack of knowledge. However, this is not always the case.

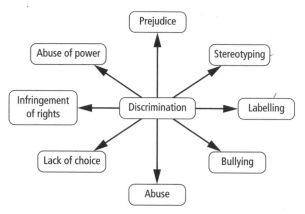

Figure 2.05 Common forms of discrimination

Prejudice, stereotyping and labelling

As you read on pages 35–36:

● prejudice is pre-conceived judgements ('pre-judgements') about people and their characteristics or behaviours

● stereotyping occurs when assumptions are made about groups of people based on information relating to just one (or very few) people.

As a result of both prejudice and stereotyping, many individuals or groups of the population end up with labels applied to them (see also page 36).

Bullying

Bullying is when a person uses his or her power or position to intimidate another. Bullying can also be classed as abuse (see also page 38), and is demonstrated through physical as well as verbal or written behaviours. Persistent bullying can cause great distress to the individual, affecting his or her ability to live a normal life and leading to associated problems such as depression, loss of self-esteem and panic attacks.

In health and social care settings, bullying occurs in a range of circumstances across all levels of care. For example, it is possible for one member of staff to bully another or for a manager to bully his or her team members. It is important to remember that all forms of bullying are discrimination and should not be allowed to go unchecked.

Dealing with bullying behaviours

When bullying occurs in the workplace, it is possible for staff to challenge this offensive behaviour and support the individual being bullied. However, bullying can also be difficult to spot and much more difficult to handle.

Reflection

1 How could you find out if an individual was being bullied by a member of staff?
2 How easy do you think it would be for the member of staff to conceal his or her actions?

Identifying bullying between staff and individuals may be difficult for a range of reasons, including:

- fear on the part of the individual
- illness
- dementia
- unwillingness by the individual or staff to acknowledge what is happening.

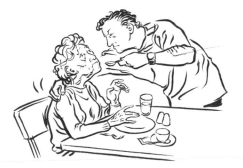

Figure 2.06 How would you respond if you thought that a colleague was bullying another person?

Suffering in silence

Emily has lived in the nursing home for three years. She knows she is a challenging individual for the nursing team because of her physical disabilities, but she tries to help them when it is necessary to move her.

Emily is worried in case Rainer is on duty this evening, because she cannot please her no matter how she tries. Emily hates the way Rainer bursts into her room and pushes and pulls her into the hoist and wheelchair to take her for dinner. Her upper arms are really sore from last night and she knows she must not complain or she will be left in her room again without a meal.

1 How does this scenario demonstrate bullying?
2 Why does Emily feel that she cannot complain?

Harassment

Harassment is a form of bullying and should be challenged immediately. Examples of harassment include:

- threatening words
- nicknames
- offensive jokes
- sexually inappropriate comments
- persistent personal criticism
- exclusion from treatment or medication.

Harassment – to continually distress, annoy, pester or trouble another person.

Reflection

More women than men suffer from harassment and bullying. Why do you think this is?

Abuse

Abuse in its wider meaning is covered on page 38, yet all forms of discrimination are abuse, whether bullying, denying a person's right to choose or applying labels to individuals. Reported cases of abuse in health and social care settings are rare; the individuals involved usually lack training and support, and are prosecuted for their part in the action. In some cases, stress due to overload of work can contribute to abusive situations.

Lack of choice

Choice is at the centre of individual empowerment. If you take away the individual's ability to choose, you take away his or her identity. People who make choices feel more in control of their lives and are generally more willing to co-operate in their healthcare. Removing individual choice is a form of discriminatory practice and is likely to result in a series of unhelpful behaviours.

Infringement of rights

All individuals are entitled by law to see their rights respected and followed. Healthcare professionals have a duty to promote the rights of individuals and to challenge those who infringe upon such rights. Protection and empowerment cannot be secured if the rights of individuals are not first established.

Understand how national initiatives promote anti-discriminatory practice in health and social care settings

UK laws provide employers and employees (including healthcare professionals) with the basic principles for dealing with people in any situation. The rules attached to each specific piece of legislation must be followed or sanctions will be applied to those breaking the law.

Key legislation

Nobody expects an individual to understand or be able to quote every law that promotes anti-discriminatory practice in health and social care settings. However, it is important for all healthcare workers to understand the basic principles of the laws that apply to their working practice, and to apply and follow these laws in every aspect of their work. Table 2.03 summarises the key legislation that applies to those working in health and social care.

Table 2.03 Key legislation that applies to those working in health and social care

Legislation	Requirements
Human Rights Act 1998 (updated 2000)	This guarantees the sixteen human rights outlined on page 32. The Act was based on the 1950 European Convention on Human Rights and Fundamental Freedoms, which aims to gain universal recognition and observance of human rights. Many countries have agreed to abide by the 66 articles identified within the convention. The Act enables all individuals to take action against authorities, including the police and government, if they feel their rights have been affected negatively. All health and social care establishments are included in this Act and must, therefore, abide by it.
Sex Discrimination Act 1975	Designed to give both men and women equal rights in relation to employment and services. It deals with both direct and indirect sexual discrimination (see pages 33–34).
Mental Health Act 1983	Protects the rights of people with mental health difficulties or learning disabilities; the intention is to protect individuals from exploitation by others. The Act also protects society from individuals behaving dangerously as a result of their mental health problems. (This creates a conflict between the individual's right to freedom and the community's right to be safe.)
Mental Health Order 1986	This covers: • the treatment of people with mental health problems in Northern Ireland • the issues involved in caring for people with learning disabilities • aspects of compulsory treatment and detaining people in hospital without their consent • issues around the protection of individuals from exploitation by others.

Legislation	Requirements
Convention on the Rights of the Child 1989	Held by the United Nations General Assembly, this reaffirmed that children's rights require special protection. The convention called for a continuous improvement in the situation of all children worldwide. Aspects of the convention are enshrined in the Children Act 1989 and Every Child Matters (see below).
The Children Act 1989	Protects children and their rights. The Act aims to ensure that children are: • protected from significant harm • supported fully if they are in care • safe and cared for suitably by the setting of standards for nurseries and residential schools.
The Children Act 2004	This Act builds on the Children Act 1989 by setting out a new framework – Every Child Matters – based around the needs of children and young people from birth to age 19 years. It laid down five aims for every child, whatever the child's background or circumstances. Each child needs to have the support he or she needs to: • be healthy • stay safe • enjoy and achieve • make a positive contribution • achieve economic well-being. The Act aims to transform children's services by bringing them together under children's trusts. The key duty in this Act is one of co-operation between all organisations involved with providing children's services.
Race Relations Act 1976 (amended 2000)	By this Act, all public sector organisations must promote racial equality. This means that they should promote equality of opportunity and good relations between people of different ethnic backgrounds. Encouraging racial hatred is unlawful and any form of discrimination on the grounds of colour, nationality or race is illegal.
Disability Discrimination Act 1995	The Act is designed to protect the rights of people with disabilities in terms of employment, access to education and transport, housing, goods and services. Under the Act, employers must not treat a disabled person less favourably than an able-bodied person. The Act places a duty on organisations to consider how they make their services fully accessible to people with a disability. Reasonable adjustments should be made and equipment provided to enable equal access.
Data Protection Act 1998	This Act is designed to protect information held about individuals. All organisations must register as a data user and follow the rules provided. These are: • data must have been collected through lawful means • the information held should only be used for the purpose agreed and relevant to the situation • the information must be stored securely • individuals must be allowed access to all their personal information on request.
Nursing and Residential Care Homes Regulations 1984 (amended 2002)	This Act places a duty on care and nursing providers to register their service and manager with the appropriate authority (for an annual fee). Local councils and health authorities then have a duty to regulate the standard of care being provided in nursing and residential care. To this end, authorities have the right to enter and inspect premises and make a series of recommendations. They also have the power to close an establishment if it fails to provide a suitable service.
Care Standards Act 2000	The National Care Standards replaced the regulation duties carried out by local authorities and health authorities under the Registered Homes Act 1984. The Care Standards Act 2000 expanded a new system for regulating health and social care provision to include domiciliary, fostering and family care as well as home care. A series of National Minimum Standards have to be applied to all services with the intention of putting the individual at the centre of the caring process.

Clearly, with Acts such as these come rights and responsibilities. For example, whilst an Act can give freedom of speech to the individual, this comes with the responsibility not to use this right to offend or discriminate against others.

Reflection

What responsibilities do you think accompany the right to life?

Codes of practice and charters

Codes of practice are designed to guide and advise health and social care workers on their rights and responsibilities. They also help individuals identify the kind of support and behaviour they can expect from the person caring for them. Most health and social care professions have a charter or code of practice which members follow. For example, the Councils for Social Care have guidelines for staff and organisations to follow.

> **Legislation, codes of practice and charters**
> Legislation, codes of practice and charters are all used as guidelines and frameworks for employers, organisations and individuals to follow to make sure that human rights are not infringed. The laws are designed to protect people from exploitation and harm, and to provide a route for seeking redress when things go wrong.

Home Life: A Code of Practice for Residential Care

First published in 1984, this is a list of 218 recommendations for monitoring the quality of social care. Many of these have now been built into regulations which inspectors check before a residential home can be registered or for a home to remain registered. Ten recommendations concerning staff qualities are shown below.

> ### Code of practice for residential care staff
>
> **148** Staff qualities should include responsiveness to and respect for the needs of the individuals.
> **149** Staff skills should match the residents' needs as identified in the objectives of the home.
> **150** Staff should have the ability to give competent and tactful care, whilst enabling residents to retain dignity and self-determination.
> **151** In the selection of staff at least two references should be taken up, where possible from previous employers.
> **152** Applicants' curriculum vitae should be checked and for this purpose employers should give

> warning that convictions otherwise spent should be disclosed.
> **153** Proprietors should consider residents' needs in relation to all categories of staff when drawing up staffing proposals.
> **154** Job descriptions will be required for all posts and staff should be provided with relevant job descriptions on appointment.
> **155** In small homes where staff carry a range of responsibilities, these must be clearly understood by staff.
> **156** Any change of role or duty should be made clear to the member of staff in writing.
> **157** Minimum staff cover should be designed to copy with residents' anticipated problems at any time.
>
> (Reproduced from *Home Life: A Code of Practice for Residential Care* with permission from the Centre for Policy on Ageing.)

Code of professional conduct for nurses, midwives and health visitors

The following extract is taken from the Nursing and Midwifery Council's (NMC) Code of Professional Conduct: Standards for Conduct, Performance and Ethics, 2004 (reproduced with permission).

> ### NMC Code of Professional Conduct: Standards for Conduct, Performance and Ethics
>
> As a registered nurse, midwife or specialist community public health nurse, you are personally accountable for your practice. In caring for patients and clients, you must:
>
> * respect the patient or client as an individual
> * obtain consent before you give any treatment or care
> * protect confidential information
> * co-operate with others in the team
> * maintain your professional knowledge and competence
> * be trustworthy
> * act to identify and minimise risk to patients and clients.
>
> These are the shared values of all the United

Kingdom health care regulatory bodies.

1.1: The purpose of the NMC code of professional conduct: standards for conduct, performance and ethics is to:
- inform the professions of the standard of professional conduct required of them in the exercise of their professional accountability and practice
- inform the public, other professions and employers of the standard of professional conduct that they can expect of a registered practitioner.

1.2: As a registered nurse, midwife or specialist community public health nurse, you must:
- protect and support the health of individual patients and clients
- protect and support the health of the wider community
- act in such a way that justifies the trust and confidence the public have in you
- uphold and enhance the good reputation of the professions.

1.3: You are personally accountable for your practice. This means that you are answerable for your actions and omissions, regardless of advice or directions from another professional.

1.4: You have a duty of care to your patients and clients, who are entitled to receive safe and competent care.

1.5: You must adhere to the laws of the country in which you are practising.

Formal polices on equality and rights

Within the healthcare sector there is a huge range of policies, guidelines and procedures to support equality and rights. You have already read through a summary of the current legislation which supports individuals and groups at a national level (see Table 2.03). In this section, you will explore the actions that can be taken at a local level. For example, the services and actions which managers and healthcare workers can become involved in, to further support those people in their employment or care.

Positive promotion of individual rights

In many healthcare settings, staff are able to contribute to the development of policies and procedures that help promote individual rights. For example, a charter in the workplace might outline the responsibilities expected from staff towards the individuals in their care, but equally it should include a section on the responsibilities of individuals towards each other and the staff who are caring for them. Remember – with rights come responsibilities!

Zero tolerance

Anytown hospital has recently put together a 'zero tolerance' policy in the A&E department, following the third attack on one of the doctors. The staff in the department have worked together with the Health and Safety Officer and Human Resources department to develop the policy, which they hope will protect staff and individuals who use the department. The main theme of the policy is that any individual displaying abusive or violent attitudes or actions towards staff or other individuals will be asked to leave.

- How does this policy demonstrate positive promotion of individual rights?

Further examples of the positive promotion of equality and rights include:
- a member of staff demonstrating good practice and mentoring others who may not be aware of the policy on equality and rights
- staff handbooks that outline rights and responsibilities for a new member of staff
- notice boards displaying key policies and guidelines.

It is a requirement by law that an organisation display health and safety regulations. In addition, an organisation's confidentiality policy may also be displayed, to reassure individuals receiving care and remind staff of best practice.

Advocacy

There are many occasions when an individual is too ill or frail to speak for him- or herself or may not have the mental ability or communication skills required. In such instances the individual is entitled to the help of an **advocate**. The advocate will speak on behalf of the person and can be:

- a fully trained and advocacy-employed person
- a member of the individual's family
- a member of staff with relevant training from an organisation that is involved in some way with the individual concerned.

> **Advocate** – someone who speaks on behalf of another person.

Whoever acts as advocate for the individual must remember that he or she is putting the views of the individual forward (not his or her own). The advocate will need to be clear about the difference between the individual's views and those of the organisation caring for him or her. In many healthcare settings guidelines are provided for staff on accepted behaviour for those acting in the role of advocate.

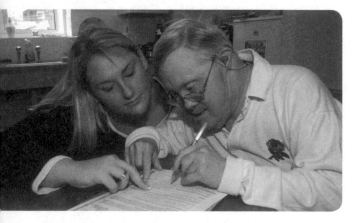

Advocates work on behalf of individuals

Work practices

Work practices must demonstrate equality and rights across the organisation at all times. All organisations will have policies and procedures that cover confidentiality, health and safety, bullying and harassment, to mention but a few. There is no point having these policies if staff and individuals do not follow the guidelines within them. A central part of healthcare training is the promotion of these policies. Staff are expected to

know the contents and demonstrate compliance at all times. Failure to do so would result in disciplinary action and, if necessary, dismissal.

Organisational policies

Having explored the role of organisational policies in maintaining and promoting equality and rights, we will now turn our attention to the contents of organisational policies.

> **Over to you**
>
> *Arrange to visit a healthcare centre, for example, a dentist or GP surgery or hospital reception, and ask for a copy of either their confidentiality policy or health and safety policy. Working with another person, identify the key aspects that would promote equality and the rights of the individual or the staff employed there.*

Staff development and training

Once a healthcare professional has qualified, he or she is expected to continue with personal and professional training to update his or her skills and knowledge. Remember, technology is developing at high speed, and a nurse or doctor could soon become outdated in his or her practice if he or she doesn't move with the times. An individual has the right to expect to have his or her treatment and care carried out to the best possible standards. In exactly the same way, it is important to recognise that training and development on equality and rights should also be updated and remain fresh in the minds of the staff employed in the organisation.

Quality issues

This is perhaps best explained as 'an organisation always striving to do better'. Maintaining the standards regarding equality and rights is difficult for any organisation, but not impossible. An organisation has to consider, for example:

- how to monitor policies
- how to update the content of policies
- what staff training is required
- how effective the policies are.

Over to you

How might a hospital trust find out if its confidentiality policy is working?

Complaint procedures

This is another example of a local policy written to support an organisation. All organisations must have a complaints procedure which will be inspected when **audits** are carried out. Although each organisation's complaints procedure will contain roughly the same information, the way they are worded will vary from one organisation to another. In general, you could expect a complaints procedure to follow the pattern shown in Figure 2.07.

Audit – in this context, the word audit is taken to mean a quality check. This would involve a detailed examination of the organisation's systems, structures and processes. The aim would be to ensure that the individual is receiving the best possible service and that the organisation involved is both efficient and effective.

Figure 2.07 Example of an organisation's complaints policy

Warmshire County Care Services
Complaints Policy

This leaflet outlines the ways you can make a complaint if you are dissatisfied with our services. If you feel that you have a complaint to make about our service or the way you have been treated then follow the simple guidelines shown below.

It is often simpler to refer your complaint to the member of staff with whom you have been dealing. He or she may be able to sort the issue out immediately for you. If you prefer not to speak to the member of staff then please ask to see his or her supervisor or line manager. Failing either of these two options you can:

- use the attached form to make a complaint
- write a letter and send it to us
- ask someone else to write the letter on your behalf and send it to us.

Our staff are here to help you and you will not be discriminated against because you have made a complaint.

- Please return this form to Warmshire County Care Services, Heaton Place, Warmshire.
- Please state your complaint below and continue on a separate sheet if necessary.
- Your complaint will be acknowledged within one week and dealt with within 28 days.

Name: ____________________
Address: ____________________
Telephone number: ____________________
Nature of complaint: ____________________

Affirmative action

This is sometimes called positive action or positive discrimination, which means favouring one individual over another because he or she is from a minority group. This is illegal in the UK under the Race Relations and Sex Discrimination Acts (see pages 52–53) unless special amendments are agreed. However, in an organisation where the individuals who make up the workforce do not reflect the people living in the local community, it is acceptable to compensate by setting targets for the employment of staff and taking positive action to meet these targets.

Positive discrimination

Maple Leaf Day Centre is based in East Wertham, where there is a high population of Asian heritage people. The individuals coming for day care are mainly from the Indian sub-continent, with one or two people from Irish backgrounds. The matron has decided that the workforce needs to better reflect the local population, so she has set a target to try to employ more nurses from Asian heritage backgrounds. She is using newspapers and local schools that she knows are accessed by the local population to advertise job vacancies. However, she knows that when it comes to appointing people, she must fill the jobs on merit only or she will be breaking the law.

Anti-harassment

Another aspect of the UK legal system is the requirement for organisations to have anti-harassment/bullying policies. UK laws aim to prevent harassment on the grounds of race, ethnicity, sex, gender, religion, sexual orientation and disability. Harassment is seen through the effects of an individual's actions on another. Thus, it is not the intentions of the person accused of carrying out the harassment that determines when harassment occurs. This could mean that the perpetrator may not realise that his or her actions are perceived as harassment.

Health and safety

Health and social care workers have a responsibility, along with their employers, to keep individuals in their care safe and free from harm. This is a legal and moral duty which should be adhered to carefully. Each organisation must have a health and safety policy and must provide staff and individuals with the information they need to follow the rules within it. For example, fire regulations must be displayed so that individuals know what to do in the event of a fire.

Over to you

Obtain a copy of the health and safety policy for the place where you are studying. Once you have made yourself familiar with its contents, develop a second policy that would meet the needs of a health centre.

Confidentiality

All organisations should have a policy that outlines their confidentiality procedures. This is usually written in such a way that it gives individuals confidence in the organisation and its staff. However, it is important to recognise that some information cannot remain confidential. This should be highlighted on the confidentiality policy so that all individuals know the circumstances in which confidentiality can be broken. Information that cannot be kept confidential is that which:

- puts the life of another individual in danger
- links to abusive or potentially abusive situations.

(For more on confidentiality, see pages 44–45.)

Human rights

With regard to human rights, it is expected that all health and social care organisations will abide by the law and ensure best practice. While there may not be a 'human rights policy' pinned to the wall, the guidelines and other organisational policies that are adopted and followed will be shown through quality practice.

How anti-discriminatory practice is promoted in health and social care settings

Active promotion of anti-discriminatory practice

Throughout this chapter we have explored the different ways that an organisation can actively promote anti-discriminatory practice. However, you need to recognise that discrimination can only be challenged and dealt with if every member of staff *actively* promotes equality of opportunity through their words and actions. Taking action against discrimination and promoting good practice is key to all health and social care work.

Identify and challenge discrimination

Whenever discrimination occurs, it should be immediately challenged and dealt with. This highlights the need for all staff and individuals to be involved in the promotion of anti-discriminatory practice.

Some organisational policies have the potential to covertly promote discrimination. For example, forms that ask for a person's 'Christian name' are not helpful to individuals who are not Christian. Some hospitals have been accused of discriminatory practice for refusing to carry out operations on people who are overweight or who smoke.

Actively promote individual rights and preferences

It is important to promote the rights and preferences of all individuals in advance of an identified need. For example, it is important to promote an anti-bullying policy for all individuals, although only a few people may need to refer to it.

Balance individual rights with the rights of others

This can be a difficult balancing act for many healthcare professionals. You need to be aware of the possible impact upon other people of promoting and securing individual rights, and consider the situation from both perspectives.

Provide support consistent with individual's beliefs, culture, key values and preferences

Healthcare workers should provide all individuals with the care and support they need to ensure their rights can be met. This includes actively promoting an individual's rights, especially when he or she cannot stand up for them.

The care value base helps to guide healthcare workers in the delivery of appropriate healthcare. The service should always (as far as possible) meet:

- individual choice
- the need for dignity and privacy
- the guidance on maintaining confidentiality
- the need for independence
- the need for protection from harm.

Following the care value base is a good starting point for meeting individual needs. However, you also need to be aware of ways in which you can respect and then meet these different needs. For example, understanding the implications of a person's religious or moral values can prevent you from offering a service that the individual could find offensive, such as serving meat to a vegetarian. When in doubt, ask the individual what he or she wants!

Personal beliefs and value systems

Your personal beliefs and value systems have the potential to impact positively or negatively on anti-discriminatory practice in health and social care settings. This can occur through a variety of different ways, as outlined below.

Culture and beliefs

The way you respond to other people is, to a great extent, based on your values, beliefs and culture. This response can affect the way healthcare professionals deal with or treat the individuals in their care.

Past events

A person's previous experiences affect how he or she works today and thinks about the future. This 'past influence' can affect, both negatively and positively, how we treat others.

Unfair assumptions

Miriam, a practice nurse, is holding the weekly Well Woman clinic at the local doctors' surgery. Before she meets her next client, she reads through her notes to see what the issues are. 'Oh no, not another teenage mum with depression,' she thinks to herself. 'She should have considered the effects of having a baby before she got pregnant. Well, she won't get much sympathy from me. I had to cope as a single mum and there were no services to help me then!'

1 How has Miriam's experiences affected her treatment of the teenage mother?

2 What might Miriam's beliefs be regarding teenage mothers?

3 How might Miriam's behaviour and attitude towards her client be improved?

Reflection

You belong to a local book club, which meets each week to review novels. You find out that one of the new people coming to work alongside you in the health centre belongs to the same club.

1 How might you behave to the three individuals you work with?

2 What are the chances of you treating one of them differently?

Socialisation

Socialisation
The process by which children and young people learn to fit into society. A person's socialisation is greatly influenced by his or her family, friends and peers.

After a person has grown up, he or she may never reflect upon the values and beliefs he or she holds about other people. In health and social care, however, it is vital to reflect upon the way we have been brought up and to examine how this might affect our treatment of others.

In addition, health and social care workers need to adopt strategies to help them overcome the assumptions they hold about people. These might include:

- getting to know the people you work with and care for; becoming aware of each person's particular culture and beliefs
- developing empathy (the ability to put yourself in someone else's situation)
- understanding why reactions occur and what lies behind them
- avoiding insensitive language; not telling jokes that could hurt another's feelings
- becoming familiar with and understanding the legal requirements surrounding equality and diversity in the UK.

Shared beliefs

Annabel has been brought up to follow the Rastafarian religion. She holds strong beliefs and follows her religious guidance closely. When she went into work this morning, she met George, who had been admitted over the weekend. George is also a Rastafarian. Annabel is very excited by this, and spends as much time as possible chatting to George.

1 George appears to have had preferential treatment. How could this situation have been better handled by Annabel?

2 How might the other individuals have felt about this situation?

Environmental influences

Environmental influences play a role in promoting anti-discriminatory practice. These might include access to a building, the availability of equipment for moving and handling individuals; also, restricted access to scanners can mean long waiting lists in some areas of the country. Such factors impact upon the individual's right to access appropriate healthcare and to be protected from harm.

Health and well-being

The health and well-being of care workers has the potential to affect the way individuals are treated and supported. For example, if a nurse is constantly taking time off work, his or her colleagues will be affected through increased workload leading to less time available to support the individuals in their care.

Care workers who need to move individuals must also protect themselves from harm. Sometimes this may mean an individual having to wait for assistance. Wherever this happens, an explanation should be given to the individual to ensure good caring relationships are maintained.

Reflective practice

To improve the effectiveness of your work, the skills and knowledge of a reflective practitioner is required. This means being able to look back at the influences in your life, finding ways of overcoming any negative aspects and promoting the positive ones. This will help ensure that all individuals receive the best possible treatments and services available to them. Daily reflections on what has gone well and what hasn't will help the development of high-quality caring skills.

Reflection

Making notes, analyse how your personal beliefs and values may influence anti-discriminatory practice. You may need to consider how you treat other people. For example:

- Do you favour some people over others?
- How do you respond to new ideas and cultures?
- What might need to change about you to ensure that you promote anti-discriminatory practice?

Explain the strategies you could adopt to reconcile your own beliefs and values with anti-discriminatory practice.

1 a) Define each of the aspects described in Figure 2.08.

b) Write one sentence about how each aspect affects the care an individual might receive in a particular health and social care setting.

2 a) Draw up a mind map of eight different groups of people that are often stereotyped (for example, older people, police); one of these groups should be people with disabilities. Identify four to six assumptions that you think are associated with each group. Use descriptive words to convey each stereotype, e.g. 'grumpy' for older people.

b) Consider the mind map you have completed.

- To what extent do the assumptions reflect the individuals you know from each group? (Hardly/ Some/ Many)
- Are most of the assumptions you have written negative?
- If you focused on the stereotype and not the individual, what would your reaction be to meeting someone, for the first time, with that label?

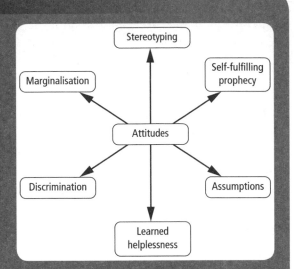

Figure 2.08 Aspects affecting the care of an individual

References and further reading

- Garcarz, W. and Wilcock, E. (2005) *Statutory and Mandatory Training in Health and Social Care: A Toolkit for Good Practice*. Oxford: Radcliffe Publishing
- Daniels, K. and Macdonald, L. (2005) *Equality, Diversity and Discrimination*. London: CIPD Publishing
- Stretch, B. (2002) Unit 1, *BTEC National Health Studies*. Oxford: Heinemann

Useful websites

The following websites can be accessed via the Heinemann website.
Go to www.heinemann.co.uk/hotlinks and enter the express code 4256P.

- British Council of Disabled People
- Commission for Racial Equality
- Disability Rights Commission
- Equal Opportunities Commission
- Stonewall: Equality and Justice for Lesbians, Gay Men and Bisexuals
- Women and Equality Unit

CHAPTER 3

Human physiology, health and disease

Key points

- Health can be defined negatively, positively, personally or holistically. Holistic views of health should focus on fulfilling potential as well as physical, mental and social health.

- The main function of respiration is to release energy from food materials to do work.

- The main function of the respiratory system is to supply oxygen for glucose oxidation and remove the waste products carbon dioxide and water.

- The main function of the digestive system is to break down large, complex food molecules into simple materials called nutrients for use in internal respiration.

- The cardiovascular system drives blood around the body. The blood is a transport medium for many substances such as simple nutrients, oxygen, water and carbon dioxide.

- The renal system removes nitrogen-containing compounds from the breakdown of protein and salts.

- The reproductive systems of males and females produce eggs and sperm which can unite to create new life.

- The nervous and endocrine systems provide a means of communication and co-ordination externally with the environment and internally between different parts of the body.

Introduction

It is vital that all learners concerned with health and social care understand how difficult it is to define health and determine the meaning of well-being; yet both these terms are used constantly in the context of care. This chapter begins with a consideration of what health and well-being might be and examines the implications of disease.

The chapter further develops your understanding of the structure and functions of the main body systems, so that you have the physiological knowledge and understanding that underpins the main features of physical care. The chapter will cover the following body systems:

- respiratory
- cardiovascular
- digestive
- reproductive
- endocrine
- renal
- musculo-skeletal
- nervous.

You will also learn about the causes, symptoms and signs of a range of associated diseases and disorders, as these aspects are fundamental to comprehending the health and well-being of individuals. Finally, you will learn about the importance of some common diagnostic techniques, such as endoscopy and ECG traces.

Definitions of health, well-being, illness and disease

Health and well-being

If you asked different people what health means to them, you would receive a multitude of responses. Many people might reply that health means 'not being ill'. This view implies that health is something that you do not think about until you become ill. Other people might suggest that health is achieved when you are at the peak of your physical, mental and emotional powers. But would this mean that if you became upset about something temporarily in your life, such as the death of a pet, you would suddenly not be healthy?

As you can see, 'health' is not an easy word to define! Some people might personalise their view of health – for example, 'when my migraine/ backache/arthritis isn't giving me trouble'. Personal views like this often relate to age, social background, circumstances, culture and experience. Some examples of personal views of health are given below.

Tariq

I am 25 years old. I have used a wheelchair for several years, after an accident at work left me paralysed. Apart from my permanent disability, I am now fully recovered from the accident. I am actively pursuing a sports career, so I train every day and take part in local events at the weekend. My goals are to compete in national events for the next two years and thereafter the Paralympics. I would say that I am in excellent health.

- What do you think is the standard by which Tariq measures his health?

The above scenarios demonstrate how each individual's view of health might link very closely with his or her moods, feelings, security and ability to carry out daily activities, whether at home, leisure or work.

Formal definitions of health

The World Health Organisation (WHO), part of the United Nations established in 1948, defined health as: 'A state of complete physical, mental and social well-being and not merely the absence of disease or infirmity.' Many health professionals criticised this definition on the grounds of idealism – what is a 'complete state of well-being'? Critics also argued that the definition implied that health didn't change throughout an individual's life. Consequently, WHO revised its definition of health as follows: 'The extent to which an individual or group is able, on the one hand, to realise aspirations and satisfy needs, and on the other hand to change or cope with the environment.'

Seedhouse (1986) proposed a definition for health as 'a foundation for achieving a person's realistic potential'.

The above definitions view health in a positive light (rather than the initial negative definition of 'the absence of illness'). They also focus on personal and physical capabilities and are strongly linked to social resources, adaptability and responsibility.

Defining well-being

If health is a complex term to define, 'well-being' proves even more enigmatic, with many health professionals still debating its meaning. Suffice to say that it is a very broad concept which generally means living a fulfilled life. Hinchliff et al (1993) describes well-being as having subjective and objective elements, as follows:

- Being well must be linked to the person feeling or believing that he or she is well.
- Some social and environmental conditions, like food and shelter, are necessary for the existence of well-being.

Defining disease and illness

The term 'disease' is generally used by health professionals when diagnosing the signs and symptoms presented by an individual for treatment, advice or care. The disease which is diagnosed is usually given a particular name. However, you may find that disease is used as a collective term (especially in some qualification specifications); further examination will determine the exact nature of the specific meaning of the term.

'Illness' describes a (usually temporary) state of being unwell and is a subjective or personal health experience. 'Ill health' describes a longer experience of being unwell, for which the cause may or may not be known.

Fundamental to the understanding of disease, illness and ill-health is an appreciation of the 'normal' physiology of body systems and anatomical features. The remainder of this chapter will focus on each of the eight body systems in turn.

> **Body system**
> A body system is a collection of organs and tissues which carry out a specific set of functions in the human body. There are seven major systems in the human body, which are listed in the introduction to the chapter on page 66.

Respiratory system

The respiratory system comprises the anatomical structures and physiological processes that take oxygen from the air into the body and transports it (via the blood) to the body's cells. Inside the body cells, internal respiration uses dissolved oxygen to release the energy from food substances; this enables essential metabolic processes to be carried out.

> **Metabolism**
> Metabolism is the sum total of all the chemical processes taking place in the body. Some processes are involved in building up complex materials from simple molecules (anabolism) while others break down complex molecules, releasing energy and leaving simple molecules (catabolism). Metabolism = Anabolism + Catabolism

The functions of the respiratory system are as follows:

1 To provide a supply of oxygen for carriage by the blood to body cells.
2 To remove the waste products carbon dioxide and water from the body.
3 To help maintain **acid-base balance** in body tissues (see also page 113).
4 To assist in **homeostasis**.

> **Acid-base balance**
> This is the normal ratio between the acidic ions and the base (or alkaline) ions that is necessary to maintain the **pH** of blood and body fluids (normal pH of blood is 7.4). All chemical reactions carried out during metabolism are governed by enzyme actions and enzymes are extremely sensitive to pH disturbances.

> **pH** – a measure of Hydrogen ions. A scale of the measure of acidity or alkalinity of a substance which ranges from 1 (strongly acidic) to 14 (strongly alkaline), with pH 7 representing neutral (neither acidic nor alkaline).

> **Homeostasis**
> The maintenance of the constant internal environment of the body in the face of changing external circumstances.

Respiration can be artificially subdivided into four sections to facilitate study; these are:

● breathing
● gaseous exchange
● blood transport
● internal or cell respiration.

Breathing

The thorax, better known as the chest, is an airtight box containing the lungs and their associated tubes – the bronchi and the heart.

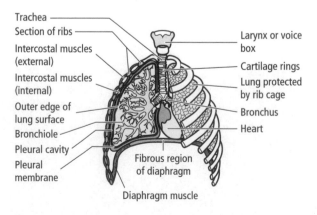

Trachea
Section of ribs
Intercostal muscles (external)
Intercostal muscles (internal)
Outer edge of lung surface
Bronchiole
Pleural cavity
Pleural membrane
Larynx or voice box
Cartilage rings
Lung protected by rib cage
Bronchus
Heart
Fibrous region of diaphragm
Diaphragm muscle

Figure 3.01 Section through the thorax to display the respiratory organs

The trachea, or windpipe, commences at the back of the throat, or pharynx, and divides into two main bronchi, each serving one lung on either side of the heart. The first part of the trachea is specially adapted to produce sound and is called the larynx or voice box. It is protected by a moveable cartilage flap, the epiglottis, which prevents food entering during swallowing. When any material, such as a crumb, manages to pass by the epiglottis, this invokes an intense bout of coughing by reflex action. This is a protective device as material entering the moist, warm interior of the lungs can initiate lung infection.

The trachea and bronchi have rings of cartilage to prevent them collapsing; those in the trachea are C-shaped, with the gap at the back against the main food tube, the oesophagus. This is because when food is masticated (chewed) in the mouth it forms into a ball shape (called a **bolus**) before swallowing. The bolus stretches the oesophagus as it passes down to the stomach and whole rings of cartilage in the trachea would hamper its progress. The gap is filled with soft muscle tissue. This means that you cannot breathe and swallow at the same time, so when feeding an individual you must allow him or her time to breathe in between mouthfuls of food.

Bolus – masticated ball of food ready for swallowing.

On entering the lung, each bronchus divides and sub-divides repeatedly, supplying every part of the lung. The tiniest sub-divisions supplying the air sacs in the lung are called bronchioles and even these are held open by minute areas of cartilage.

The inner lining of the trachea and bronchi is composed of mucus-secreting **goblet** cells and ciliated, columnar **epithelium** cells. Mucus is the sticky white gel which traps dust particles that may enter with the air, and cilia are microscopic filaments on the outer edges of cells. Cilia 'beat' towards the nearest external orifice causing the flow of mucus (with its trapped dirt particles) to leave via the nose or the throat. Many respiratory diseases cause an abundance of watery mucus to be secreted resulting in productive coughs or runny noses.

Goblet cells – mucus-producing cells.

Epithelium (or epithelial tissue) – lining tissues which exist on external and internal surfaces of organs, such as the skin, bladder and vagina as well as the interior of blood vessels and body cavities. Multi-layered epithelia such as the skin may provide protection but other single-celled epithelia such as the lung alveoli enable substances to pass through by diffusion or osmosis.

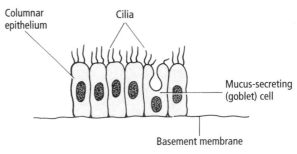

Figure 3.02 Mucus-secreting cells (goblet cells) and ciliated cells lining the trachea and bronchi

The lungs themselves have a pink, spongy feel and are lined on the outside by a thin, moist membrane known as the **pleura**. The pleura is continued around the inner thoracic cavity so that the two pleural layers slide over one another with ease and without friction. The surface tension of the thin film of moisture does not allow the two layers to pull apart but does allow them to slide. This means that when the chest wall moves in breathing, the lungs move with it.

Pleura – membranes covering the lungs and inner chest wall.

Over to you

Wet the rim of a drinking glass and place it on a sheet of damp glass – feel the surface tension between the two objects because of the moisture. It is much easier to slide the glass around than pull it off.

Pleurisy is a serious inflammation of the pleura. There are two types:

- *'wet' pleurisy is when fluid collects between the two layers*
- *'dry' pleurisy is when there is no fluid yet the layers are roughened and inflamed.*

Individuals with dry pleurisy find it very painful to breathe, while those with wet pleurisy have difficulty breathing because of the space taken up by the accumulated fluid.

Forming the thoracic wall outside the pleura are the bones of the rib cage and two sets of oblique muscles joining them together. These are the external and internal intercostal muscles (*inter* means between and *costal* means ribs). The action of these muscles enables the rib cage to move upwards and outwards during inspiration and downwards and inwards during expiration.

A sheet of muscle called the diaphragm forms the floor and lower boundary of the thorax. The diaphragm is dome-shaped with the highest, more fibrous, part in the centre and the muscular, fleshy fringes firmly attached to the lower ribs.

The only way that air can enter or leave the air-tight cavity of the thorax is via the trachea. Rhythmic breathing is controlled by the respiratory centre in the brain; this process is shown in Figures 3.03 and 3.04.

When a gunshot or stab wound occurs in the chest wall, another opening for air into the chest is formed. Air can now enter through the wound more easily than through the trachea and the surface tension of the pleura is destroyed. The lung collapses to a much smaller size and is virtually useless. Individuals can live quite well with only one lung – but, in this type of injury, there is likely to be shock and loss of vital oxygen-carrying blood, so the individual's life would be threatened. First aid treatment is to place a large pad over the wound as quickly as possible to prevent air entering and the lung collapsing. Emergency transport to a hospital must be ordered quickly.

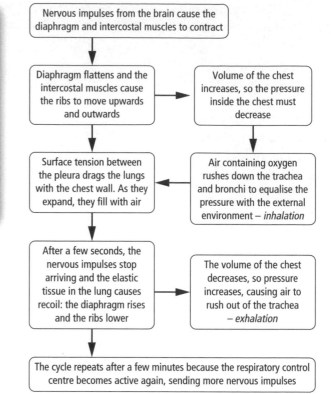

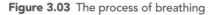

Figure 3.03 The process of breathing

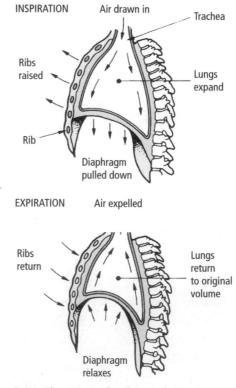

Figure 3.04 Changes in the thorax during inspiration and expiration

Gaseous component	Inspired air (breathed in)	Expired air (breathed out)
Oxygen	20 per cent	16 per cent
Nitrogen	80 per cent	80 per cent
Carbon dioxide	0.04 per cent	4 per cent
Water vapour	Depends on climate	Saturated (100 per cent)

Table 3.01 The composition of inspired (or inhaled) and expired (or exhaled) air

Over to you

Make a list of the similarities and differences between inspired and expired air. These changes in composition of the air must have occurred in the lungs.

Gaseous exchange

The bronchioles end in thousands of tiny air sacs, each of which contains a cluster of single-layered alveoli, rather like a bunch of grapes on a stem. The walls of the alveoli consist of very thin, flat, simple squamous epithelium (see Figure 3.05) and each is surrounded by the smallest blood vessels known as capillaries. The walls of the capillaries are also composed of simple squamous epithelium, in a single layer. This means that air entering the alveoli during breathing is separated from the blood by only two single-layered, very thin walls. There are elastic fibres round the alveoli enabling them to expand and recoil with inspiration and expiration respectively. A film of moisture lines the inside of each alveolus and here the air gases pass into solution.

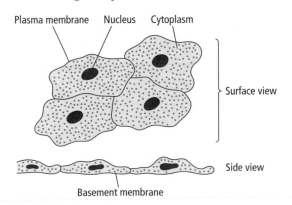

Figure 3.05 Simple squamous epithelium

The role of diffusion in gaseous exchange

Although the largest component of air is nitrogen (see Table 3.01) and this too passes into solution, it plays no part in the process of respiration. The other gases in inhaled and exhaled air (oxygen, carbon dioxide and water vapour) exchange through the process of diffusion.

Diffusion
The passage of molecules from a high concentration of molecules to a low concentration of molecules.

Diffusion occurs in liquids or gases because the molecules are in constant random motion. It is an overall 'equalling up' of a situation where you have a lot of molecules meeting a few molecules.

Diffusion will stop in time, as the numbers of molecules become more evenly distributed. When this occurs, there is said to be equilibrium. (Note: this does not mean the molecules stop moving, only that there are equal numbers of molecules passing in both directions, resulting in no overall gain or loss.) In the human body, where diffusion is a common method of transport, the state of equilibrium is not desirable as overall transport will cease. To prevent equilibrium being attained, the high concentration must be continually kept high and the low concentration must also be maintained.

The purpose of breathing is to keep the oxygen concentration high and the carbon dioxide concentration low in the alveoli so that gaseous exchange can occur.

● Breathing in fresh air at regular intervals

replenishes the high concentration of oxygen molecules in the lungs; the oxygen then diffuses into the blood inside the lung capillaries (where oxygen concentration is low) and travels to the body's cells for metabolism.

- With carbon dioxide and water, the situation is reversed: the high concentration is in the blood returning to the lungs from the body's cells; since the concentration is low in the refreshed air in the lungs, the gases diffuse out of the bloodstream and into the lungs. In this way, diffusion removes the waste products of metabolism (carbon dioxide and water) from the blood, which are then excreted in the expired air from the lungs.

The temperature of the incoming air will clearly be that of the environment, but the nose, throat and trachea rapidly warm this air and, after being in the lungs for a short time, it is virtually at body temperature when breathed out.

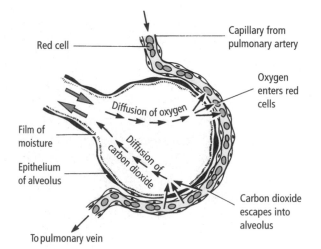

Figure 3.06 Gaseous exchange in the alveoli

Over to you

1 *Using Table 3.01 on page 71, showing the composition of inspired and expired air, and your knowledge of diffusion, explain how water vapour behaves in the lung alveoli.*

2 *An old-fashioned method of establishing whether someone was breathing was to place a cold surface like a mirror in front of the mouth and nose. Can you explain the scientific rationale behind this?*

Blood transport

Having gained access to the blood inside the lung capillaries, the dissolved oxygen rapidly attaches itself to the red pigment known as haemoglobin inside the red blood cells, forming a bright red oxyhaemoglobin. This is then carried in the blood to the body tissues and cells. No body cell is very far away from a capillary, except the cells in hard bone and firm cartilage that are nourished by diffusion.

Cells are continuously using up oxygen in respiration so there is always a lower concentration of oxygen than in the blood. This means that oxygen released from the haemoglobin is able to diffuse out of the tissue capillaries down a concentration gradient into the cells. Carbon dioxide and water are waste products of a cell's metabolism and are in high concentration in the cells. You will recall that carbon dioxide is virtually zero in lung capillary blood so these materials move from the cells into the blood.

Carbon dioxide and water form a weak acid called carbonic acid, which **ionises** into hydrogen carbonate and hydrogen ions with the assistance of the **enzyme** carbonic anhydrase (also present in red blood cells). Most carbon dioxide and water, however, moves out of the red blood cells and is carried (as hydrogen carbonate ions) in the watery **plasma** of blood, although some remains in the red blood cells.

Ionise – to be converted into ions. An ion is an electrically-charged particle, having either a positive or negative charge.

Enzyme – biological catalyst promoting the rate of chemical change. Catalyst molecules are themselves unchanged at the end of a reaction and can be used over and over again.

Plasma – a yellowish fluid that is the liquid part of blood; it is mainly water in which various substances are carried.

This chemical reaction is easily reversed, so that when in the presence of a low carbon dioxide environment, such as the lungs, the carbon dioxide and water are released and eliminated through breathing. Expired air, therefore, contains more water and carbon dioxide than inspired air.

$$H_2O + CO_2 \leftarrow H_2CO_3 \leftarrow H^+ + HCO_3^-$$

Water + Carbon   Carbonic   Hydrogen   Hydrogen
     dioxide   acid   ions   carbonate
                                    ions

Internal, or cell, respiration

Internal respiration of cells is the breaking down of glucose with the use of oxygen to produce carbon dioxide and water, but most of all to release energy from the glucose molecule.

$$C_6H_{12}O_6 + 6O_2 = 6CO_2 + 6H_2O + ENERGY$$

Glucose + Oxygen   Carbon   Water
                         dioxide

The energy is utilised by the cells in their different metabolic processes, such as muscle contraction, hormone manufacture and enzyme production, etc. The actual processes in internal respiration are very intricate and involve many enzymes and complex molecules; the above equation is a summary.

Control of breathing

The respiratory centres in the brain alternately excite and suppress the activity of the **neurones** supplying the respiratory nerves (mainly the phrenic nerve to the diaphragm) causing inspiration and expiration. Nervous receptors, sensitive to chemicals dissolved in the blood (particularly oxygen, carbon dioxide and hydrogen ions), are located both centrally and peripherally in the body. These chemical receptors, known as chemoreceptors, initiate reflexes when they are stimulated, sending nerve impulses to the respiratory centre. These change breathing activity, to restore the concentrations of the chemicals. This is part of homeostasis in the body.

Neurones – an alternative name for nerve cells.

The main factors affecting breathing and respiration are:

- exercise
- emotion
- altitude
- release of **adrenaline**, such as in frightening circumstances.

Adrenaline – a hormone produced by the adrenal glands which boosts the heart and breathing rates and increases the strength of the heartbeat.

All of the above increase the rate of ventilation or breathing to an appropriate level and, when the stimulating factor is removed, ventilation returns to normal. Lower breathing rates result from conditions such as hypothermia, hypothyroidism (abnormally low thyroid hormone) and drugs such as morphine and barbiturates.

Over to you

Figure 3.07 represents a vertical section through the thorax. Identify labels A–G and describe their purpose.

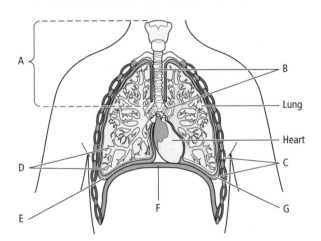

Figure 3.07 Vertical section through the thorax

Common illnesses and disorders of the respiratory system

Asthma

This condition is more correctly termed bronchial asthma, to distinguish it from cardiac asthma which is a condition associated with heart failure.

Bronchial asthma is characterised by recurring episodes of breathlessness, a feeling of tightness in the chest and wheezing. It can be mild, moderate or severe at different times of the day or night. Although many adults suffer from asthma, it is more commonly a disease starting in childhood and often clearing up in early adult life; however, it can begin at any age. During a severe attack, there is distress, sweating and rapid heart rate with the victim often unable to talk. Sometimes there is a bluish colour to the lips (where the skin is very thin) and face due to poor oxygenation of the blood.

No cause for asthma can be found in some people but others have an allergic reaction to an inhaled substance, known as an allergen. Common allergens include:

- pollens
- house dust and dust mites
- animal fur, feathers or skin flakes
- food or drugs.

Attacks can be triggered by stress, anxiety, exercise (particularly in winter), tobacco smoke or air pollutants.

Asthma is not directly inherited but there is a strong tendency for the condition to run in families. Smoking during pregnancy exerts an influence and while there is no evidence that environmental pollution causes asthma, it can certainly worsen the condition. Approximately 1 in 10 children in the UK has asthma.

General principles of treatment

Inhalers containing a fine aerosol spray of a drug which relaxes the muscle of the bronchi, called bronchodilators, are used to treat an attack of asthma. Long-term treatment with corticosteroids is often employed in chronic asthma. These are similar to a naturally occurring group of hormones from the adrenal cortex. They are useful in treating inflammatory conditions where there is no obvious source of infection.

Bronchitis

Inflammation of the bronchi produces a productive cough with yellow/green sputum or phlegm, raised temperature, wheezing and shortness of breath. It may be an **acute** infection, coming on suddenly, or a **chronic** infection resulting in narrowing of the bronchi and bronchioles and accompanying destruction of the alveolar walls; this is known as emphysema.

> **Acute** – illness which flares up suddenly and is not long-lasting.
> **Chronic** – illness which is deep-seated and long-lasting.

Acute bronchitis is often associated with a cold or influenza but may also result from air pollution. The main cause of chronic bronchitis is smoking tobacco products although air pollution can be a major factor in industrial areas. Chronic bronchitis is often associated with a condition called emphysema where the alveolar walls break down to create larger areas. This results in a reduced surface area for oxygenation and makes breathing faster and more difficult. Chest infections are common with this condition, especially in the winter months.

> **Did you know?**
>
> *Emphysema is a very common condition in the UK, affecting more males than females.*

Dai

I used to be a coal miner in South Wales; the work was hard and dangerous. Dust and heat were a problem, but after work all the lads would go for a few pints to refresh themselves. In those days, we all smoked – everybody did. I smoked one twenty packet each day; I knew it wasn't very good for me. After I was made redundant and the mine closed down, I was out of work for a few years and then got another job in a quarry, still dusty and hard! I had to take early retirement when I was 45 years old because my breathing was terrible and I got a lot of phlegm on my chest every winter. It hasn't got any better – in fact it has become worse and I have had to give up smoking on the specialist's instructions. He said that he would not treat me if I didn't, so there was no choice really. I can only go out in a wheelchair now and I have heart trouble too. I have an oxygen cylinder by my bed for difficult days. Life isn't much fun these days.

1 Discuss the factors that have contributed to Dai's health problems.

2 Examine how Dai's lifestyle has influenced the onset and progression of his condition.

3 Dai was a smoker for most of his life. Should he be denied treatment by the NHS specialist?

4 Do you think that men like Dai should receive compensation from the government?

General principles of treatment

Inhalers similar to those used in asthma may relieve breathlessness, and oxygen therapy may be necessary. Antibiotics are used for infective bronchitis and the individual should prevent further damage by not smoking and avoiding polluted areas.

Smoking is harmful to individuals for the following reasons:

- The bronchi are narrowed and this, rather like asthma, interferes with the air flowing into and out of the lungs.
- Less oxygen is available to the body cells because the carbon monoxide in cigarette smoke attaches firmly to the haemoglobin in the red blood cells, thereby excluding oxygen.
- Cilia, responsible for the flow of mucus and, therefore, the elimination of dirt and other particles from the respiratory tract, are destroyed.
- Gaseous exchange is less efficient.
- Increased mucus production, the accumulation of dust and the destruction of cilia lead to smoker's cough.
- There is a greater risk of infection.
- Elasticity of the lungs is reduced leading to emphysema.

Cystic fibrosis (CF)

This disorder is also known as mucoviscidosis for it is characterised by the production of very thick (*viscid*) mucus (*muco-*) that is unable to flow easily and lubricate the intestines, nose, mouth, throat, bronchi and bronchioles. CF remains a serious disorder causing chronic lung infections and an impaired ability to absorb fats and other nutrients from food. People with CF are affected from birth and, previously, most sufferers died in childhood. Today, with daily physiotherapy, effective medication and the opportunity for transplants if necessary, the outlook is greatly improved.

CF is caused by inheriting two recessive **alleles** for the condition, one from each parent.

It is therefore a genetically inherited disorder.

> **Allele** – half a gene. Each gene, responsible for a characteristic, consists of two alleles, one from each parent. The alleles may be similar or different, dominant or recessive. Dominant alleles always show in the individual when present; a recessive allele will only show when both alleles are recessive.

Some individuals develop early symptoms of CF but others may not show any signs of the disease for a long time. Typically, there are recurrent infections, particularly of the upper respiratory tract and of the chest, and these can cause lung damage. Motions are often putty-coloured, greasy and 'smelly'. This is due to the sparsity of pancreatic enzymes. Sweat glands often do not function well and sweat is extra salty; this may give rise to heatstroke in hot weather. Infertility can occur in both sexes and the condition may be diagnosed in adult life as a result of investigations by infertility clinics. Children may be classed as 'failures to thrive' and growth may be impaired. The condition affects about 1 in 2000 children and is more common in the white Caucasian population.

General principles of treatment

Physiotherapy to aid the flow of mucus in the chest and appropriate antibiotic treatment to avoid further lung damage is important. Pancreatic enzymes are provided to aid food digestion. In some cases a heart-lung transplant may be considered to replace damaged lungs.

Cardiovascular system

The cardiovascular system is the main transport system of the body, carrying oxygen, nutrients such as amino acids (nitrogen-containing compounds), glucose and digested fats, hormones, antibodies and the waste products carbon dioxide and urea.

The heart

The heart is a muscular pump which forces blood around the body through a system of blood vessels, namely arteries, veins and capillaries. Blood carries dissolved oxygen to the body cells and at the same time removes the waste products of respiration (carbon dioxide and water). However, blood is also important in distributing heat around the body, hormones, nutrients, salts, enzymes and urea.

The adult heart is the size of a closed fist. It is located in the thoracic cavity between the lungs and protected by the rib cage.

Test yourself

1   Explain the role of the pleura in breathing.

2   Define the following terms:

   • diffusion

   • equilibrium

   • homeostasis.

3   Outline how respiratory gases are carried in the blood.

4   Describe how air enters and leaves the lungs.

5   The composition of alveolar air in the lungs is different to inspired or expired air composition. From your knowledge of gaseous exchange, suggest what the composition might be, giving reasons for your answers.

6   Why are the alveoli specially adapted for gaseous exchange?

7   Explain why gaseous exchange does not occur in the trachea, bronchi and bronchioles.

8   Explain why chest problems arise in cystic fibrosis.

9   State three effects of long-term smoking on the respiratory system.

10 Describe the signs and symptoms of asthma.

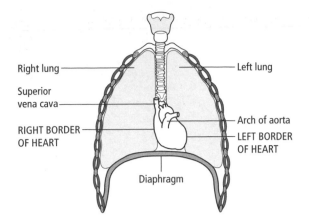

Figure 3.08 The location of the heart in relation to the thorax

The heart is surrounded by a tough membrane – the pericardium – that contains a thin film of fluid to prevent friction. The heart is a double pump, each side consisting of an upper chamber (the atrium) and lower chamber (the ventricle). Each of the four heart chambers has a major blood vessel entering or leaving it. Veins enter the atria and arteries leave the ventricles.

> **Reflection**
>
> *It is useful to remember that:*
>
> - *Atria have veins entering and ventricles have arteries leaving – in each case, A and V, never two As or two Vs.*
> - *Arteries are blood vessels that leave the heart while veins take blood towards the heart.*

Circulation to and from the heart

The right side of the heart pumps deoxygenated blood from the veins to the lungs for oxygenation. The left side pumps oxygenated blood from the lungs to the body. The circulation to and from the lungs is known as the pulmonary circulation and that around the body is the systemic circulation referring to body systems.

The two sides of the heart are completely separated by a septum. The blood passes twice through the heart in any one cycle and this is often termed a double circulation. A schematic diagram showing the double circulation with the heart artificially separated is shown in Figure 3.09.

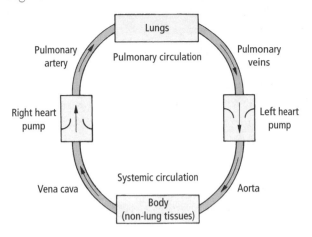

Figure 3.09 Schematic diagram showing the double circulation of the heart

In the pulmonary circulation, the pulmonary artery carrying deoxygenated blood leaves the right ventricle to go to the lungs – you will realise that it must divide fairly soon after leaving the heart because there are two lungs to be supplied, hence the right and left pulmonary arteries. The pulmonary veins (there are four of them) bring oxygenated blood to the left atrium.

The main artery to the body leaving the left ventricle is the aorta; the main vein bringing blood back to the heart from the body via the right atrium is the vena cava. The vena cava has two branches: the superior vena cava returning blood from the head and neck, and the inferior vena cava returning blood from the rest of the body. In many diagrams of the heart, these are treated as one vessel.

It is important that the blood flows in one direction only through the heart, so it is supplied with special valves to ensure that this happens. There are two sets of valves between the atria and the ventricles, one on each side. Sometimes these are called the right and left atrio-ventricular valves but the older names are also used – the bicuspid (left side) and tricuspid valves. These names refer to the number of flaps, known as cusps, that make up the valve; the bicuspid having two and the tricuspid having three cusps.

Each cusp is fairly thin so, to prevent them turning inside out with the force of the blood flow, they have tendinous cords attached to their free ends and these are tethered to the heart muscles of the ventricles by small papillary muscles. The papillary muscles tense just before the full force of the muscle in the ventricles contracts; in this way, the tendinous cords act like guy ropes holding the valves in place.

Reflection

It is easy to remember the position of the valves between the atria and the ventricles because TRIcuspid is RIghT, so the bicuspid valve must be left.

The two large arteries, the pulmonary and the aorta, also have exits guarded by valves; these are called semi-lunar valves (because the three cusps forming each valve is half-moon shaped). When the blood has been forced into the arteries by the ventricular muscle contractions, the blood must not be allowed to fall back into the ventricles when they relax. These valves can also be called the pulmonary and aortic valves.

The valves make a noise when they close but not when they open – rather like clapping your hands. These noises are often called heart sounds and can be heard through a stethoscope placed over the heart. The noises sound rather like 'lubb, dup, lubb, dup'; 'lubb' is the sound of the atrio-ventricular valves closing and 'dup' is the sound of the semi-lunars closing. In some people, there may be a swishing sound between heart sounds and this is called a murmur. Some murmurs are significant while others are not; they are due to disturbed blood flow.

Over to you

In pairs, use a stethoscope to listen to each other's heart sounds and identify the 'lubb' and 'dupp'. Try to count the exact heart rate using this method, remembering that one pair of sounds equals one beat. Carry out some mild exercise and listen again.

The *myocardium* is the name for the heart muscle. The *endocardium* is the name of the smooth endothelial lining of the cavities.

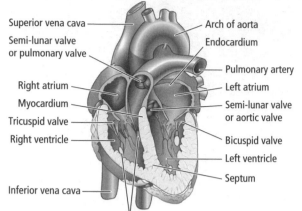

The *chordae tendineae* and *papillary muscles* tie the edges of the valves to the ventricular wall and stops the blood from flowing backward.

Figure 3.10 Vertical cross-section through the heart

Did you know?

When you view a heart diagram or picture, you should be aware that you are looking at it the opposite way round, i.e. the right side of the heart diagram represents the left side of the heart, and vice versa. If you get confused, pick up the diagram and place it over your heart facing outwards.

The structure and function of cardiac muscle

Heart muscle is cardiac muscle, composed of partially striped, interlocking, branched cells. It is myogenic, which means capable of rhythmic contractions without a nerve supply. However, the atrial muscle beats at a different pace to the ventricular muscle, so it needs a nerve supply to organise and co-ordinate the contractions so that the heart is an efficient pump. The heart muscle has its own blood supply from the coronary arteries and veins.

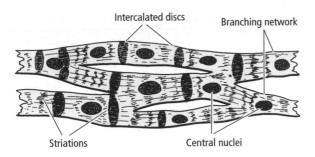

Figure 3.11 Microscopic diagram of heart muscle

The muscular walls of the atria are much thinner than the ventricular walls, as the flow of blood is aided by gravity and the distance travelled is merely from the atria to the ventricles. The ventricles are much thicker than the atria, but also different. The right ventricle is about one-third the thickness of the left ventricle because this has to drive oxygenated blood around the whole of the body, including the head and neck which is against the force of gravity.

Over to you

From the knowledge gained so far, estimate the distance that blood from the right ventricle has to travel and compare this to the effort that the left ventricle has to exert to drive blood as far as your toes. This is the reason for the difference in thickness between the two ventricles.

Arteries and veins

Arteries leave the heart and supply smaller vessels known as arterioles which, in turn, supply the smallest blood vessels, the capillaries. Arteries usually carry oxygenated blood. Veins carry blood towards the heart, picking up blood from capillaries and smaller veins known as venules.

Each type of blood vessel has structural and functional differences, as outlined in Table 3.02 and Figure 3.12.

Arteries	Veins	Capillaries
Carry blood away from heart to organs	Carry blood to heart from the organs	Connects arteries to veins
Carry blood under high pressure Thick, muscular walls Round lumen	Carry blood under low pressure Thin, muscular walls Oval lumen	Arterioles and capillaries cause greatest drop in pressure due to overcoming the friction of blood passing through small vessels
Usually contain blood high in oxygen, low in carbon dioxide and water	Usually contain blood low in oxygen, high in carbon dioxide and water	Delivers protein-free plasma filtrate high in oxygen to cells and collects up respiratory waste products of carbon dioxide and water
Large elastic arteries close to the heart help the intermittent flow from the ventricles become a continuous flow through the circulation	Veins in limbs contain valves at regular intervals and are sandwiched between muscle groups to help blood travel against gravity	Walls are formed from a single layer of epithelium cells

Table 3.02 The functional differences of blood vessels

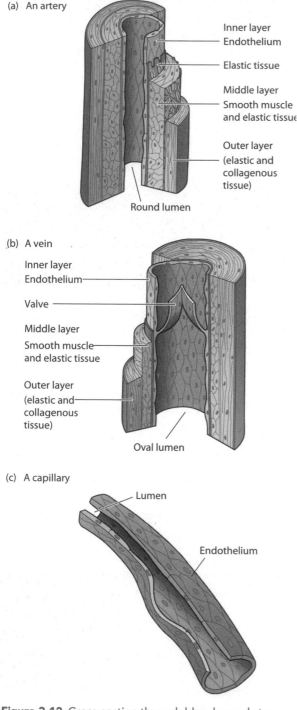

(a) An artery

Inner layer
Endothelium

Elastic tissue

Middle layer
Smooth muscle
and elastic tissue

Outer layer
(elastic and
collagenous
tissue)

Round lumen

(b) A vein

Inner layer
Endothelium

Valve

Middle layer
Smooth muscle
and elastic tissue

Outer layer
(elastic and
collagenous
tissue)

Oval lumen

(c) A capillary

Lumen

Endothelium

Figure 3.12 Cross-section through blood vessels to show their structure

Each organ has an arterial and venous supply bringing blood to the organ tissues and draining blood away respectively. A simple diagram of the blood circulation to the body organs is shown in Figure 3.13.

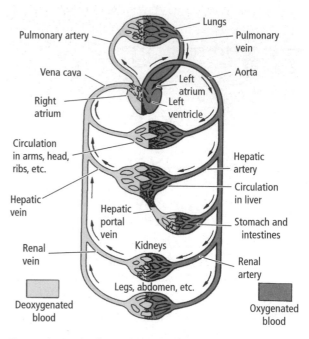

Pulmonary artery
Lungs
Pulmonary vein
Vena cava
Aorta
Left atrium
Right atrium
Left ventricle
Circulation in arms, head, ribs, etc.
Hepatic artery
Circulation in liver
Hepatic vein
Hepatic portal vein
Stomach and intestines
Renal vein
Kidneys
Renal artery
Legs, abdomen, etc.
Deoxygenated blood
Oxygenated blood

Figure 3.13 The human circulatory system

The linking vessels supplying the cells of the organ tissues are the capillaries, with walls composed of a single layer of squamous epithelium. A protein-free plasma filtrate is driven out of the capillaries to supply the cells with oxygen and nutrients (protein molecules are generally too large to leave the capillary network).

Type and general function of blood cells

Plasma

Blood consists of straw-coloured plasma in which several types of blood cells are carried. Plasma is mainly water in which various substances are transported, such as dissolved gases like oxygen and carbon dioxide, nutrients like glucose and amino acids, salts, enzymes and hormones. There is also a combination of important proteins, collectively known as the plasma proteins, which have roles in blood clotting, transport, defence and the regulation of **osmosis**.

> **Osmosis** – the movement of water molecules from a high concentration to a low concentration through a partially permeable membrane. The partially permeable membrane is usually the cell membrane of single-layered epithelial cells.

Erythrocytes

The most common cells by far in the plasma are red blood cells, also known as erythrocytes. These are very small cells with a bi-concave shape and elastic membrane (as they often have to distort to travel through the smallest capillaries). Erythrocytes have no **nucleus** in their mature state (hence their shape), providing a larger surface area for exposure to oxygen. They are packed with haemoglobin, which gives them (and blood) a red colour. In oxygenated (arterial) blood, the oxyhaemoglobin is bright red, but after the dissolved oxygen is delivered to body cells, the reduced haemoglobin (in venous blood) is dark-red in colour. Due to the absence of nuclei, erythrocytes cannot divide and have a limited lifespan of around 120 days.

> **Nucleus** – a membrane-bound structure that contains the cell's genetic information and controls the cell's growth, function and reproduction.

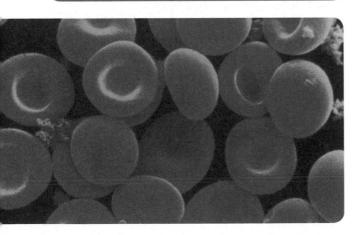

Human blood viewed under an electron microscope

Leucocytes

White blood cells, or leucocytes, are larger, nucleated and less numerous. There are several types but the most numerous are granulocytes (also termed polymorphs, neutrophils and phagocytes), which are so-called because they contain granules in their cytoplasm as well as lobed nuclei. They are capable of changing their shape and engulfing foreign material such as bacteria and carbon particles; this process is known as **phagocytosis**. A granulocyte acts rather like an **amoeba** and is sometimes said to be amoeboid. Granulocytes are, therefore, very important in the defence of the body.

> **Phagocytosis** – process by which leucocytes change shape and engulf foreign material.
> **Amoeba** – a single-celled microscopic animal living in water which moves by changing shape by flowing.

> **Did you know?** .
> *The number of granulocytes rises significantly in infections, so a blood count can often be a valuable pointer to an infection in an undiagnosed illness.*

Smaller white blood cells are lymphocytes, with round nuclei and clear cytoplasm; they assist in the production of antibodies to neutralise the **antigens** on **pathogens**. Antibodies are, chemically, globulins, which are types of plasma protein carried in the plasma. In a completely different way, lymphocytes also contribute to the defence of the body.

> **Antigen** – a substance that causes the immune system to produce antibodies against it. Antigens are proteins (or sometimes carbohydrates) inserted into the surface coats of pathogens.
> **Pathogen** – any disease-causing micro-organism, virus, bacterium or fungus.

Larger than the lymphocytes are monocytes, also with large round nuclei and clear cytoplasm. They are very efficient at phagocytosis of foreign material and, like granulocytes, can leave the circulatory blood vessels to travel to the site of an infection. They begin phagocytosing pathogens very rapidly.

Usually classed with the white blood cells are thrombocytes, more commonly called platelets. Not true cells, they are products of much larger cells which have broken up. They play an important role in blood clotting.

The cardiac cycle

The cardiac cycle comprises the events taking place in the heart during one heart beat. Taking the average number of beats in a minute to be 70, then the time for one beat or one cardiac cycle is 60 seconds divided by 70 beats, which works out at 0.86 seconds. You must remember that this is based on an average resting heart rate. When the heart rate rises to, for example, 120 beats during moderate activity, the cardiac cycle will reduce to 0.5 seconds. As you can see, the higher the heart rate the smaller the cardiac cycle, until a limit is reached when the heart would not have time to fill between successive cycles.

Using the resting figure of 70 beats per minute, we can represent the cardiac cycle in a time frame of 0.1 second boxes to study the events occurring in the heart. This is shown in Figure 3.14. The shaded boxes signify when contraction is occurring; relaxation time is left blank. The atria and ventricular activity is shown on separate lines.

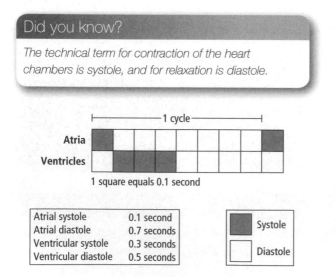

1 square equals 0.1 second

Atrial systole	0.1 second
Atrial diastole	0.7 seconds
Ventricular systole	0.3 seconds
Ventricular diastole	0.5 seconds

■ Systole
□ Diastole

Figure 3.14 Timed events in the cardiac cycle; systole and diastole

The events in the cardiac cycle can be described in stages, as follows:

- Both atria contract forcing blood under pressure into the ventricles.
- Ventricles bulge with blood and the increased pressure forces the atrio-ventricular valves shut (giving rise to the first heart sound – 'lubb').
- Muscle in the ventricular walls begins to contract; the pressure on the blood inside rises, forcing open the semi-lunar valves in the aorta and pulmonary artery.
- Ventricular systole forces blood into the aorta (left side) and pulmonary artery (right side). These arteries have elastic walls and begin to expand.
- As the blood leaves the ventricles, the muscle in the ventricular walls starts to relax. For a fraction of a second, blood falls backwards, catching the pockets of the semi-lunar valves and making them close; this gives rise to the second heart sound, 'dupp'.
- With the ventricles in diastole, the atrio-ventricular valves are pushed open with the blood that has been filling the atria. When the ventricles are about 70 per cent full, the atria contract to push the remaining blood in rapidly and, thus, the next cycle begins.

You can see that when the chambers are in diastole and relaxed, they are still filling. The cycle is continuous; with a high heart rate it is the filling time which is shortened. The heart chambers are never 'empty'; as they slowly relax, increasing the capacity, blood enters. Never forget that in a healthy heart, both atria and both ventricles contract at the same time.

Over to you

Construct a diagram similar to Figure 3.14 but with an enhanced heart rate of 120 beats per minute. Notice how little time the heart has to fill in diastole; this is why the heart rate has an upper limit (this is different between individuals).

Cardiac output

The cardiac output is the quantity of blood expelled from the heart in one minute. To calculate this you need to know the quantity of blood expelled from the left ventricle in one beat (known as the stroke volume) and the number of beats in one minute (or the heart rate). The average individual has a stroke volume of 70 cm^3 and a heart rate of 60–80 beats per minute. An individual who trains regularly might have a lower heart rate but a higher stroke volume.

Differences in lifestyle

Heather is a sprinter and has trained every day since she entered her teen years while Samantha enjoys watching TV and only occasionally goes night-clubbing. Explain the figures in Table 3.03 below with respect to their lifestyle and calculate their cardiac output.

Control of the cardiac cycle

The heart is controlled by the **autonomic nervous system**. This has two branches, namely the sympathetic nervous system and the parasympathetic nervous system (see also pages 128–129). These two systems act rather like an accelerator and a brake on the heart.

- The sympathetic nervous system causes each heartbeat to be increased in strength and the heart rate to rise. It is active during muscular work, fear and stress, and is boosted by the hormone adrenaline (the 'fight or flight' response; see also pages 110 and 127).
- The parasympathetic nervous system calms the heart output and is active during peace and contentment.

Autonomic nervous system – consists of sympathetic and parasympathetic branches serving internal organs and glands. There is no conscious control over this system.

Did you know?

Palpitations are forceful, often rapid heart beats that an individual is aware of. They are most commonly due to an active sympathetic nervous system plus adrenaline secretion during times of fear or aggression.

The sympathetic and parasympathetic nervous systems supply a special cluster of excitable cells in the upper part of the right atrium, called the sino-atrial node (S-A node) or, in general terms, 'the natural **pacemaker**'. An interplay of impulses from the sympathetic and parasympathetic nerves acting on the S-A node regulate the activity of the heart to suit circumstances from minute to minute, hour to hour and day to day. Every few seconds, the S-A node sends out a cluster of nerve impulses across the branching network of atrial muscle fibres to cause contraction. The impulses are caught by another group of cells forming the atrio-ventricular node (A-V node) and relayed to a band of conducting tissue made of large, modified muscle cells, called **Purkinje fibres**. The transmission of impulses is delayed slightly in the A-V node to enable the atria to complete their contractions and the atrio-ventricular valves to start to close.

Pacemaker – artificial device for controlling the heart rate.
Purkinje fibres – modified muscle fibres forming the conducting tissue of the heart.

	Heather	Samantha
Stroke volume (cm^3)	95	72
Resting heart rate (beats/minute)	62	72
Cardiac output (cm^3/min)		

Table 3.03 Heart statistics for Heather and Samantha

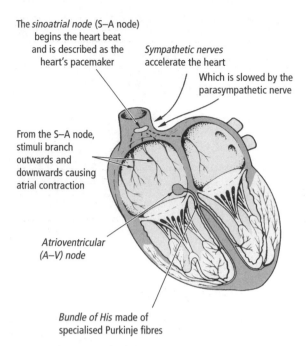

The *sinoatrial node* (S–A node) begins the heart beat and is described as the heart's pacemaker

Sympathetic nerves accelerate the heart

Which is slowed by the parasympathetic nerve

From the S–A node, stimuli branch outwards and downwards causing atrial contraction

Atrioventricular (A–V) node

Bundle of His made of specialised Purkinje fibres

Figure 3.15 Control of the cardiac cycle

Heart valves are located on a fibrous figure-of-eight between the atrial and ventricular muscle masses. The first part of the conducting tissue (the **bundle of His**) enables the excitatory impulses to cross to the ventricles. The bundle of His then splits into the right and left bundle branches, which run down either side of the ventricular septum before spreading out into the ventricle muscle masses. Impulses now pass very rapidly so that the two ventricles contract together forcing blood around the body organs.

> **Bundle of His** – a strand of conducting tissue that bridges the fibrous ring between the atria and ventricles.

Any interference in the conducting system, possibly as a result of a blocked coronary artery causing tissue death, can result in a condition called heart block. This can mean that some parts of the heart beat at a different rhythm.

Cardiovascular disorders

Changes in blood pressure

Blood pressure (BP) is the force exerted by the blood on the walls of the blood vessels. It is generated by the walls of the left ventricle during contraction.

> **Did you know?**
>
> *Although new units were devised some time ago to measure blood pressure in kiloPascals (kPa), you will find that most establishments in the UK still measure BP in the old units of millimetres of mercury (mmHg), although mercury is not used any longer in BP measuring equipment or sphygmomanometers because it is poisonous. The units are mmHg because Hg is the chemical symbol for mercury.*

At first sight, blood pressure recordings look like a fraction, e.g. 120/80 mmHg (the so-called 'average' BP for a young adult) but this is only a way of displaying an upper systolic reading when the ventricles are contracting and a lower diastolic reading when they are relaxed.

The highest blood pressure is found in large arteries close to the heart, such as the aorta, the carotid arteries and the arteries in the arms. There is a gradual drop in BP as the blood is forced through the medium and small arteries and the arterioles. The veins have little BP and blood has to be assisted back to the right atrium by skeletal muscle pressure in the limbs and the presence of valves to prevent backflow.

> **Reflection**
>
> *You are lying in bed; your head, heart and legs are in the horizontal plane and the alarm clock rings. When you leap out of bed, your head is uppermost and your legs reach the floor – your BP has to adjust within a fraction of a second.*
>
> - *What will happen if it takes longer?*
> - *Why do you think that older people are advised to sit up in bed slowly for a few minutes before swinging their legs to the floor?*

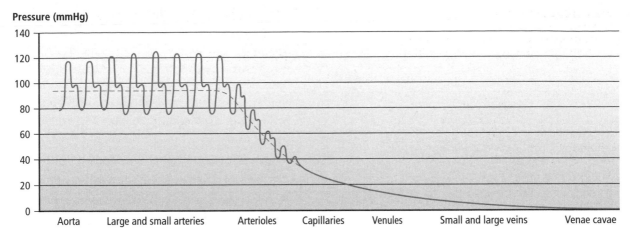

Figure 3.16 Graph showing the variations in blood pressure in the circulation

Hypotension

This is the technical term for low blood pressure with dizziness and fainting episodes. Many healthy people have a lower BP than average for people of their age and have no symptoms of hypotension. Others may have some underlying disorder that causes hypotension. The most common type is postural hypotension, caused by suddenly sitting or standing up.

Hypertension

This condition is characterised by an abnormally high blood pressure at rest. The World Health Organisation (WHO) defines hypertension as a BP consistently above 160/95 mmHg, but many people are classed as mildly hypertensive if their BP is over 140–160/90–95 mmHg.

The condition affects 10–20 per cent of people in the UK and is most common in middle-aged and older men. Many people, including young adults, are unaware that they have hypertension so doctors advise that clients should have their BP measured at regular intervals. Raised BP can lead to strokes and heart disease, both of which are life-threatening conditions.

For many people with hypertension there is no identified underlying cause; this is often referred to as essential hypertension. In other cases, causes may be identified – as you will see on pages 86 and 114.

Coronary artery disease

When the coronary arteries are narrowed or blocked, the heart muscle is starved of blood and this may cause chest pain, known as angina pectoris. It is commonly brought on by exertion and relieved by resting. During increased activity the heart muscle demands more blood to compensate for the extra effort but cannot receive it due to the narrowness of the vessels. The chest pain may be a dull ache or feeling of pressure spreading to the arms (particularly the left side), neck or back. The arteries are narrowed due to the formation of fatty deposits, or plaques, on the arterial walls. These are termed atheromatous plaques and are commonly associated with hardening of the arterial walls, a condition commonly known as atherosclerosis.

You have already learned about the value of monitoring blood pressure to detect early signs of hypertension and subsequent heart disease and strokes. Many general practitioners (GPs) will carry out a blood pressure check on a client attending for something quite unrelated. People are advised to have at least one annual blood pressure check; these should be more frequent for clients with a family history of heart disease or where there is a borderline hypertensive state.

Heart attack

Heart attack, coronary thrombosis (blood clots in the coronary arteries) or myocardial infarction (death of a wedge-shaped piece of cardiac muscle) tend to be synonymous. The narrowed coronary arteries have finally become blocked and the client suffers chest pain, often severe, similar to angina but not relieved by resting. Atherosclerosis causes the inner lining of the arteries to become roughened, predisposing the blood to clot and finally close off the blood supply to the tissues after the blockage. If a major coronary artery or one of the larger branches is blocked, the client may die. When a smaller branch is closed off, the client may survive the heart attack with effective treatment.

When the causes of malfunction can be identified, they usually fall into two broad categories: genetic disposition to hypertension or coronary heart disease and lifestyle choices.

Genetic disposition

People with a family history of heart disease and strokes, particularly before the age of 50 years, are recommended to have their cholesterol levels checked regularly because of genetic or inherited influences. Some families are known to have metabolic disorders that give rise to high levels of blood lipids, or fats, particularly cholesterol, causing life-threatening disorders.

Lifestyle choices

- *Diet* – it has long been thought that diets rich in animal fats and dairy produce are a major factor influencing both raised cholesterol levels and atherosclerosis. In turn, a high-fat diet is also associated with obesity and being overweight – another factor influencing the development of heart disease and hypertension.
- *Alcohol* – long-term heavy drinking is associated with coronary heart disease, hypertension, heart failure and strokes. In addition, alcohol contains 'empty calories' which provide no nutritional benefits but contribute significantly to obesity or being overweight.
- *Smoking* – many people immediately think of lung cancer when they think of the harmful effects of smoking, but coronary heart disease might be considered a more important effect. Young adults smoking 20 cigarettes daily are three times more likely to develop coronary heart disease than non-smokers, and the risk increases significantly with more cigarettes smoked. Other arteries supplying body parts are also affected, particularly the leg arteries (peripheral arterial disease) and the brain (strokes).
- *Exercise* – overweight and obese 'couch potatoes' are more likely to develop heart disease than people who exercise regularly and, therefore, use up energy from fats in the diet.
- *Stress* is another important influence in heart disease although most doctors think that this is secondary to the factors listed above. People with a 'type A' personality (see also Chapter 4, page 137) are described as self-critical, always striving towards goals, feeling a sense of time urgency, taking on too much and being easily aroused to anger. These characteristics are thought to increase the risk of heart disease and hypertension, but these people are also busy and active. There is some evidence that depression, grief, redundancy or other personal crises affects the progress of cardiovascular disorders.

Peter

I went to Tunisia on holiday after some very hectic weeks running my small business. My wife insisted that we didn't cancel the booking although I felt that it was a critical time for the business. However, I was receiving calls on my mobile phone so was able to keep in touch every day and make important decisions. The flight had been traumatic as there had been a terrorist scare when someone left a bag when he went to the lavatory. Anyway, three days

Diagnosis

Various methods of obtaining information about the structure of the heart and the way in which it functions have helped doctors to diagnose cardiac disorders for many years. Although listening to the heart sounds and counting the heart rate provided valuable information, modern techniques such as electrocardiography (ECG), chest X-rays, echocardiography, angiography, CT scanning, MRI, cardiac catheterisation and specialised blood tests have meant that the study of the heart has developed into a whole new branch of medicine known as cardiology.

Many people are loosely familiar with the procedure for obtaining electrocardiogram traces. Like the monitoring of blood pressure, electrocardiograms can be carried out almost anywhere because machines can be light and portable. There is also the facility of attaching a form of tape recorder to the client so that continuous 24-hour recordings can be obtained.

The electrical activity of the heart is detected by electrodes attached to the chest, wrist and ankles. You will recall that the S-A node (under the guidance of the sympathetic and parasympathetic nerves; see page 83) sends out rhythmical impulses that excite the atrial muscle and then follows the conducting tissue around the heart. It is this activity that the electrodes are recording, immediately before the heart muscle masses contract. Many heart disorders produce abnormal electrical activity and the ECG is, therefore, a useful tool for diagnosis.

Heart disorders that can be detected by ECG include:

- coronary thrombosis
- coronary artery disease
- heart muscle disorders (cardiomyopathy)
- arrhythmia (variation of rhythm, such as **fibrillation** and heart block)
- ectopic beats (extra beats).

As the ECG trace is timed and recorded, unusual heart rates, known as tachycardia (faster than normal) and bradycardia (slower than normal) can be identified.

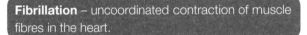

Fibrillation – uncoordinated contraction of muscle fibres in the heart.

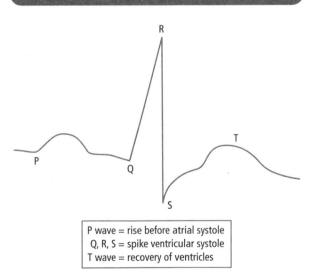

P wave = rise before atrial systole
Q, R, S = spike ventricular systole
T wave = recovery of ventricles

Figure 3.17 Normal ECG (electrocardiography) reading

Treatment

Treatment of a heart condition is any measure that will prevent or cure a disorder or relieve symptoms to obtain a better quality of life. Many heart treatments also involve accompanying changes in lifestyle. Heart surgery has evolved over the last fifty years; before then it was rarely done and dangerous. Modern medicine has now made heart treatment very successful.

Heart by-pass surgery

This is more commonly known as a coronary artery by-pass operation. The by-pass is made using a length of leg vein joined to the aorta at one end and the coronary artery beyond the blockage at the other. The surgeon will have viewed a cardiac **angiogram** previously to ensure that the individual's heart is suitable for surgery. Some people have more than one blockage so a double or triple by-pass is performed. When the client's leg veins are not suitable, synthetic tubing can be used.

> **Angiogram** – an X-ray photograph of blood vessels, taken after injecting the vessels with a substance opaque to the rays.

There are often two surgical teams for the operation, one working on the leg and the other on the heart. The individual is placed on a heart-lung machine which replaces the functions of both the heart and the lungs while the repair is carried out. The operation takes several hours and the client has to be deemed well enough to undergo the surgery. Care in an ICU (intensive care unit) for about 10–12 days follows the operation. This type of operation is now carried out worldwide and over 10,000 by-pass operations are performed annually.

Heart pacemakers

You have learned about the S-A node and its rhythmical excitation producing the heartbeat (see page 83); the pacemaker is used when the S-A node is malfunctioning or when there is an interference with the conduction of natural impulses. It is an artificial device implanted into the client's chest to maintain a regular rhythm. A pacemaker allows the individual to lead a normal life and batteries last many years; replacement batteries involve just a minor operation. Advanced pacemakers can adapt the rhythm to exercise.

When fitting a pacemaker, an insulated wire is guided through a major vein so that the electrode end lies within the heart muscle. The battery end is located in a pocket of skin under the collar bone or abdomen.

Heart transplant

Transplantation means replacing a diseased part of the body, usually an organ, with a part from another individual, alive or recently deceased. This sounds like a simple technique to regain full or near full function; however, unless the donor individual is a very close blood relative, the body's immune system treats the donated part as foreign material and begins to destroy it. This destruction process is called rejection.

In the UK, heart transplants can only come from donors who have been pronounced clinically dead. The donor heart is kept carefully in chilled saline and is transported to the recipient deemed most suitable to receive it. He or she will have been 'tissue-typed' on joining the waiting list for transplant surgery. By matching tissue types of donor and recipient as closely as possible, the risk of rejection is reduced. No two people other than identical twins have identical tissue types, but close relatives often have similarities. Antigens on the surface of body cells, most particularly on leucocytes, are identified and recorded as a tissue type.

During the operation, the individual is attached to a heart-lung machine to maintain the blood supply to vital organs. Nearly all the diseased heart is removed and the new donor heart is connected to all major blood vessels. The individual must then be placed on an immunosuppressive drug regime, chief of which is the drug cyclosporine; the client will remain on this regime for the remainder of his or her life. Infection must be guarded against because of the reduced immunity, so the individual must be given clear instructions on how to proceed when infection is suspected.

Lifestyle changes

When coronary arteries are affected by atherosclerosis, it is highly likely that other arteries are affected, such as those supplying the legs and the brain. It is therefore advisable to make appropriate lifestyle changes.

- The client should be encouraged to eat a healthy, balanced diet consisting of complex carbohydrates such as wholegrain foods, fresh fruit and vegetables, fish, white meat, fibre and water. Conversely, the individual should avoid the heavy consumption of most fat, particularly animal fat, and convenience foods loaded with salt, sugar and fat. A high-fat and high-sugar diet also causes obesity, another factor in promoting hypertension and heart disease.

- The client can be assisted and supported to stop smoking, for example, by help lines, chewing gum, patches and/or lozenges. The situation regarding smoking and its dangers must be clearly explained – smoking raises blood pressure and increases atheromatous deposits in blood vessels (see also page 85), as well as damaging lung tissue. The client must be monitored during the period – mostly, this should have taken place before treatment commenced.

- Alcohol consumption should be kept within recommended limits or preferably to occasional use only, for it also raises blood pressure and causes palpitations leading to coronary heart disease.

- A sensible exercise regime should be undertaken with professional guidance, to reduce fatty deposits, keep body weight in balance and stimulate the circulation and respiratory function.

- It is almost impossible to have a stress-free life and, indeed, a small amount of stress is beneficial from time to time; however, stress should not be continuous. An organised life without rush and bother should be the aim and, for some people, this might involve reducing hours at work, less responsibility and more delegation.

Heart murmur

Josh is 14 years old, small for his age and has never been interested in playing sport. Now he is at secondary school, sports sessions are more intensive and he finds it impossible to participate much because he gets breathless and feels ill. The school nurse has spoken to his parents and advised them to consult health professionals. The doctors feel that Josh may have a congenital malformation in his heart, as they have heard a murmur in his heart sounds. Further investigation is required: Josh is to have a cardiac-catheterisation where blood samples will be taken for analysis.

1 What is a murmur? What can it indicate?
2 The result of the cardiac-catheterisation is that the blood samples on the left side of Josh's heart have a lower oxygen level than normal. No problems have been identified with Josh's respiratory function. Explain how blood on the left side of the heart could have a lower oxygen level than normal.
3 When the heart chambers are displayed using radio-opaque material, a small open defect in the atrial septum can be seen. Using your knowledge of the heart structure, describe the normal flow of blood through the heart and how Josh will have been affected by this 'hole' in the septum.
4 Josh has had surgery to repair the heart structure. In the cardiac rehabilitation centre, he has been given advice for the care of his heart and his adult lifestyle. Explain why Josh has been given advice on blood pressure monitoring, diet, exercise, smoking, drinking and stress levels.

The digestive system

The purpose of the digestive system

The purpose of the digestive system is to break down the large, complex molecules that make up food into small molecules capable of being absorbed through the wall of the gut or alimentary canal into the bloodstream. Once in the blood, these small molecules act as raw materials to build body structures or for energy release during internal respiration. Energy is needed to do work, such as breathing, the heart pumping blood around the circulation, the transmission of nerve impulses, and so on.

The role of enzymes in food breakdown

In order to break down large, complex food molecules at body temperature without the use of harmful chemicals, such as acids and alkalis, the body produces 'magical' substances called enzymes.

Enzymes

Enzymes are biological catalysts – substances that can act within living organisms to enable the break down or building up of other chemicals to proceed at a different rate compatible with life. The enzymes themselves are unchanged at the end of the reactions or tasks they facilitate. Because they are catalysts, relatively few molecules of enzymes are required to break down lots of large food molecules.

Enzymes are specific to the material on which they act (called a **substrate**). For example, a protease acts on protein only and a lipase acts on lipids, or fats, only. You may have noted that adding *–ase* at the end of the enzyme name signifies that it is an enzyme and this usually follows the name (or part of the name) of the substrate. Not all enzymes follow this way of naming, but most do.

Substrate – the substance or substances on which an enzyme acts.

Special features of enzyme reactions

Enzymes are sensitive to temperature and work best, or optimally, at body temperature. At low temperatures they work very slowly, if at all; and at high temperatures they become distorted (called denatured) and permanently stop working. This sensitivity to heat is because enzymes are themselves proteins.

> **Reflection**
>
> *Think about the protein in foods that you consume. Fish, meat and eggs do not alter their consistency when kept in a refrigerator – but when cooked at high temperatures, they change permanently.*

Enzymes are sensitive to the acidity or alkalinity of their surroundings, known as pH (see also page 68). Some digestive enzymes, like pepsin (also known as gastric protease), work well in an acidic environment; the stomach lining secretes pepsin and hydrochloric acid for maximum efficiency in breaking down proteins. Lipase, on the other hand, prefers alkaline conditions, so the pancreas secretes alkaline salts, such as sodium hydrogen carbonate, to provide optimal conditions. Salivary amylase prefers neutral, or pH 7.0, conditions (*amylum* is the Latin name for starch, so amylase works on starch).

> **Macro- and micronutrients**
>
> The main bulk of the human diet consists of protein, fat and carbohydrate, so these are called macronutrients. They provide heat energy which is measured in calories or joules. Vitamins and mineral salts are only required in tiny amounts and are called micronutrients. They do not provide energy, but are important in energy release processes, oxygen carriage, metabolic rate, red blood cell formation, and so on.

Gross structure of the alimentary canal

The alimentary canal is a tube that extends from the mouth to the anus. It is dilated, folded and puckered in various places along its length. You will need to know the names of the various regions of the alimentary canal, their main purpose and the outcomes of their activities. Many glands are associated with the alimentary canal and have important roles to play in digestion.

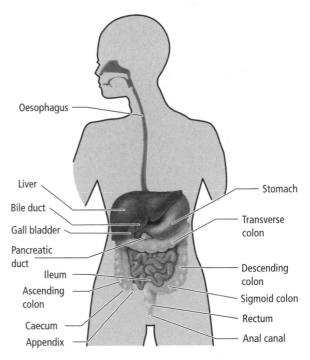

Figure 3.18 The human alimentary canal

Mechanical digestion

Ingestion is the act of taking food and drink into the mouth. There, it is mixed with saliva and chewed (or masticated) by the action of the tongue and teeth. This has the effect of rolling the food into a small ball known as a bolus, which is then swallowed. This process is called mechanical digestion and is an important part of physically breaking the food down at an early stage. Saliva contains an enzyme known as salivary amylase, which begins the digestion of carbohydrates.

Hard to chew

An older person with no teeth is given a meal containing grilled steak. As there is hardly any mechanical digestion, lumps of meat will not be properly digested when they leave the stomach.

Digestion in the stomach

The stomach is the widest part of the alimentary canal, tucked mainly behind the rib cage under the diaphragm on the left side. It receives food from the mouth by way of the oesophagus, or gullet. The swallowed bolus remains in the oesophagus for a few seconds only and no enzymes are secreted here, although salivary amylase from the mouth will continue to act on the food during this brief journey. The oesophagus is mainly a muscular transit for food boluses.

Food can remain in the stomach for up to three hours; a protein meal will remain there the longest. During this time, the strong stomach walls roll and churn the food around and pour on secretions from the gastric glands. The resulting paste-like material is called chyme. Gastric glands produce gastric juice that contains gastric protease and hydrochloric acid and works on proteins. In babies, another enzyme, rennin, solidifies and digests milk protein. The pH of the stomach is pH 1–2, which is strongly acidic.

The stomach empties the chyme in spurts through the pyloric sphincter, a thick ring of muscle which alternately contracts and relaxes.

Digestion in the small intestine

The next part of the alimentary canal is the small intestine, so-called because of its small diameter. It is around 6 metres (20 feet) in length.

The duodenum, liver and pancreas

The first C-shaped part of the small intestine is the duodenum. It is mainly concerned with digestion, which is helped by two large glands that pour their secretions or juices into this area: the liver and the pancreas.

The liver is a large dark-red organ occupying the top right half of the abdomen and partly overlapping the stomach. It has a multitude of vital functions in the body, one of which is to produce bile. Bile contains no enzymes but important salts that cause the **emulsification** of fats. You will recall that protein and carbohydrate have already experienced enzymic action. Lipids (fats) do not mix readily with water, so the enzymes have only a small water/lipid surface on which to work. Emulsification in the duodenum results in the fats forming millions of tiny globules, so that enzymes can work efficiently over a massively enlarged water/lipid surface area.

Emulsify – the mixing of two liquids which do not readily make a smooth mixture, such that one is dispersed within the other as tiny droplets, e.g. water and oil.

Bile also contains bile pigments – bilirubin and biliverdin. These are the waste products of degraded haemoglobin from old, broken red blood cells, and they give the brown colour to faeces. Bile is secreted continuously by the liver and temporarily stored in a sac called the gall bladder. When a lipid-rich meal arrives, the gall bladder releases bile into the small intestine.

The pancreas is a slim, leaf-shaped gland,

located between the intestines and the stomach, close to the duodenum. It secretes enzyme-rich pancreatic juice as well as the alkaline salts referred to previously. Pancreatic enzymes go to work on all three macronutrients.

The intestinal wall of the duodenum also contains glands which secrete enzyme-rich juices that continue the digestive process on all macro-nutrients. This juice is often called *succus entericus*. These enzymes work either on the surface or inside the epithelial lining cells.

The ileum

The remainder of the small intestine, known as the ileum, is mainly concerned with the absorption of the now fully digested food. It is specially adapted for this by its long length, folded interior and lining covered in many thousands of tiny projections called villi.

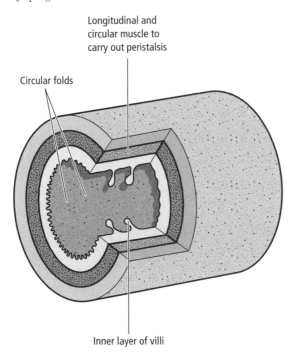

Figure 3.19 Section through the small intestine

Epithelial cells of villi are covered in microvilli, projections so small that they can only be detected using an electron microscope. These adaptations increase the surface area for absorption of nutrients from digested food to enormous proportions. Each villus is lined by columnar

cells and goblet cells only one-cell thick, with an internal extensive capillary network and a blind-ended branch of the lymphatic system called a lacteal. The chief products of protein and carbohydrate digestion (amino acids and simple sugars like glucose) pass into the capillary network; this drains to the liver via the hepatic portal vein, or portal vein. Fats (now fatty acids) pass into the lacteal and the lymphatic system, and eventually into the general circulation. Glycerol, also a product of fat digestion, passes into the portal vein.

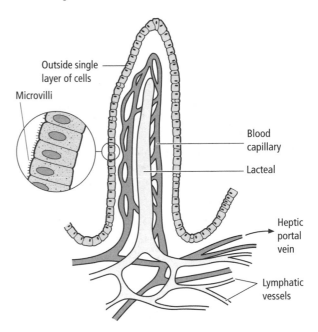

Figure 3.20 Structure of a villus

> ### Did you know?
>
> *A portal vein is one which begins in capillaries (in the villi) and ends in capillaries (in the liver). Most blood vessels only have capillaries at one end.*

Peristalsis

Food and chyme move down the alimentary canal by a process known as peristalsis. Note in Figure 3.21 the two sheets of muscle surrounding the tube – one sheet runs in a circular fashion around the tube while the other runs down the tube. Behind the bolus or chyme the inner circular muscle contracts (and the longitudinal muscle relaxes), pushing material in front of it. This is rather like your fingers pushing toothpaste up the tube. In front of the material, the circular muscle relaxes and the longitudinal muscle contracts, to hold the tube open to receive the food. Two sets of muscles acting in this way are said to be antagonistic. Mucus is secreted by enormous numbers of goblet cells in the gut lining, to reduce friction as chyme and waste is moved along by peristalsis.

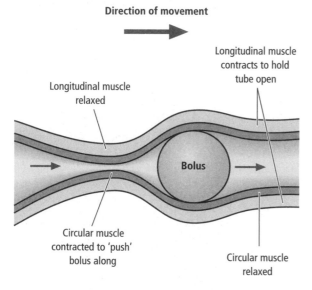

Figure 3.21 Peristalsis

The caecum and appendix

In the right-hand lower corner of the abdomen, the small intestine meets the large intestine. There are biological remnants at this point – the caecum and the appendix, a large structure with a worm-like appendix at the end. While these serve a useful purpose in grass-eating animals, they no longer serve any function in the human body. However, the appendix can become inflamed or pustulous, resulting in a life-threatening condition known as appendicitis.

The large intestine

The large intestine, or colon, runs up the right side of the abdomen then turns to travel across to the left side of the body before ending in a short tube called the rectum which opens to the exterior in the centre of the lower buttocks. The opening is guarded by a muscular sphincter, the anus.

Most of the large intestine has a puckered appearance because the longitudinal muscle splits into three bands and the circular muscle bulges out between these bands. During the journey down the alimentary canal, many glands have poured watery juices onto the chyme. The body cannot afford to lose too much water so the purpose of the large intestine is to slow down the passage of food waste so that water can be reabsorbed. (The absorption of nutrients has already occurred in the small intestine.) In this way, the motion, or faeces, becomes semi-solid. The motion can then be eliminated by muscular action of the rectum and relaxation of the anus at a convenient time. There are no enzymic juices in the large intestine.

Location	Gland and juice	Contents	Substrate	End product	Other comments
Mouth	Saliva/ salivary glands	Salivary amylase	Carbohydrate: starch	Disaccharides: double sugar molecules	Mechanical digestion; bolus formed. Neutral pH.
Oesophagus	None	None	None	None	Salivary amylase still acting on short journey.
Stomach	Gastric glands/ gastric juice	Pepsin (gastric protease)**, hydrochloric acid; rennin in babies	Protein	Amino acids and peptides (like double amino acids)	Acid pH for pepsin to work. Food churned into chyme. Bacteria in raw food killed by acid.
Small intestine a) Duodenum	Intestinal glands/ intestinal juice (succus entericus)	Peptidase; various carbohydrases	Peptides; 'double' molecule sugars or disaccharides	Amino acids; glucose and other simple, soluble sugars	Slightly alkaline pH (pH 8)
b) Liver – an associated gland, not part of alimentary canal	Liver/ bile	No enzymes; bile salts; bile pigments	None	None	Bile salts important in emulsifying lipids. Converts small intestine contents from acid to alkaline.
c) Pancreas – an associated gland, not part of alimentary canal	Pancreas/ pancreatic juice	Pancreatic amylase; lipase; pancreatic protease** (formerly called trypsin); alkaline salts	Lipids or fats; carbohydrates; proteins and peptides	Glycerol and fatty acids; glucose; amino acids	An important digestive gland. Salts convert acidic stomach secretions to alkaline so that enzymes work optimally.
d) Ileum	None	None	None	None	Main area for absorption of the end-products of digestion via millions of villi.
Large intestine a) Colon	None	None	None	None	Main area for reabsorption of water.
b) Rectum	None	None	None	None	Muscular walls expel semi-solid faeces through anus at periodic intervals.

(**Gastric protease and pancreatic protease are secreted as inactive precursors; they become activated by other substances once they are mixed with chyme in the lumen (hole) of the tube.)

Table 3.04 Summary of the main digestive processes, locations and outcomes

Faeces contains:

- cellulose (fibre or roughage) from plant cell walls (fruit and vegetables)
- dead bacteria – those killed initially by the hydrochloric acid in the stomach, as well as those, usually harmless, bacteria living in the large intestine
- scraped-off gut lining cells.

The colour of faeces is due to bile pigments (see also page 92).

Over to you

You have just eaten a meal of fish and chips. Write an account of the processes involved in the digestion of this meal.

Where nutrients from food go once they enter the bloodstream

When the nutrients from food have been absorbed in the small intestine, they take two routes through the body, as follows:

- Amino acids (from proteins), simple sugars (from carbohydrates) and glycerol (a product of fat digestion) pass via the capillaries of the villi into the hepatic portal vein, which continues to the liver.
- Fats (now fatty acids) pass into the lacteal and the lymphatic system, and eventually into the general circulation.

Amino acids

Amino acids travel via the bloodstream to areas of need in body cells. They are nitrogen-containing compounds important in making enzymes, some hormones, plasma proteins, new cells (growth) and in repair processes. Surplus amino acids are broken down in the liver as they cannot be stored. Some parts of the molecules are used for energy but the nitrogen-containing part and any surplus is converted into urea and excreted by the kidneys (see also pages 109–116).

Glucose

Glucose is mainly transported to cells to be broken down during internal respiration for energy release. Any surplus is either stored in liver and muscles as glycogen or converted into fat to be stored around organs or under the skin. The hormone insulin, also produced by the pancreas, is vital for these storage conversions (see also page 118).

Glycerol and fatty acids

Glycerol is either used for energy or for reconverting fatty acids into a form of fat which can be stored. Fatty acids travel from the lacteals through the lymphatic system into the main veins of the neck; this circuitous route enables smaller quantities of potentially harmful lipids to enter the circulation gradually.

Common disorders of the digestive system

There are various conditions associated with malfunction of the digestive tract. Understanding the processes of digestion and absorption and the functions of the large intestine will enable you to analyse the signs and symptoms associated with such disorders. The general causes of disorders of the digestive system are dietary and psychological factors. Some types of gastric ulcer have been found to be the result of a bacterial infection, which is easily treated with an antibiotic.

Irritable bowel syndrome

This disorder is aptly named, for it is characterised by bouts of abdominal pain and disturbance of bowel habit such as constipation and diarrhoea. The abdomen can feel distended or bloated and a little relief is gained from passing wind or faeces. Intermittent pain and excessive wind are common features. Malnourishment tends not to occur, but there is clearly poor absorption of water during bouts of diarrhoea. Sufferers often have poor appetite during such bouts and this, together with diarrhoea, may lead to weight loss.

Irritable bowel syndrome seems to appear in early and middle adulthood, affecting more females than males. It is one of the most common conditions affecting the digestive tract. People with this disorder show no abnormalities of the intestine and are usually not underweight or malnourished. There may be some disturbance of the muscle walls of the intestine, but the actual cause is unknown; some doctors believe that anxiety and stress is a major factor in its development.

Treatment

Irritable bowel syndrome has no cure but dietary changes (including a high-fibre diet) and measures to relieve anxiety and stress can be sought. The individual may need help from professionals to identify and deal with the source of anxiety; psychotherapy or counselling may help and, in appropriate cases, this can be supported with drugs to combat anxiety.

The quality of life of those with irritable bowel syndrome can be so affected that, as a last resort, people elect to have part of the large or small intestine removed. This operation occurs in two main ways, as follows:

- Part of the diseased colon is removed and the open end brought to the surface of the skin where an artificial opening, or stoma, is made. A lightweight bag is attached by adhesive strips to the skin to receive the faeces; this is known as a colostomy. The bag is easily changed after a motion. It is a serious operation and a stoma nurse supports the individual before and after the operation in the management of the stoma and bag, as well as any dietary and lifestyle changes. Faeces discharge once or twice a day. After recovery and training, the individual should be able to lead a normal life.
- An ileostomy is a similar procedure, but this time the ileum is brought to the surface.

Over to you

Using your knowledge of the digestive system, identify the differences between the management of a colostomy and an ileostomy.

Gastric ulcers

Also known as peptic ulcers, these can occur in the stomach, lower end of the oesophagus and duodenum (sometimes called a duodenal ulcer). A patch of lining, usually around 1 cm (0.4 inches) across, is eroded away to leave a raw area; this is often thought to be due to excess hydrochloric acid. Most individuals are in middle adulthood when they develop gastric ulcers. A gnawing pain in the abdomen (which can be so severe as to wake the person), burping, weight loss and feeling bloated are the usual symptoms, although some individuals will have no symptoms at all.

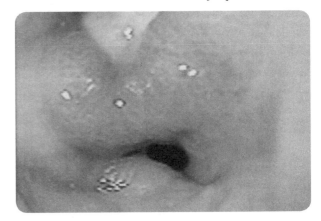

Gastric ulcer

Gastric protease, or pepsin, is an enzyme that digests protein when activated by hydrochloric acid. Body structures, including the stomach wall, are mainly made of protein but are normally protected by a thick mucus. This protection may break down allowing ulceration if there is:

- too much acid produced
- a decrease in mucus secretion
- an inherited family disposition to ulcers
- reliance on the aspirin group of drugs
- smoking
- irritation by alcohol, caffeine or bile
- a bacterial infection
- psychological stress.

Treatment

Treatment of gastric ulcers includes the following:

- *Lifestyle changes* – many people are able to heal ulcers themselves by changes in lifestyle. For example, avoiding irritants of the stomach lining (see above list), not smoking, eating smaller and more frequent meals.
- *Medication* – if the cause is thought to be acid over-secretion, there are antacid medicines to neutralise the acid, blockers to stop acid being produced, and drugs to form a protective coat over the ulcer. If bacterial infection is present, antibiotics will effect a cure in most cases.
- *Surgery* – when all other treatment fails and the ulcer is affecting the quality of life of the individual, a partial gastrectomy may be performed (removal of the part of the stomach containing the ulcer).

Gall stones

One-fifth of women have gallstones at post-mortem, demonstrating that this is a common disorder. Men are less affected. Gall stones are more likely to occur with a cholesterol-rich diet, so are also associated with obesity. Some doctors believe that not eating for long periods may cause bile to stagnate and form stones.

Gall stones are formed when too much cholesterol is passed into bile by the liver, causing solid lumps to form (precipitation). The most common forms of gall stones are made up of cholesterol, although bile pigments and calcium salts may also be found. Many gall stones cause no symptoms until they become stuck in the bile duct, which causes intense pain in the upper right area of the abdomen (known as biliary colic) and sometimes nausea and vomiting.

When there is a reduction in the quantity of bile entering the duodenum, fats will not be fully emulsified, enzymatic digestion will be reduced and fats will pass out of the body in faeces. However, since the condition is painful, there is not likely to be much weight loss unless there is a long wait for treatment.

Treatment

With gall stones, an individual needs to ensure that his or her diet is not unduly high in sugar and fat and to maintain the ideal weight for his or her height. Clearly, if overweight or obese, the individual would be advised to alter the diet and take more exercise.

Removal of the gall bladder may be necessary if there are repeated attacks of biliary colic. This will cure the majority of cases of gall stones.

> ### Did you know?
>
> *The outcomes of most disorders of the digestive tract have common features, such as pain, loss of weight and poor absorption of nutrients and/or water. Early stages of most cancers anywhere in the body do not result in pain, but mostly loss of weight and often fatigue.*

> ## Shirley
>
> I am 56 years old and married with four teenage children. I have to admit that I am overweight but not obese. Since my pregnancies, I have found it difficult to lose weight although I have tried many slimming diets. For a few months now, I have had an uncomfortable feeling in my stomach and have felt bloated, so I started taking those yoghurt drinks advertised on TV. Yesterday, I felt sick and vomited several times, and felt an awful pain in my stomach, slightly to the right and upwards. I felt dreadful and my husband called the ambulance. I am now in hospital and have had drugs to relieve the pain. I still feel uncomfortable in my tummy and the doctors are putting me on a waiting list for an operation. I had an X-ray and they say that I have a lot of 'stones' which must be removed.
>
> 1 Explain Shirley's condition using words that she can understand.
> 2 What factors have contributed to Shirley's condition?
> 3 Outline the normal physiology of the alimentary canal in the area concerned.

Endoscopy

With the development of endoscopy (see below), where the gut can be visually examined and samples of lining tissues taken for **biopsy** without surgical intervention, diagnostic techniques have undergone a major revolution. Previously, reliance was placed on X-rays with radio-opaque meals and enemas, and exploratory surgery known as laparotomies. These techniques are still in use today but endoscopy has greatly reduced the need for these procedures.

> **Biopsy** – examination of cells, tissue or fluid which has been surgically removed, in order to form a diagnosis.

> **Endoscopy**
> The collective term for viewing a cavity or tube with a flexible, fibre-optic tool. The tool, known as an endoscope, can have many attachments for cutting, grasping, snaring and removing cells or tissue for pathological examination. Many endoscopes have cameras attached to the lens and images can be viewed on-screen.

When an endoscope is used for viewing the stomach, it is known as a gastroscope; when viewing the colon, it is called a colonoscope.

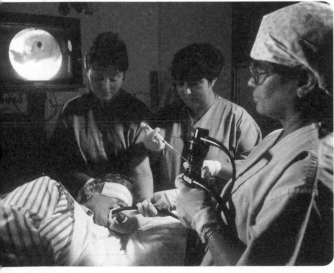

An endoscope

Variations in endoscopy

Gastroscopy

The client is asked to fast for at least 6 hours prior to the examination, so that the stomach is empty. A sedative drug and local anaesthetic throat spray is given to ease the discomfort and ensure relaxation as the gastroscope is passed down the throat into the stomach. A gastric ulcer will be visible to the doctor.

Colonoscopy

To empty the colon, laxative drugs are provided and the client is requested to drink several litres of a special cleansing agent. The client is offered a sedative drug to help ease the discomfort and facilitate relaxation. The colonoscope is passed through the anus and the flexible tube can be threaded through the various parts of the large intestine. Small benign (non-cancerous) growths called polyps can be removed and evidence of inflammation noted. An individual with irritable bowel syndrome will have a colonoscopy to eliminate more serious colon conditions.

1   Write a short account of the characteristic features of enzymes.

2   What is meant by mechanical digestion?

3   Describe the way food and chyme is moved through the alimentary canal.

4   Explain how protein food such as fish is digested in the alimentary canal.

5   Explain how toxins (poisons) such as those produced by bacterial food poisoning are eliminated by the digestive system.

6   Describe how the stomach lining is protected from hydrochloric acid.

7   How is the structure of the ileum adapted for its functions?

8   Explain the role of the digestive system in conserving water in the body.

9   Outline the role of the pancreas in digestion.

10 Draw and label a diagram of the alimentary canal.

The reproductive system

The reproductive system consists of the organs and tissues that are essential to producing offspring to ensure continuity of the species; these differ from male to female. Both the male and female reproductive systems contain **gonads** for the production of **gametes** and various tubes and tissues for ensuring fertilisation of the female ovum by a male sperm to form an embryo. The female also has organs for nurturing the developing child until birth.

Gonads – organs which are also sex glands; they produce gametes and hormones. They are the ovaries in females and the testes in males.

Gamete – sexual reproductive cell; it cannot develop further unless united with a gamete of the opposite sex. The male gamete is a spermatozoon (sperm); the female gamete is an ovum (egg).

Only one set of chromosomes

It is important to know that each body cell has in its nucleus a set of coded instructions in clusters, called **genes**, which are carried on **chromosomes**. There are normally 23 pairs of chromosomes (a total of 46) in each human cell. However, a human gamete carries only one set of 23 chromosomes.

This is why a gamete cannot develop further unless fused with a gamete from the opposite sex. On fusion with another gamete, the full complement of chromosomes (23 pairs) is restored and the resulting **zygote** can develop into another human being. (Gametes from other species carry different numbers of chromosomes.)

Gene – a unit of inheritance responsible for passing on specific characteristics from parents to offspring through constituent alleles. Chemically, alleles and genes are composed of deoxyribonucleic acid, or DNA.

Chromosome – long, thread-like structure located in the cell nucleus made of two parallel strands, which plays an important role in cell division. Genes are located on chromosomes.

Zygote – formed during fertilisation, when the nuclei of the ovum and sperm fuse; the start of a new human life.

Structure of the female reproductive system

The female reproductive system is located in the pelvis and comprises the ovaries, fallopian tubes (or oviducts), uterus and vagina.

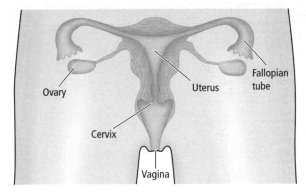

Figure 3.22 The female reproductive system

Ovaries are oval-shaped bodies that produce the female gametes (ova) and female sex hormones (oestrogen and progesterone). The ovaries contain ova (eggs) in an unripened state, each surrounded by a single layer of cells. This is known as a follicle. Each follicle has the ability to mature during one menstrual cycle and release the ovum, with the potential for fertilisation. A baby girl is born with thousands of immature follicles. During a woman's fertile years (typically between 12 and 45 years of age), only about 400–500 of these follicles will ripen and produce eggs; a few of these may be fertilised.

Close to each ovary is an oviduct, otherwise known as a fallopian tube, with finger-like processes called *fimbriae* closely applied to its surface. Once an ovum is released from the ovary, it will enter and travel down the oviduct towards the uterus, or womb. Muscular movements of the fimbriae may assist this process.

The uterus is an inverted, pear-shaped muscular organ with a special lining called the endometrium. The thickness of the endometrium varies at different parts of the female sexual, or menstrual, cycle. The muscle, or myometrium, is able to contract and relax as well as retract or shorten the length of the muscle fibres. This is important during childbirth. The uterus nourishes and anchors the embryo and foetus during pregnancy and the muscular walls expel the foetus in childbirth.

The lower end of the uterus protrudes into the vagina and is called the cervix. This is a tight muscular ring with a small opening, normally sealed by a plug of mucus. The vagina is an extensible muscular tube capable of accommodating the male penis during sexual intercourse.

When a zygote is formed from the fusion of the two gametes, it undergoes rapid cell division and after a few days becomes an embryo. After eight weeks of development, the embryo is now called a foetus.

Structure of the male reproductive system

The male reproductive system comprises:

- testes in skin sac called scrotum
- epididymes
- sperm ducts (or *vas deferentia*)
- urethra
- penis
- associated glands, known as the prostate gland and the seminal vesicles.

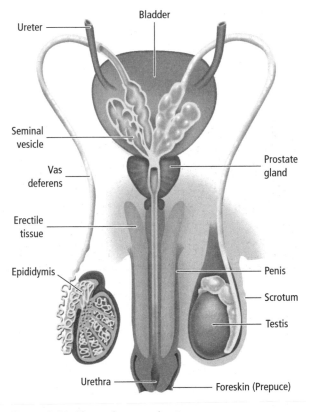

Figure 3.23 The male reproductive system

Like the ovary, the testis produces both male gametes (spermatozoa) and male sex hormones. It is divided internally into a number of sections, each containing masses of coiled seminiferous tubules in which the sperm are formed. Cells between the coiled tubes – the interstitial cells – produce testosterone, the sex hormone in males. Unlike the ovary, sperm are formed continuously, often into old age.

Did you know?

It is not unheard of for some men to father children when they are close to 90 years of age.

Sperm cannot form properly at body temperature (37°C), so the testes hang outside the body cavity in a skin sac called the scrotum. Once formed, the sperm are released into the lumens (central holes) of the seminiferous tubules and into the epididymis to mature, before emerging into the vas deferens (sperm ducts) of each side. During sexual intercourse, sperm are moved by rhythmical contractions down the vas deferens to the urethra, deep inside the penis. During this journey, the prostate gland and the seminal vesicles add their secretions: the prostate gland provides sugars and protein for the sperm and the seminal vesicles provide sugars such as fructose that activate the sperm. The resulting fluid is known as semen.

Did you know?

The vas deferens is cut and tied in a vasectomy, a form of male sterilisation. This means that although ejaculation is still possible during sexual intercourse, there are no spermatozoa to effect fertilisation. It is possible to perform a vasectomy-reversal operation, but a successful pregnancy will occur only in about half of these cases.

The penis consists of the urethra and columns of special erectile tissue. Both urine and semen pass down the urethra (but never at the same time). Erectile tissue has large spaces within which fill with blood when the man is sexually aroused, so that the penis becomes stiff and erect. This facilitates entry of the penis into the vagina and assists in depositing semen close to the cervix, at the top of the vagina. In the unexcited, so-called flaccid or limp state, this is impossible.

Basic functions of the reproductive system

The menstrual cycle

After **puberty**, ovarian follicles may come under the influence of follicle-stimulating hormone (FSH) produced by the pituitary gland at the base of the brain. Each month, FSH stimulates about 20 immature follicles to grow and produce the sex hormone oestrogen. One of these developing follicles will outstrip the rest (called the 'dominant follicle') and release an ovum about 14 days later; this is known as ovulation. The remaining follicles will atrophy (waste away).

Puberty – time of life when the secondary sexual characteristics develop and the capability for sexual reproduction becomes possible, usually between the ages of 10 and 17 years.

The follicular cells surrounding the ovum of the dominant follicle have multiplied rapidly and produce a lot of oestrogen. The whole follicle measures about 1 cm in diameter just before ovulation. Raised oestrogen levels inhibit FSH by a **negative feedback mechanism**; this allows another pituitary hormone, luteinising hormone (LH), to flourish. LH causes ovulation and then converts the remaining follicular cells in the wall of the ruptured follicle into a glandular structure called the **corpus luteum**. Secretions from the corpus luteum are rich in another sex hormone, progesterone. As progesterone increases in concentration, it inhibits LH (by another negative feedback mechanism), allowing FSH to increase once again and stimulating about 20 more immature follicles into growth.

Gonadotrophins

The two pituitary hormones involved in the menstrual cycle are:

- follicle-stimulating hormone (FSH), which acts on the ovary causing follicle growth
- luteinising hormone (LH), which stimulates ovulation and formation of the corpus luteum.

These hormones are said to be gonadotrophins, which means 'acting on gonads' (the ovaries and testes).

The role of oestrogen and progesterone

Oestrogen and progesterone are ovarian or female sex hormones that prepare the female body for pregnancy if the ovum is fertilised. They do this by acting on the breasts and endometrium of the uterus.

Oestrogen promotes growth of cells and progesterone promotes gland formation (endometrial glands nourish the embryo until a blood supply is formed and breast glands produce milk after birth). In the first half of the menstrual cycle, when oestrogen is produced from follicle cells, the endometrium builds up in thickness. After ovulation, when progesterone increases and oestrogen declines, the newly thickened endometrium becomes glandular, ready to nourish any developing zygote.

After about three and a half weeks, when no fertilisation has taken place, the corpus luteum in the ovary begins to decline and oestrogen and progesterone levels in the blood drop significantly. The thick, glandular endometrium cannot survive without these hormones and begins to peel away with small loss of blood. This is known as menstruation, and the whole cycle is called the menstrual cycle (although the female sexual cycle is a more correct term).

For study purposes, although not so precise in real life, the cycle is deemed to start at day 1 and finish at day 28, menstruation lasts 5–7 days and ovulation occurs on day 14.

Figure 3.24 The menstrual cycle

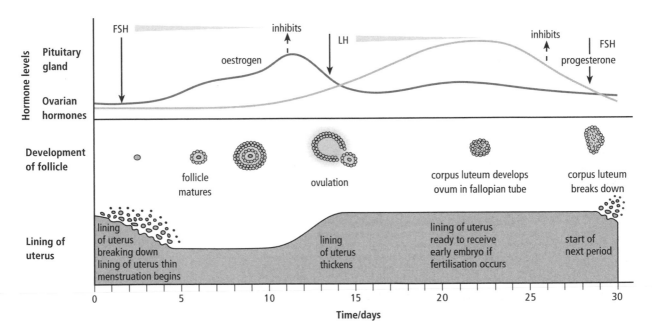

Fertilisation

For fertilisation to take place, sexual intercourse should take place in the period around ovulation. The ovum remains fertile usually for around 24 hours after ovulation, and is normally fertilised about one-third of the way down the fallopian tube. Sperm survive only about 48 hours or less in the female reproductive tract.

During foreplay, caressing and kissing, both partners become sexually aroused. Feelings are very strong and powerfully driven by nature. The male's penis becomes hard and erect as the erectile spaces fill with blood, and the female's vagina becomes slippery with mucus. The male inserts his penis into the vagina and generally thrusts up and down until a climax or orgasm is reached; ejaculation of semen takes place high in the vagina just below the cervix.

The ejaculate is only about 3 cm^3 in volume, but this contains around 300 million spermatozoa – and only one is needed to fertilise the ovum. However, many spermatozoa fall out of the vagina and the journey through the cervix and fallopian tubes is hazardous; consequently, out of this huge number, only about 100 sperm ever reach the vicinity of the ovum. The sperm try to penetrate the few layers of follicular cells still surrounding the ovum (called the 'corona radiata'). When one sperm manages to get through the corona radiata and ovum membrane, a chemical reaction occurs to the cell membrane and further sperm cannot pass through.

Did you know?

It has been said that the journey a sperm takes to reach an egg is equivalent to a person swimming the Atlantic Ocean if it consisted of treacle not water. Yet we are all here to prove that this amazing journey happens many times every day!

The successful sperm leaves its tail behind and its nucleus moves towards the nucleus of the ovum; when they meet, the two nuclei fuse. This is the moment of fertilisation, or conception. After a short rest, the fertilised ovum, now called

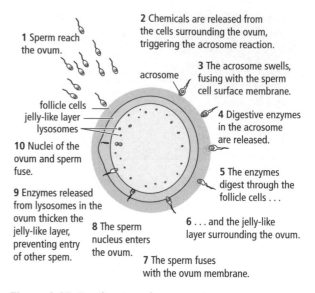

1 Sperm reach the ovum.

2 Chemicals are released from the cells surrounding the ovum, triggering the acrosome reaction.

acrosome

3 The acrosome swells, fusing with the sperm cell surface membrane.

follicle cells
jelly-like layer
lysosomes

4 Digestive enzymes in the acrosome are released.

10 Nuclei of the ovum and sperm fuse.

5 The enzymes digest through the follicle cells ...

9 Enzymes released from lysosomes in the ovum thicken the jelly-like layer, preventing entry of other spem.

8 The sperm nucleus enters the ovum.

6 ... and the jelly-like layer surrounding the ovum.

7 The sperm fuses with the ovum membrane.

Figure 3.25 Fertilisation of an ovum by a spermatozoon – the moment of conception

a zygote, starts to divide – first two cells, then four, then eight, and so on, until a ball of cells is formed. Meanwhile, this ball of cells continues to travel down the fallopian tube; it takes a week to reach the endometrium of the uterus.

Pregnancy

On arrival in the cavity of the uterus, the zygote will come to rest on a patch of thick, glandular endometrium and begin to burrow down using new finger-like processes. By the eleventh day after ovulation, the burrowing or implantation is complete and the ball of cells is buried deep in the endometrium. The female is pregnant but this is a dangerous moment for the new life: as the time of menstruation approaches, there is the risk that it will be swept away by the loss of endometrium and blood. To prevent this, a hormone produced by the embryo, human chorionic gonadotrophin (HCG), is released into the mother's uterine blood. This stimulates the corpus luteum into further growth and more oestrogen and progesterone is produced to prevent menstruation. The enlarged corpus luteum of pregnancy maintains the endometrium for the first twelve weeks by which time the embryo and its coverings (amnion and chorion) have grown and a placenta has been formed –

a special structure which helps to maintain the pregnancy and nourish the developing child.

The role of the placenta

The placenta has many functions, one of which is to secrete large amounts of oestrogen and progesterone and to relieve the corpus luteum of its burden by the twelfth week of pregnancy. Sometimes the placenta is not mature enough to produce the high levels of oestrogen and progesterone at twelve weeks; when this occurs, there is a subsequent fall in the levels of these hormones and the endometrium begins to break down. This is called a miscarriage and the pregnancy will stop. This is why the third month is a critical time in pregnancy.

The placenta and **umbilical cord** form an indirect link with the blood vessels of the mother's uterus so that:

- the foetus is able to move but is anchored to the uterus
- oxygen, glucose, amino acids, hormones, vitamins and mineral salts, etc. can pass from the mother's blood to the foetus
- carbon dioxide, urea and other waste products can pass from the foetus to the mother's blood to be eliminated.

Umbilical cord – long, 'rope-like' structure containing umbilical blood vessels which connects the foetus to the placenta.

All the beginnings of the major organs have been formed by the eighth week of pregnancy, including a beating heart. The organs grow and develop further during the remaining 32 weeks of pregnancy. The mother's breasts enlarge under the influence of oestrogen and progesterone, and are prepared to produce milk within a few days of the birth.

Ultrasound

During pregnancy, it is common practice for the mother to visit her local hospital for one or more ultrasound scans. This procedure uses high-frequency sound waves to check the development of the foetus inside the womb. A gel is applied to the skin of the abdomen and a transducer (device that transfers energy from one source to another) is then gently moved to and fro across the skin's surface. Sound waves bounce off soft tissue and fluid-filled organs, and the echoes are converted into images on a viewing screen. An ultrasound is easy to perform, causes no pain and is safer than X-ray. It enables the development of the foetus to be checked throughout the pregnancy and any abnormalities or problems identified.

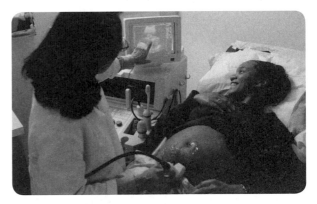

Ultrasound scan in pregnancy

Over to you

Ask a parent you know if you can have a photocopy of his or her baby's ultrasound scan – an enlarged copy would be even better. Try to identify parts of the foetus, the placenta and umbilical cord. It is quite difficult sometimes! Perhaps several peers could bring in photocopies to give you more experience in the interpretation of ultrasound scans.

Birth

Close to 40 weeks' **gestation**, birth occurs. The foetus is usually head-down in the pelvis and is said to be 'engaged'. Oestrogen and progesterone levels fall and a new pituitary hormone, oxytocin, causes muscular contractions of the uterine wall. The contractions start slowly (about every 20 minutes) and then become more frequent (every 2–3 minutes).

Gestation – the period of development from conception to birth; a technical term for the duration of pregnancy.

The first stage of labour

The first stage of labour is to widen the cervix (called dilatation); this takes between 4 and 12 hours. At some point, the mucus plug is released from the cervix (a 'show') and this is followed by the release of the amniotic fluid in which the foetus has been lying ('the waters breaking'). The uterus, cervix and vagina now form a continuous birth canal.

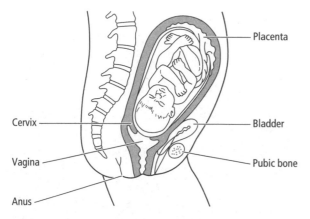

Figure 3.26 The first stage of labour showing the cervix partially dilated; it will soon be fully dilated, forming a continuous birth canal with the uterus and vagina. The waters have not yet broken and the baby's head is engaged

The second stage of labour

The second stage of labour begins as strong contractions aided by the mother pushing with her abdominal muscles. This helps the baby's head, the widest part of the baby, to be pushed out of the cervix into the vagina. The head is the widest part of the baby, as the shoulders can flex. The rest of the baby follows quite quickly – the second stage lasting, generally, from 10–60 minutes. The baby takes a few breaths or cries to re-oxygenate the blood after the journey through the birth canal. The umbilical cord connecting the baby to the placenta is clamped and cut.

The third stage of labour

The third stage of labour is the delivery of the placenta. This takes place after a short rest interval, when contractions re-commence. The placenta has peeled away from the slack uterus and passed down the birth canal. It is carefully examined to ensure that it is whole – any remnants inside the uterus may cause infection.

Infertility

One in every 4–6 couples in the UK is infertile – unable to produce children or offspring or achieve conception. To become pregnant, there are certain fundamental requirements:

- the female must be able to produce heathy ova
- the male must be able to produce mature, mobile spermatozoa in sufficient quantities
- sexual intercourse must take place
- there should be no obstruction for the sperm to reach the ovum in the fallopian tube
- a spermatozoon must be capable of fertilising the ovum
- the zygote must be able to implant in the uterus
- the embryo must be healthy
- the hormonal requirements must be adequate for further development
- the pregnancy must be maintained by the appropriate hormonal environment.

Approximately 40 per cent of infertile couples have problems in both partners; the remainder is equally split between male and female infertility.

> **Reflection**
>
> *Once a woman reaches 35 years, her chances of conceiving naturally are significantly reduced. However, many people are now choosing to start a family later in life, for various reasons including: marrying later; waiting until a career is well established; the financial pressures of owning a home and raising a family. If this trend continues there may be a further decline in the UK birth rate.*
>
> *Statistics show that there are around 14 births per thousand people (1992). This is a moderate birth rate but the death rate is also falling and people are living longer. The UK population is,*

Causes of infertility in males

The most common cause of infertility in males is lack of healthy sperm. Sperm may be weakened, short-lived, abnormal, sparse or completely lacking. This can be the result of:

- inflammation of the testes
- mumps
- cystic fibrosis
- sexually transmitted diseases
- smoking, drugs and other toxins.

Failure to deposit the semen high in the vagina as a result of impotence is also common.

Impotence

This is the failure to reach or maintain an erection to carry out sexual intercourse. It is the most common sexual dysfunction in males. Psychological causes may stem from depression, anxiety, guilt, stress and fatigue. Physical disorders such as diabetes, endocrine or neurological malfunction and alcohol dependence can also result in impotence. Side effects of certain drugs can include this effect.

Causes of infertility in females

- The most common cause of infertility in females is a failure to ovulate. The cause of this may be unknown, hormonal imbalance, stress, ovarian cyst or cancer.
- Fallopian tubes may become blocked because of previous inflammation, sexually transmitted disease or congenital abnormalities.
- One or both fallopian tubes may have been removed due to ectopic pregnancy (see below).
- Uterine conditions such as endometriosis (a very painful condition in which patches of shed endometrium lodge elsewhere), fibroids (benign muscular tumours in the uterine wall) and 'hostile' mucus in the cervix (which produces antibodies to the partner's sperm).

Ectopic pregnancy

Ectopic means 'abnormal placement'; in ectopic pregnancy, the implantation of the zygote takes place somewhere outside the uterus. This may be in the abdomen or pelvis or, most commonly, in the fallopian tube. An ectopic pregnancy can be life-threatening to the mother as rupture of the tube, shock and internal or vaginal bleeding can occur. Ectopic pregnancy is most likely to occur where there is an abnormality in the uterus or fallopian tube, or when infection has caused a blockage of the tube.

Over to you

From your knowledge of the menstrual cycle and pregnancy, suggest why ectopic pregnancies might occur and why they are so dangerous.

Treating infertility

About 50 per cent of couples treated for infertility will become parents. Treatment varies with the cause. The principle is to introduce sperm to the ova by avoiding mechanical or psychological barriers. In some cases, this means mixing ova with semen outside the body.

Male infertility treatment

Men who cannot produce spermatozoa cannot become fathers other than by adoption or artificial insemination by a donor (AID). The anonymous donor's semen is screened for micro-organisms and a careful medical history is taken to ensure that the donors are in good health and as free from physical and mental disorders as possible.

For men with a low sperm count, artificial insemination using their sperm (AIH) can be tried. AIH is also used where there is impotence or antibodies hostile to sperm in the vaginal mucus.

Female infertility treatment

If there is the failure to ovulate, specific drugs can stimulate ovulation. Fallopian tubes, uterine abnormalities or fibroids can sometimes be repaired or removed.

In vitro fertilisation (IVF) is fertilisation of an ovum by a spermatozoon in a culture medium (nutritive substance used in a laboratory), after which the fertilised egg is implanted in the uterus to continue normal development. In vitro means glass, referring to the glass dishes in which fertilisation takes place. IVF is a complex treatment which involves:

- fertility drugs to stimulate ova to maturity; this can be monitored by ultrasound scanning
- removal of mature ova by laparoscopy (a laparoscope is a type of endoscope inserted through a skin incision in the abdomen)
- fertilisation with semen outside the body in a culture medium followed by a short delay and incubation and examination to see whether embryos are developing
- implantation of several embryos in the uterus through the vagina; unwanted ova or zygotes can be freeze stored for other attempts.

IVF success rates are improving but few women become pregnant straight away. IVF can be tried several times but the procedure is expensive.

A similar procedure called gamete intra-fallopian tube transfer (GIFT) involves obtaining ova as for IVF and, after examination, replacing them with a sample of semen in the fallopian tube. This is both less expensive and less complicated than IVF.

Ashwan

Tony and I have been married for ten years; we are both reaching 40 years of age. We have a nice home and our own business is doing well. We have been trying to have a baby for the past three years and have now decided to seek professional help. After providing a sample of semen, Tony has been told that his sperm count is bordering on low, and I am going for a special X-ray of my womb tomorrow.

1 Explain the possible causes of infertility.
2 Why is it necessary for Ashwan to have an X-ray of her uterus?
3 The result of the special X-ray shows a distorted uterine cavity. The consultant believes that this is due to several fibroids.
  Explain why both investigation results have affected the chances of having children.
4 Tony and Ashwan have both had their physical health checked and blood tests for hormone levels. Explain the role of hormones in reproduction.
5 Explain the choices of treatment for Tony and Ashwan and explain the principles and value of each one relevant to this couple.

1 Explain the differences between a body cell and a gamete.

2 Name the male and female gonadotrophins.

3 Differentiate between a zygote, embryo and foetus.

4 Identify the functions of the placenta.

5 What is responsible for ovulation?

6 Describe the stages of the birth process.

7 Where does fertilisation usually take place?

8 Explain why the third month of pregnancy can be a critical time.

9 Vasectomy is one way that sexual partners can use to prevent pregnancy. Explain how this is achieved.

10 Explain why the uterus is not ready to receive an embryo for implantation at the time of fertilisation.

The renal system

The renal system is essential for life as it plays a major role in:

● elimination of the waste products of metabolism from the body

● maintenance of the correct water balance in the body

● maintenance of the acid-base balance in the body.

The renal system is, therefore, very important in homeostasis – maintaining the internal environment of the body (see also pages 112–113).

Gross structure of the renal system

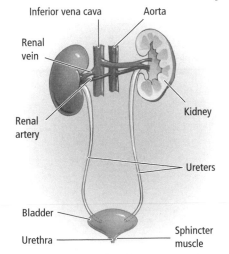

Inferior vena cava   Aorta

Renal vein

Renal artery

Kidney

Ureters

Bladder

Urethra

Sphincter muscle

Figure 3.27 The renal system

The renal system comprises two kidneys, their tubes known as ureters, the bladder and the urethra.

● The kidneys lie on the posterior, or back wall, of the abdomen, above the waist and partly protected by the lowest ribs. There is a kidney on each side of the vertebral column.

● The bladder is a central pelvic organ which collects urine.

● The kidneys are connected to the bladder by two ureters, which are tubes about 20–30 cm (8–12 inches) in length. Both bladder and ureters have a lining of transitional epithelium surrounded by muscle and fibrous tissue.

● The bladder is connected to the exterior by the urethra, a tube through which urine is expelled. The urethra is much longer in males than females. In males, the urethra just below the bladder is completely surrounded by the prostate gland; it also forms part of the penis (see also pages 101–102).

The kidneys

The kidneys are bean-shaped organs and are relatively large, measuring approximately 10–12 cm (4–5 inches) in length. They are surrounded by a capsule of fibrous tissue and body fat for protection. A small adrenal gland caps each kidney; these secrete the hormone adrenaline (see also page 83). Each kidney is supplied by a branch of the aorta known as the renal artery. The renal vein returns blood to the vena cava.

Within each kidney, the arterial blood vessel breaks up into small branches, which supply approximately one million units called nephrons. These are the filtering units of the kidney. A cross-section diagram of a kidney illustrates two distinct parts (see Figure 3.28): the darker, outer part of the kidney is the renal cortex and the paler, inner section is the renal medulla.

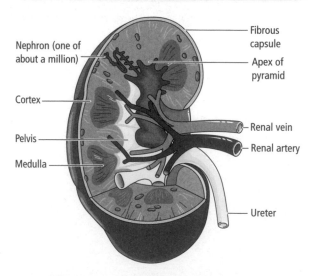

Figure 3.28 Cross-section diagram of a kidney

Labels: Nephron (one of about a million); Cortex; Pelvis; Medulla; Fibrous capsule; Apex of pyramid; Renal vein; Renal artery; Ureter

The functions of the renal system

Although there are some minor functions of the renal system, the two major tasks are:

- to produce urine in order to eliminate excess water and salts and the waste products of metabolism
- to effect homeostasis.

Urine production

Urine production comprises three distinct processes:

- ultra-filtration
- non-selective reabsorption
- selective re-absorption.

These processes take place in the millions of nephrons found in each kidney.

Structure and function of a nephron

The first part of a nephron is a cup-shaped Bowman's capsule, made of single-layered squamous epithelial cells and into which a tangle of capillaries, called a glomerulus, fits very closely (see Figure 3.29). The capillaries emanate from arterioles that branch off the renal artery. The capillaries through which blood enters the glomerulus are known as afferent capillaries; those which take blood away from the glomerulus are the slightly smaller efferent capillaries.

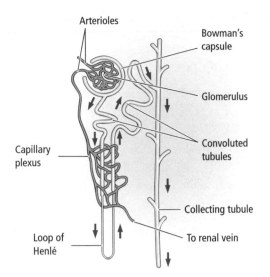

Arterioles

Bowman's capsule

Glomerulus

Convoluted tubules

Capillary plexus

Collecting tubule

Loop of Henlé

To renal vein

Figure 3.29 Structure of a nephron

Ultra-filtration

In the glomerulus, the efferent capillaries are narrower than the afferent capillaries. This means that a 'traffic jam' of blood under high pressure occurs. Because of the high pressure, water and other small particles are forced through the walls of the glomerulus into the Bowman's capsule; larger blood cells and proteins are too large to filter through the walls of the glomerulus and remain in the blood. This process is known as ultra-filtration. The resulting filtrate has a similar composition to plasma and is known as glomerular filtrate. It contains water, glucose, amino acids, salts, fatty acids and urea.

- Amino acids (compounds containing nitrogen) result from protein digestion. They cannot be stored in the body as raw material, so when there is a surplus it is broken down chemically to from urea, containing nitrogen, and other materials.
- Urea is produced in the liver and eliminated from the blood by the kidneys to be excreted in urine. Urea is always dissolved in plasma but, if levels increase significantly, it acts as a poison.

Non-selective reabsorption

The glomerular filtrate now passes from the Bowman's capsule into the renal tubule. This is sometimes called the first convoluted tubule because it is intricately wound. This tubule is closely associated with a capillary network (the capillary plexus) formed via the efferent capillary from the glomerulus (see Figure 3.29). As the glomerular filtrate flows down the renal tubule, the following is reabsorbed by the blood in the capillary plexus:

- all the filtered glucose and amino acids (these are too important to the body cells to be passed out in urine)
- seven-eighths of the water and salts (mainly sodium and chloride ions).

> **Did you know?**
>
> *Ultra-filtration and reabsorption are non-selective processes. In other words, they will happen even if the body contains raised levels of water or salt.*

> **Did you know?**
>
> *When blood pressure falls due to shock or haemorrhage (bleeding), BP is too low to cause ultra-filtration and almost no urine is produced. This is a protective device because further loss of water and salts through urine production would cause serious dehydration and possibly death.*

The filtrate that remains in the renal tubule is reduced in water and salts and contains increased concentrations of urea. It now passes into a long loop of Henlé (see Figure 3.29). The loops of Henlé are sandwiched in the medulla between the last parts of the nephron – the collecting ducts (see Figure 3.29).

Selective reabsorption

Each loop of Henlé leads into a second convoluted renal tubule and it is here that the filtrate is first tailored to suit the requirements of the body. An important hormone from the pituitary gland, anti-diuretic hormone (ADH), allows water to be reabsorbed through the tubular cells. When the body needs water to be conserved, such as after sweating on a hot day or after intense physical activity, ADH secretion is high and water is reabsorbed into surrounding capillaries. When there is a surplus of water, for example, after drinking lots of fluids or with absence of sweating on a cold day, ADH secretion is minimal. In this case the tubular cells act rather like waterproofed tubes and the excess water is passed into the urine. In a similar but more complex way, another hormone from the adrenal glands, called aldosterone, regulates the sodium ions in the body.

Filtrate now moves on to the collecting ducts, and these join together to run into the base of the kidney and the ureters. The collecting ducts are sandwiched in the cortex in a high sodium area formed in the loops of Henlé. In the presence of ADH, water passes out of the filtrate (by osmosis) causing further concentration; the remaining filtrate can now be termed urine.

Composition of urine

This varies according to diet, climate and state of health. Urine is a clear, amber-coloured watery solution of urea (2 per cent), salts and minor nitrogen-containing substances such as creatinine and uric acid. There should be no glucose, blood cells or protein in urine from an individual with good health. Analysis of urine is routinely carried out to test kidney function.

Urine leaves the kidneys via the ureters, moving partly by peristalsis and partly aided by gravity to the bladder, where it is stored temporarily. The bladder holds about 0.5 litres (0.9 pints) of urine before sending nerve impulses to the spinal cord to signal the emptying reflex. Urine then leaves via the urethra at periodic intervals. The base of the bladder is guarded by a muscular sphincter under conscious control.

Homeostasis

Tissues and organs can function efficiently only within a narrow range of variables such as temperature, pH (acidity/alkalinity), blood pressure, blood glucose, heart rate, respiratory rate and osmo-regulation (water concentration). Receptors (receiving cells) in the body must be able to detect external and internal changes and transmit the information to a control centre (most often, the brain) which then corrects the deviation by means of effectors (action cells or 'doing' cells), usually gland secretions or muscular responses. This is known as negative feedback as the change is damped down or reduced to return the system to normal behaviour.

Osmo-regulation

You have already learned how water is regulated by the kidneys and the action of ADH. Osmo-receptors in the brain monitor the osmotic pressure of the nearby blood flow. When the blood becomes more dilute (low osmolality), the osmo-receptors are not stimulated and little ADH is produced, leaving surplus water to pass out in the urine. When osmolality rises, osmo-receptors are stimulated and cause ADH secretion from the pituitary, water is reabsorbed and osmolality returns to normal.

Regulation of pH

Regulation of the pH of body fluids is partly carried out by the lungs and the kidneys. The process comprises several complex chemical reactions. Relatively small but significant quantities of acids enter the body each day; some from food and drink, such as vinegar and citrus fruit, others as a by-product of metabolism. The deeper parts of the kidney cortex have a special sodium-concentrating process located in the loops of Henlé. This conserves ions like sodium and disposes of excess hydrogen ions (acidic ions) by secretion from the second renal tubule. Under these conditions, urine becomes acidic.

> ### Did you know?
>
> *Diabetes mellitus (mellitus means 'sweet') is a medical condition caused by insufficient insulin, a hormone produced by the pancreas. Insulin assists glucose to move through cell membranes for internal respiration. When insulin is lacking, blood sugar levels become abnormally high. The first renal tubule cannot reabsorb the extra glucose, so urine becomes loaded with the surplus (there is no glucose in normal urine). Glucose is an osmotically active substance and consequently attracts water with it. An untreated diabetic will, therefore, produce lots of urine (polyuria) loaded with glucose (glycosuria) and be constantly thirsty (polydipsia).*

Renal dysfunction

Types of renal dysfunction

Renal failure

This condition arises when the kidneys cannot effectively remove waste products like urea, excess salts and water from the blood and expel them from the body in urine. It also occurs when water, salts and blood pressure are not regulated by the kidneys. The condition can be acute, resulting from shock or haemorrhage, or chronic, causing progressive, long-term damage. Signs and symptoms might include:

- decreased urine production
- fatigue
- weakness
- raised blood pressure
- nausea, vomiting and loss of appetite.

Renal infection

Any obstruction to the flow of urine will cause urine to stagnate and become a focus for infection, known as pyelonephritis. Thus, kidney infection may result from the following:

- kidney or ureteric stones (see below)
- enlarged prostate gland in males
- tumours
- congenital defects.

In females in particular, bacterial infection of the kidneys may result from cystitis (an inflammation of the bladder) because the infection has spread from the bladder and up the ureters to the kidneys. The female ureter is short and close to the vaginal and anal orifices, so these can be sources of infection. Cystitis is more common during pregnancy. Back pain and high temperatures result from pyelonephritis.

Kidney stones or calculi

Various chemicals (for example, calcium) can precipitate out of filtrate/urine and form hard bodies known as calculi or kidney stones. Some doctors think that stones may result from dehydration, particularly in hot weather or following infection. Males appear to be more vulnerable to this condition than females. Kidney stones can exist without symptoms, but stones in the ureters and bladder can be excruciatingly painful to pass.

Prostate enlargement

Although not strictly part of the renal system (because of its role in the male reproductive system), enlargement of the prostate produces urinary problems due to its position encircling the urethra at the base of the bladder. Prostatic enlargement occurs mainly in men in middle to later adulthood. Although prostatic cancer is a possible cause, it is more often a benign enlargement without a known cause.

Symptoms include:

- difficulty in passing urine (*dysuria*)
- reduced flow of urine
- dribbling from an overfull bladder progressing to incontinence

Sudden abdominal pain with only a few drops of urine produced indicates acute retention of urine. This is a life-threatening condition requiring emergency treatment. As previously mentioned, obstructed flow of urine and stagnation can lead to kidney infection.

Causes of renal dysfunction

The causes of renal problems vary, from infection to long-term use of painkillers and allergic reactions. Some causes are as yet unknown.

Diabetes

Diabetes mellitus is an endocrine disorder where the pancreas fails to produce enough effective insulin. Type I diabetes commonly begins in young people and is a life-threatening illness if left untreated; it is treated by insulin injections. Type II diabetes is usually found in older, overweight individuals and can be controlled by tablets or even diet.

Diabetes is a condition that can affect blood vessels in many parts of the body, including the small arterioles that supply the kidney glomeruli. These vessels may even be partly obstructed resulting in renal failure and hypertension. High levels of blood glucose also predispose to bacterial infection and this may result in pyelonephritis.

Raised blood pressure

Hypertension causes kidney damage and kidney damage causes hypertension – a vicious circle. Hence, raised blood pressure from an unknown cause can cause kidney damage that leads to even higher BP.

Lifestyle factors

You have already learned about the effects of lifestyle on raised blood pressure (see page 85); most of the points previously raised are appropriate to renal disease. Not having regular blood pressure or blood glucose checks may lead to diabetic or renal damage. Drinking plenty of water is important for kidney function.

Raghav

I am overweight and developed hypertension as a complication of Type II diabetes. What I didn't bargain for was the combined effect on my kidneys. Now I have to go for blood cleaning, called dialysis, three times every week for at least four hours. The return journey to the hospital adds another two hours to each dialysis, and I am so tired when I come home that I have to sleep. Day gone! I have lost half my life and seriously wonder if it is all worth it. To make matters worse, my wife is threatening to walk out on me. She's struggling to cope with my 'renal diet' – restricted protein, fluid and potassium-containing food. She gets very confused about what I can and cannot eat.

1 Explain how diabetes can affect the kidneys.
2 Explain the physiological principles relevant to kidney function that lie behind the renal diet.
3 Discuss how renal disease affects the quality of life for the individual and his or her immediate family.

Diagnosis of renal disorders

There are more ways to diagnose disorders of the renal system than most body systems. These include 'normal' X-ray techniques plus those with radio-opaque materials and ultrasound scanning. Blood and urine samples can reveal abnormal chemical constituents, and endoscopy through the urethra can be undertaken to assess the interior of the urethra and bladder.

Blood tests

In addition to routine blood tests, there are tests to show how much of certain nitrogenous substances, such as creatinine and urea, is 'cleared' from the blood and eliminated in urine. The results are useful when compared with normal figures.

Urine dipsticks

There is now a wide range of dipsticks for testing the presence of protein, blood, glucose, bile and pH in urine. The sticks are chemically treated to show a colour change when the appropriate substance is present. Some sticks are able to show a range of colours to indicate the concentration of substances.

Management of renal disorders

Urethroscopy

This is a type of slim endoscope used for viewing the interior of the urethra. A cystoscope visualises

the bladder and both can be used for removing obstructions such as prostatic enlargement polyps and benign tumours.

Dialysis

When kidney function is poor and/or failing, dialysis is used to 'take over' the functions of the kidney. This is usually seen to be a temporary measure, short- or long-term, until transplantation can occur. Although transplants are expensive, the operation is a one-off cost whereas dialysis, also expensive, is a continuous cost every year. Dialysis occurs alongside dietary restriction and medication.

There are two main types of dialysis: haemodialysis and CAPD (continuous ambulatory peritoneal dialysis).

- Haemodialysis involves attaching the individual to a kidney machine for at least four hours a day, three or four times a week. The person will require a 'fistula' operation several months beforehand; this is usually in the arm. A fistula is an artificial connection between an artery and a vein, into which the needle attachment to the kidney machine is made. Multiple layers of special membrane material separate the client's blood from dialysing fluid in the kidney machine. Any substance (waste products, toxic materials and excess water) needing to be removed from the blood is in low or zero concentration in dialysate so that the substance passes across by diffusion and osmosis. Any substance not requiring elimination can be kept at a high concentration in the dialysate. The dialysate runs to waste and the 'cleaned' blood is returned to the client. A few individuals have home kidney machines but most haemodialyse in hospital.
- CAPD uses the inner lining or peritoneum of the abdomen as the dialysing membrane and the dialysate is introduced through a special tap and catheter. The process takes about one hour to complete (twice a day), i.e. empty the old dialysate and introduce the fresh. The client may walk about with the dialysate

inside (hence use of the word 'ambulatory') and continue with work. Although peritoneal dialysis can take place in hospital, most individuals carry out CAPD at home and work.

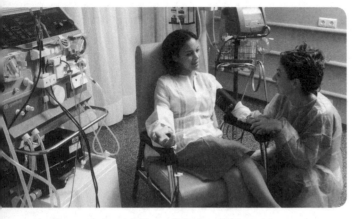

Person using a kidney dialysis machine

Kidney transplant

In the UK, most transplant organs are only available from recently deceased persons or close relatives. The composition of the recipient individual's **antigenic** make-up is determined from blood tests and matched to a donor's make-up so that they are as closely matched as possible. This process is called 'tissue-typing'. Failing kidneys are usually left in place and the new kidney placed in the pelvis and connected to the bladder by the donor's ureter. The donor blood vessels are connected to branches of the lower aorta and vena cava. The client begins immuno-suppressant therapy to prevent rejection and monitoring is carried out by urinalysis, blood tests and ultrasound scanning. The chief danger of rejection is in the first few months after the transplant. More than 80 per cent of transplants are successful enabling the individual to live a normal life while continuing on immuno-suppression.

> **Antigenic** – types of inherited protein markers existing on the surface of an individual's body cells; blood cells are usually used as these are easy to obtain.

Kidney failure

After many years on medication for high blood pressure, Graham was surprised to learn that his lethargy, poor appetite and fatigue was considered by his doctors to be due to failing kidneys. Doctors advised that he should have a fistula put in his arm ready for dialysis in the future. Eighteen months later, Graham started haemodialysing three times each week. He had dietary restrictions of protein, salt and potassium-rich foods as well as water.

1 What is the relationship between high blood pressure and kidney failure?
2 What is the nature and purpose of a fistula?
3 Explain how urine is produced by a normal kidney.
4 Explain how haemodialysis can replace some kidney functions.
5 Explain why fluid and dietary restrictions are necessary in an individual undergoing dialysis.
6 Evaluate the benefits of dialysis and kidney transplant as methods of treatment.

Test yourself

1 Draw and label a diagram of a nephron.
2 Explain the process of ultra-filtration.
3 Why are proteins present in blood but not found in urine?
4 Explain why glucose is filtered from the blood yet not found in urine.
5 Why is glucose found in the urine of diabetics?
6 Explain how water is regulated by the kidneys.
7 Describe the principles behind dialysis procedures.
8 Explain the importance of tissue-typing both donor and recipient before a kidney transplant takes place.
9 Explain why urinary problems are common in older men.
10 Explain the relationship between blood pressure and kidney damage.

The endocrine system

Endocrine glands produce hormones that travel to their target organs via the blood circulation to effect a change. Hormones are by nature proteins or **steroids** which are secreted by endocrine glands straight into the blood stream. Many are controlled through a negative feedback process while others, like insulin, may be controlled by levels of the chemicals they control, such as glucose. Major endocrine glands are scattered throughout the body.

> **Steroid** – substance from a lipid/fat base using cholesterol as a source.

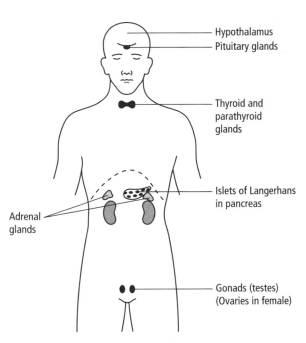

Hypothalamus
Pituitary glands

Thyroid and parathyroid glands

Islets of Langerhans in pancreas

Adrenal glands

Gonads (testes) (Ovaries in female)

Figure 3.30 Major endocrine glands

Major effects of the more common hormones

You have already learnt about some important hormones and their actions when reading about the other body systems. The actions of these and other major hormones are covered in Table 3.05 on page 118. (The table is not complete; there are many local and more systemic hormones beyond the scope of this chapter.)

How hormones produce effects in the body

Hormones are generally secreted in short bursts until the level in the blood builds up. If the endocrine gland is not stimulated to produce its hormone, there is often a very low level of hormone or none at all in the blood.

Similarities and differences with the nervous system

Hormones control and co-ordinate other body systems in a similar way to the nervous system, but the way in which they do this is different:

- hormone action is much slower than nerve impulses in effecting change
- hormones tend to be used for long-term changes whereas nerve impulses tend to be used for rapid changes
- hormones themselves are chemical molecules whereas nerve impulses are electro-chemical phenomena
- hormones travel through the bloodstream and are, therefore, potentially available to all body cells. Nerve impulses can only arrive where cells have nerve supplies.

For a particularly dramatic effect, hormones and nerve impulses can work in tandem, such as in an emergency and during childbirth.

Disorders of the endocrine system

Hormone disorders may arise from too little or too much hormone being secreted. They generally arise over quite a long period of time and close family members frequently don't notice the subtle changes until later on.

Hormone	Endocrine source	Target organ(s)	Effects
Adrenaline – secreted in 'fight or flight' conditions	Adrenal gland, located above the kidney on each side	Heart and blood vessels	Increases heart rate and strength of each beat. Narrows arterioles to the skin and organs of the digestive tract. Increases calibre of muscle arterioles.
		Liver	Converts glycogen to glucose for increased energy supplies.
		Respiratory centre in brain	Faster, deeper breathing to increase oxygen intake and carbon dioxide elimination.
Thyroxine – regulates the rate of metabolism	Thyroid gland, positioned over the trachea in the neck	Body cells. Particularly influential in skeletal growth and brain development.	Stimulates the rate of metabolism in almost all body cells – particularly internal respiration. A lack of thyroxine in childhood produces stunted growth and poor cognitive function. (Note: Thyroxine requires dietary iodine for its production and iodine is often added artificially to food products in geographical areas deficient in iodine.)
Insulin	Pancreas	Liver	Converts glucose to glycogen and fat for storage. Has the opposite effect to adrenaline.
Anti-diuretic hormone	Pituitary gland	Kidney nephrons	Increases the permeability (leakiness) of the latter parts of the nephron tubules so that water is absorbed back into the bloodstream and thus conserved. Secreted in large amounts in hot climates.
Follicle stimulating hormone	Pituitary gland	Ovary	Causes growth of immature follicles in the ovary at the start of the menstrual cycle.
		Testis	Stimulates sperm production at puberty.
Luteinising hormone	Pituitary gland	Ovary	Stimulates ovulation and the formation of the corpus luteum.
		Testis	Stimulates interstitial cells between the seminiferous tubules to secrete testosterone.
Oestrogen	Ovary and placenta	Female sexual organs and breasts	Responsible for the secondary sexual characteristics such as breast growth, body hair, onset of menstruation, etc. Promotes endometrial growth and maintains a pregnancy.
Progesterone	Ovary and placenta	Uterus and breasts	Promotes glandular development in a thickened endometrium and in breasts. Maintains a pregnancy.
Testosterone	Testis	Male sexual organs; musculo-skeletal system.	Responsible for secondary sexual characteristics in males – voice breaking, body hair, penis growth, muscular development, etc.

Table 3.05 Major effects of the more common hormones

Sylvia

I live with my mother, Agnes, who is now in her 60s. I thought she was ageing pretty rapidly because she had slowed up in lots of ways and she couldn't seem to grasp using money any longer. Her hair had gone quite wild, wiry and very dry, and she had trouble with dry skin too. We spent a small fortune on special shampoos, facial moisturisers and laxatives! She was always cold, even when the weather was warm, and she slept a great deal.

It crossed my mind that my mother might be in the very early stages of Alzheimer's disease, but I felt really guilty thinking that so convinced myself that it was just the effects of ageing. When my sister came to visit from New Zealand after a two-year break, she was astonished at the change in our mother in that short period and insisted on getting her checked at the doctors. A week later, the doctor called to tell my mother that she had a hormone disorder and left a prescription for tablets. Since she started taking the medication, the change in her has been remarkable – she's back to her old chirpy self. I feel awful about missing something so serious.

1 Can you identify the hormone disorder that Agnes has? Give reasons for your answer.
2 Why did Sylvia not notice her mother had developed a health problem?
3 Explain the characteristic features of hormone action.

Test yourself

1 It can be important to conserve water in the body when the weather is hot. Describe the role of the endocrine system in water conservation.

2 Explain how blood sugar levels vary with hormone activity.

3 Differentiate between the nervous and endocrine systems in bringing about communication and co-ordination.

4 Describe the hormonal influences of the menstrual cycle.

5 Adrenaline is an important hormone in adapting the human body for emergency action. What are the key features arising from adrenaline secretion?

6 Name the major endocrine organs.

7 State the function of thyroxine.

8 Diabetes mellitus is characterised by a higher than normal blood glucose level. Explain how this arises.

9 Name the hormones secreted by the placenta.

10 Explain how secondary sexual characteristics are influenced by hormones.

Musculo-skeletal system

The musculo-skeletal system comprises:

- the axial skeleton – the bones that lie in the midline of the body (the skull, spinal column, ribs and sternum)
- the appendicular skeleton – the limb bones and their respective girdles
- skeletal muscle, which is attached to the bones of the skeleton.

Support

The musculo-skeletal system supports body weight against the downward pull of gravity.

Did you know?

A person's height is greater at the beginning of the day than at the end of the day. That is why it is important to take height measurements in a research study at the same time each day. This effect is due to gravitational pull, so the skeleton is important in preventing body organs becoming progressively compressed.

In ideal posture, the body weight is evenly distributed about the skeleton, but this is difficult to maintain, particularly with movement. The skeletal muscles exert muscle tone or firmness and are continually contracting minutely to maintain this even distribution. The musculo-skeletal system also gives support to other structures in the body. For example:

- the rib cage supports the lungs so that breathing can take place efficiently
- the brain is supported by the base of the skull.

Muscle tone

Tone is when a few muscle fibres contract in turn to give firmness to the muscle. In sleep, muscles still have tone. In an unconscious state, muscle tone is lost and muscles become soft and floppy. In such circumstances, it is very important to prevent the soft tongue from flopping back and covering the airway. This would cause asphyxiation and death if not quickly relieved.

Over to you

Stand perfectly still with your arms by your sides for several minutes. Notice how you appear to sway slightly both backwards and forwards and from side to side. This is your muscle tone correcting the pull of gravity.

Types of muscle tissue

There are three types of muscle in the body, as shown in Table 3.06 below.

Muscle type	Structure	Function
Cardiac muscle	Short, striped cylindrical cells which branch repeatedly.	Can contract without a nerve supply. Enable atria and ventricles of the heart to contract and drive blood around the circulation.
Involuntary muscle	Spindle-shaped cells with central nuclei.	Contracts walls of blood vessels and internal organs when stimulated by nervous impulses.
Voluntary muscle	Long, striped cylindrical cells which have many nuclei.	Contracts strongly when stimulated by nervous impulses to provide voluntary movement.

Table 3.06 Types of muscle tissue

Cardiac muscle

Cardiac muscle is a specialist type of muscle tissue found only in the wall of the heart (see also page 79). It functions without conscious effort. You have already learned how cardiac muscle contracts and relaxes to drive blood around the circulation (see pages 77–78).

Involuntary muscle

Involuntary muscle is not attached to the skeleton. It is also known as smooth, unstriped or unstriated muscle. This type of muscle provides slow contractions over long periods of time. You have already learned how peristalsis moves food, chyme and waste through the alimentary canal (see pages 93–94). Other examples of involuntary muscles include those which cause the pupils of the eye to dilate and contract in response to light, and those which cause contractions of the womb during labour.

Voluntary muscle

Voluntary muscle is attached to the skeleton and works in response to conscious direction, i.e. at will. It is also called skeletal, striped or striated muscle. Voluntary muscle consists of contractile muscle fibres packed closely together. One end of the muscle is the origin and the other is the insertion; the ends are tendinous or fibrous and attached to bone. Contraction of voluntary muscles creates skeletal movement by reducing or increasing the angle at a **joint**.

> **Joint** – place where two or more bones meet.

Movement

At least two voluntary muscles are involved in moving and replacing a bone. Muscles can only pull, never push, so one muscle contracts to displace the bone and another is needed to return the bone to its original position. These muscles are said to act **antagonistically**.

> **Antagonists** – pair of muscles which have opposite actions.

To cause movement, muscles must act across a joint. When a muscle contracts it shortens, effecting movement by pulling on the bone beyond the joint. The origin of the muscle remains fixed while the insertion moves towards it, thus reducing the angle of the joint.

Figure 3.31 shows movement of the forearm caused by muscles flexing and returning (extending).

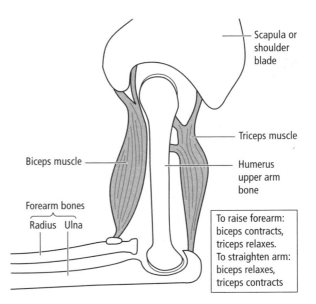

Figure 3.31 Movement at the forearm

Types of joints

There are three groups of joints which permit different types of movement; some allow no movement at all. These are:

- fibrous joints (non-moveable)
- cartilaginous joints (slightly moveable)
- synovial joints (freely moveable).

Most joints are of the synovial type; an example is shown in Figure 3.32 on page 122.

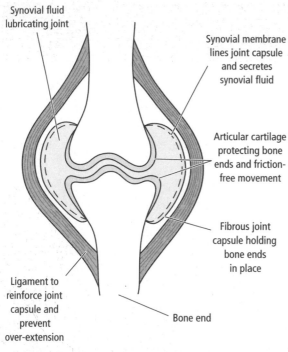

Synovial fluid
lubricating joint

Synovial membrane
lines joint capsule
and secretes
synovial fluid

Articular cartilage
protecting bone
ends and friction-
free movement

Fibrous joint
capsule holding
bone ends
in place

Ligament to
reinforce joint
capsule and
prevent
over-extension

Bone end

Figure 3.32 Diagram of a synovial joint

Somatic nervous system

Movement is fundamental to all animal life – it enables the finding of food, water and shelter and facilitates reproduction. For voluntary muscle to contract, it must receive nerve impulses from a nerve supply. These nerves are part of the somatic nervous system (somatic means 'of the body').

Protection

Protection of many vital organs is carried out by the skeleton. Some of the major organs of body systems and their protective skeletal parts are shown in Table 3.07.

> **Bone – a living tissue**
> Bone consists of a calcified protein network containing living cells (osteoblasts and osteoclasts) that constantly lay down new bone and remodel other areas; it is as much of a dynamic living tissue as blood or skin. Limb bones and some others are hollow and contain marrow where red blood cells, platelets and granulocytes are manufactured.

Disorders of the musculo-skeletal system

As movement is essential to a good quality of life and the ability to carry out the activities of daily living, any disorder of movement will severely affect the individual's physical, emotional and mental health.

Table 3.07 Major organs of body systems and their protective skeletal parts

Body system	Organ protected	Part of the skeleton
Nervous system	Brain	Cranium of the skull
	Spinal cord	Spinal column
	Sense organs – eye, ear, nose, tongue	Skull
Respiratory system	Lungs and bronchi	Rib cage, spinal column and sternum
Cardiovascular system	Heart and major blood vessels	Rib cage, spinal column and sternum
	Spleen	Rib cage
Renal system	Kidneys	Rib cage and spinal column
	Bladder	Pelvis
Digestive system	Liver	Rib cage
Reproductive system	Ovaries, uterus	Pelvis

Arthritis

Pain, stiffness and swelling of one or more joints is known as arthritis. There are several different types of arthritis; two of the most common forms are described below.

Osteoarthritis

This is the most common arthritic disease, generally affecting people in middle and later adulthood. It arises from wear and tear on the joint, overgrowth of bone at the joint edges and thinning or absent areas of the articular cartilage. Friction, stiffness and pain are experienced with movement and the bone ends become worn away. Large weight-bearing joints are often the first to show degeneration although previously injured joints can display arthritic changes earlier.

Anything that causes extra wear and tear on joints is a contributory factor for osteoarthritis, such as:

- being overweight or obese
- occupational hazards, i.e. footballer or other sport professional, dancer, window cleaner, typist
- skeletal deformities or misalignment of bones
- injuries to joints or joint inflammations
- normal ageing process (over 60 years).

Many of these are lifestyle factors.

Rheumatoid arthritis

Rheumatoid arthritis can occur at any age, even in childhood. Joints become red, inflamed and swollen during attacks and there may be a slightly raised temperature and other aches and pains. Small joints like those in the fingers, wrists and toes are typically affected. The frequency and severity of attacks can vary and the condition is more common in females.

Rheumatoid arthritis is considered to be an **auto-immune disease**, possibly triggered by a streptococcal bacterial infection in childhood. In this case, the synovial membrane (see Figure 3.32) becomes inflamed and thickened and this may spread to the underlying cartilage.

Auto-immune disease – disease in which the individual develops antibodies against his or her own tissues.

Diagnosis

X-rays can confirm both types of arthritis together with the signs and symptoms of the condition. In osteoarthritis, bone overgrowths and increased density of bone ends are significant.

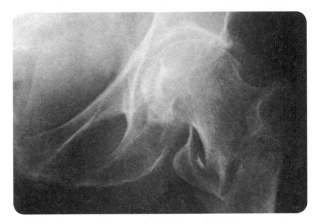

X-ray showing osteoarthritis

Osteoporosis

Bone consists of a protein background of collagen on which calcium salts become impregnated. Collagen provides a degree of flexibility while the calcium salts give bone its hardness. In osteoporosis, the collagen background becomes reduced making the bone brittle and more liable to fractures. The dysfunction is most common in women after the menopause because oestrogen (now in decline) is not present in sufficient quantities to maintain the consistency of bone. However, the condition can occur in both sexes as a natural part of the ageing process. Other causes include heavy smoking and drinking (lifestyle causes), poor calcium intake and hormonal disorders. There is also a genetic influence as daughters of mothers with osteoporosis are at greater risk.

Diagnosis

X-rays and sometimes blood tests are used to diagnose osteoporosis.

Treatment of disorders of the musculo-skeletal system

Common medications

- Painkiller (analgesic) drugs such as aspirin and non-steroidal anti-inflammatory drugs (NSAID) such as ibuprofen are used to treat arthritic pain and stiffness. Corticosteroids may be injected into joints to provide relief.
- Hormone replacement therapy (HRT) with or without calcium tablets can be used to treat osteoporosis.

Joint replacement

The medical term for this is arthroplasty. It is undertaken when a joint is unstable, very painful and deformed or diseased. Hips and knees are the most common joints to be replaced, by plastic or metal artificial joints that are cemented in place after the diseased joint and its socket have been removed. Shoulder, elbow and finger joints are also replaced on a regular basis. Antibiotic cover ensures there is no subsequent infection.

Physiotherapy

In most musculo-skeletal disorders, exercise and physiotherapy is important to prevent joint stiffness, ease pain and keep muscles active.

- Arthritis sufferers are encouraged to take non-weight bearing exercise such as swimming.
- Exercise is particularly beneficial for building bone and long, brisk walks are recommended for clients with osteoporosis.
- Physiotherapy exercises can be active, to strengthen particular muscle groups, or passive, where the therapist moves the part, to keep joints mobile.
- Other treatments may involve massage, infra-red heat treatment and hydrotherapy (exercising in water).

Ajay

I am 62 years old. I have complained of aches and pains in my bones for several years, but during the past two years the pain in my left hip has become so severe that I am now quite inactive and reliant on a walking stick. I played county cricket in my younger days, but because I am so inactive these days I am putting on weight. I recently visited my GP, who arranged for me to have X-rays at the local hospital. I will see her again in three weeks; in the meantime she has prescribed analgesic drugs to relieve the pain.

1 Identify the likely cause of Ajay's pain.
2 Which two factors have contributed to Ajay's condition?
3 Why has Ajay's GP sent him for X-rays?
4 What changes will the GP or radiologist expect to see in the X-rays to support the diagnosis?
5 Why is it important for Ajay to become more active?

Test yourself

1 Name the three types of muscle in the human body and state one location for each type.
2 Why is it necessary to have at least two muscles to effect a movement?
3 Name three organs protected by the skeleton.
4 Differentiate between the axial and appendicular skeletons.
5 Explain the changes that take place in a joint affected by osteoarthritis.
6 What is meant by muscle tone?
7 Why is an individual's height less at the end of the day than at the beginning?
8 Which blood cells are manufactured in bone marrow?
9 Outline the features of osteoporosis.
10 What is bone made of?

The nervous system

The nervous system is responsible for receiving and interpreting sensation, activating muscles and many glands, and regulating activities of the internal organs.

Nerve cells, or neurones, are highly specialised cells capable of transmitting **impulses**. Neurones have lost their ability to divide and, therefore, to reproduce. This is important as people never make new neurones despite the large numbers that cease to function every day as the human body ages. Since the human body has billions of neurones to start with, the loss is trivial until later adulthood is reached, when brain function starts to stutter a bit. Poor lifestyle choices associated with illegal drugs, smoking and alcohol consumption, for example, increase the number of failing neurones.

> **Nerve impulse** – an electro-chemical burst of activity, often known as an action potential.

Structure and function of neurones

Neurones have long protoplasmic extensions known as nerve fibres, along which impulses pass. In the sophisticated human nervous system, most nerve fibres are encased in a fatty sheath of myelin; these may be called myelinated fibres. The effect of the myelin is to speed up the transmission of nerve impulses many, many times; for example, speeds of 100 metres per second are quite common.

The nucleated part of the cell is often referred to as the cell body. Cell bodies are found only in the peripheral white matter of the brain, the grey matter of the spinal cord, and in clusters known as ganglia just outside the spinal cord.

Axons and dendrons
Nerve fibres carrying impulses away from the cell body of the neurone are called axons and those carrying impulses towards the cell body are dendrons. In the human body, impulses can travel in one direction only.

Neurones have been differentiated into three types depending on their function and the direction of impulse transmission.

Sensory neurones

Also called receptor neurones, these carry impulses into the central nervous system (brain and spinal cord) from specially adapted cells known as receptors. These cells can convert sensations of pain, pressure, touch and temperature into nerve impulses that then travel along the sensory neurones with which they are closely associated. Sensory neurones have long dendrons and short axons.

Motor neurones

Also referred to as effector neurones, these have long axons and short dendrons. They carry nerve impulses from the central nervous system to muscles and glands, causing them to either contract or secrete.

Relay neurones

Also called connector neurones, these have short axons and dendrons and, as their name suggests, carry impulses from one neurone to another. They are common in the spinal cord.

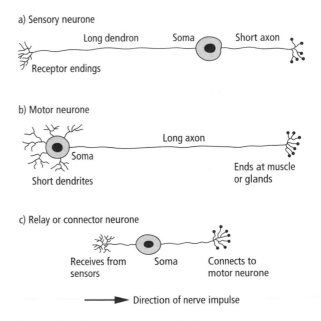

Figure 3.33 Sensory, motor and relay neurones

The transmission of information by nerve pathway

Synapses are minute spaces between adjacent nerve fibres or cell bodies. If sufficient impulses arrive, either in quantity or over time, a special chemical called a neurotransmitter is secreted into the synapse allowing the impulses to pass onwards in one direction only. The neurotransmitter is secreted from the swollen end of an axon. The most common transmitter is acetylcholine. The function of the synapse is to allow only 'serious' bursts of impulses to travel onwards. It acts rather like a security guard at a gate.

There is an enormous number of impulses bombarding the nervous system every minute – sights, sounds, smells, tastes, the touch of clothes and furniture, temperature, etc. The body needs to filter out much of this information and respond only to some. The synapses carry out this selection process extremely well.

Reflex action

Using an example of a common occurrence, for example, pricking a finger, the following sequence will occur:

1 A pain receptor in the skin of the finger is stimulated and an impulse is generated.
2 The impulse passes to the dendron of a sensory (receptor) neurone then travels through the cell body (in the ganglia) to a short axon close to the spinal cord.
3 The sensory axon synapses with the dendron of a relay neurone; the impulse passes through the cell body and axon.
4 The relay axon synapses with the dendron of a motor neurone in the grey matter of the spinal cord; the impulse travels through the motor neurone cell body and away via the axon.
5 The motor axon synapses with the appropriate muscle, which contracts and the finger is withdrawn rapidly.

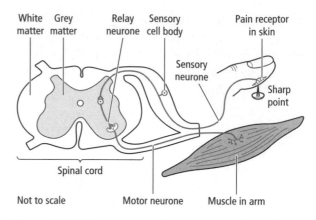

Figure 3.34 Nerve pathway illustrating pricking a finger with a sharp point

If you can imagine this journey, you will realise that the sensory dendron and the motor axon must be very long – depending on the length of the arm, they could be over a metre in length! Equally the sensory axon, relay fibres and motor dendron must be very short as they all exist inside the spinal cord.

When injury happens as in the example of pricking one's finger, a person may shout out, look at the damage and even shed some tears. Relay neurones are responsible for the connections to the brain allowing the person to react, but by this time the arm will have been removed to minimise damage. For this reason, only two or three neurones have been involved in communicating the pain and effecting the necessary action. Synapses delay the passage of impulses by a few milliseconds, so the fewer the number of synapses the quicker the reaction. Such a reaction into and out of the spinal cord is called a reflex action – it is a rapid and automatic response to a stimulus.

The functions of the nervous system

The functions of the nervous system can be summed up in two words: communication and co-ordination.

To function efficiently, the various regions and organs of the body must transfer information from one source to another and enable events to work in a co-ordinated way. For instance, there is no point in preparing to pour digestive juices into the alimentary canal if there is no food in the digestive tract for it to act upon. Generally speaking, these are also the functions of the endocrine (or hormonal) system, but the nervous system tends to react more quickly than the hormonal system. Hormones travel via the circulating blood so there might be over a minute between production of a hormone and its effect. In a life-threatening emergency this method of communication is too slow and considerable damage might be sustained. Travelling via nerve fibres, however, is much faster and is, therefore, preferred in actions requiring almost immediate effect. For example, reproductive processes such as menstruation and childbirth can be controlled by hormones, but preparing to run from an aggressive dog needs an instant response and is controlled by nervous pathways.

The somatic and autonomic nervous systems

Although the nervous system is a whole body system, for study purposes it is often split into the somatic nervous system and the autonomic nervous system.

- The somatic nervous system is further broken down into the central and the peripheral nervous systems. The central nervous system (CNS) is the brain and spinal cord. The peripheral nervous system (PNS) supplies the rest of the body.
- The autonomic nervous system (ANS) is further divided into the sympathetic and parasympathetic nervous systems.

Figure 3.35 demonstrates these divisions.

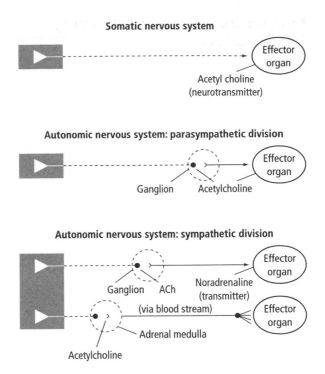

Figure 3.35 The components of the nervous system

The autonomic nervous system mainly acts involuntarily; i.e. the system is not controlled by will or conscious thought. Heart rate, peristalsis of the muscles in the alimentary tract moving food, and outpouring of adrenaline are not events you can control – they happen automatically.

The somatic nervous system acts mainly under your control and is said to be voluntary. When you need to move skeletal muscles to brush off a fly, lift a spoon to your mouth or clean your teeth, you are in control.

Voluntary movement

Running transversely across the outer wrinkled surface of the brain is a noticeable cleavage, or central sulcus, dividing two important areas of the cerebral cortex. In front of the sulcus, on each side, is the centre for motor or muscle control, and behind it is the centre for receiving sensation – the sensory cortex.

Voluntary movement begins in the motor cortex, where the body image is represented upside down. The right cerebral hemisphere controls the left side of the body and vice versa.

The muscles requiring very precise control, such as the face, tongue and hands, have much larger areas allocated on the cortex surface than those controlling less precise movements, such as the back muscles; this is despite the fact that the muscles associated with less precise movements are mainly larger muscles.

The nerve fibres, or axons, leaving the motor neurones in the motor cortex form a thick nerve fibre pathway. This crosses over to the other side in the medulla then passes down the white matter of the spinal cord to the appropriate level for the spinal nerve to emerge and supply the relevant muscles. At this level, the appropriate fibres pass into the H-shaped grey matter of the spinal cord to synapse with the lower motor neurones and pass to the muscles. When the spinal cord is severed in an accident, the areas below the division become numb and the muscles are paralysed.

Although the term 'voluntary movement' is used freely, there is massive input at the unconscious level from other neurones in the body. For example, the cerebellum controls information about muscle co-ordination, the position of the body and balance, and the sensory cortex receives information from receptors in joints and muscles.

The autonomic nervous system

Autonomic nerves differ from somatic nerves in that they do not pass directly to the organ concerned; instead, they synapse with another neurone then continue to the organ concerned. In the sympathetic branch of the ANS, these synapses lie in a chain of ganglia close to the spinal cord; in the parasympathetic branch, the synapses are usually in the wall of the organ concerned.

The sympathetic and parasympathetic nervous systems both send branches to many organs, but not all. For example, the sympathetic nervous system sends a branch to the adrenal medulla and the kidneys, but the parasympathetic nervous system does not.

In Figure 3.37, you will notice the different distribution of the two branches of the ANS:

- the sympathetic branch emanates from the thoracic and upper lumbar spinal cord sections
- the parasympathetic branch emerges from the underside of the brain via the cranial nerves and the sacral sections of the cord.

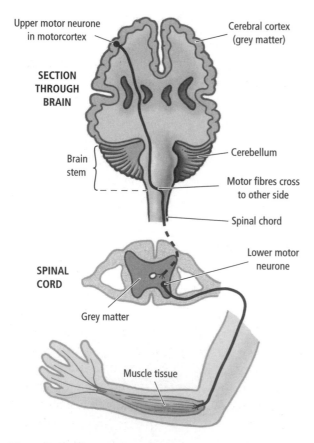

Upper motor neurone in motorcortex

Cerebral cortex (grey matter)

SECTION THROUGH BRAIN

Brain stem

Cerebellum

Motor fibres cross to other side

Spinal chord

SPINAL CORD

Lower motor neurone

Grey matter

Muscle tissue

Figure 3.36 The motor pathways

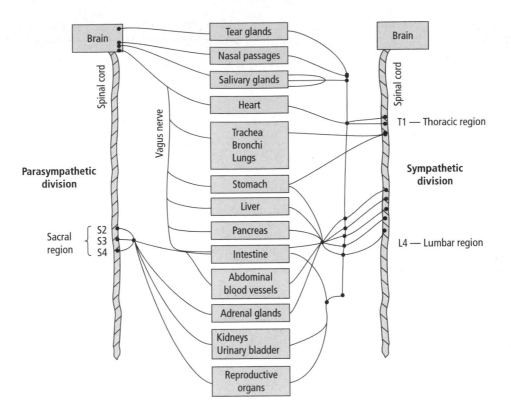

Figure 3.37 Structure of the autonomic nervous system

Disorders of the nervous system

Parkinson's disease

Strictly speaking, this is a disease of the nervous system, but many of the signs and symptoms affect the musculo-skeletal system. The first signs are tremors of hands, arms or legs which are more noticeable at rest. Later, there is stiffness and weakness of the muscles followed by a fixed, so-called 'wooden' expression on the face, a rigid, stooped posture and a shuffling type of walk. Movements are slowed; muscles have more tension and there is often accompanying depression.

A definitive cause is not known, but certain psychological medications and illegal drugs can lead to this condition. Cardiovascular disease and a rare brain infection are also known to be predisposing factors. Levadopa, converted to dopamine in the body, is used to treat Parkinson's disease.

Multiple sclerosis (MS)

Previously known as disseminated sclerosis, this is a disease of the nervous system with signs and symptoms affecting the musculo-skeletal system. The condition is marked by periods of remissions and relapses; the frequency of both is highly variable and it is not unknown for someone to be diagnosed as having MS and not suffer another attack. Generally, the signs and symptoms vary with the part of the brain affected by patchy demyelination (loss of myelin sheath; see also page 125). Individuals may present with dragging of one leg affecting walking, double vision, or loss of sensation or muscle power. Females are affected slightly more than males and it commonly affects young adults.

Although the definitive cause of MS is unknown, there is a strong genetic influence as relatives of people with MS are eight times more likely to develop symptoms. Environment is also important as the disease seems to be one associated with temperate clients; some theorists believe that a virus contracted in early life may play a role. Others classify this condition as an auto-immune disease.

People with MS should lead as active a life as possible and exercise to strengthen muscles. Steroid drugs may be used to reduce symptoms.

Debbie

I was pregnant with my third child when I experienced such tiredness that I could hardly drag myself around. Nobody seemed to have any idea what was wrong with me. It didn't get any better after Tim was born and my parents lived with me to help for six months as my husband was away at sea. I kept having medical appointments and some tests which didn't seem to reveal anything, and then one day my world fell apart when the doctor told me I had MS. I was only in my thirties and had three young children; it was awful. I am not aware of previous family history of the disease. I still teach part-time and manage most household tasks, though I do have a cleaner. I do not know what the future holds but I am on a new drug which seems to suit me and all I can do is hope for the best. I could end up using a wheelchair permanently or die quite young. However, I try to keep cheerful – although some days it is difficult because I worry for my children.

1 Explain what is meant by patchy demyelination in the brain.

2 What is the purpose of myelin in the nervous system?

3 Why are the symptoms of multiple sclerosis difficult to diagnose?

Test yourself

1 Describe the differences between sensory/receptor and motor/effector neurones.

2 Explain how impulses cross synapses.

3 Explain the difference between the somatic nervous system and the autonomic nervous system.

4 What is a ganglion?

5 Why does a stroke affecting the right side of the brain affect the left side of the body?

6 Which branch of the nervous system is closely associated with ganglia?

7 Differentiate between voluntary and involuntary movement.

8 Where does voluntary movement begin?

9 Where are neuronal cell bodies located?

10 Which parts of the body are supplied by motor neurones?

References and further reading

After you have read this chapter, you will need to dip into various sources to find extra information as there will not be a single source covering most of the topics. Many long-term illnesses have supporting organisations that supply extra material and can be found by typing the name of the condition into a search site on the Internet; examples include www.howstuffworks.com, www.ask.co.uk, www.netdoctor.co.uk.

Useful sources

- *Nursing Times* magazine
- *Health Matters* magazine
- British Medical Association (2005) *Complete Family Health Guide*. (2nd ed.). London: Dorling Kindersley
- Stoppard, M. (2005) *Dr Miriam Stoppard's Family Health Guide*. London: Dorling Kindersley
- GCE level Human Biology/Biology text books
- VCE Health and Social Care textbooks

Relevant websites

The following websites can be accessed via the Heinemann website.
Go to www.heinemann.co.uk/hotlinks and enter the express code 4256P.

- BBC health
- Department of Health
- Government statistics
- National Institute for Health and Clinical Excellence
- Health Protection Agency
- BUPA private healthcare

CHAPTER 4

Psychology and health

Key points

- Although physical health and illness are often associated with the functioning of body systems, the mind plays a powerful role. Psychology provides insight into the relationship between stress and illness.

- The stress response activates a number of body functions and can be useful in the short-term. Prolonged stress can contribute to ill-health.

- A sense of control in health and illness is important; it can modify the stress response and improve a variety of health outcomes. Personality type is significant for this sense of control or lack of it.

- There are many reasons why people adopt and maintain a healthy lifestyle or fail to do so. Health professionals can use a model of behaviour to assess (and influence) the decisions people make about personal health measures.

- The experience of, and response to, pain varies from person to person. A psychological approach to pain response and pain management includes an understanding of both the physiology and psychology of pain.

- The way people deal with illness and/or diagnosis may include a series of stages, some beneficial, others less so. When adapting to illness, different coping behaviours as well as the availability of information are associated with different outcomes. The adoption of the sick role is an important aspect of the psychological experience of being ill.

- Anxiety reduction methods are important in both lessening psychological distress, and controlling or alleviating the physiological effects of illness.

- Substance abuse is explained in psychological terms with reference to the two common addictions to smoking and alcohol.

Introduction

Psychology is the study of mind, feelings and behaviour, and covers many aspects of human life. Within the diverse field of psychology, there are several different areas of study. These include the following:

- *Neuropsychology* investigates the role of genes, how the brain works and its relationship to bodily, cognitive and emotional functioning.
- *Abnormal psychology* involves the study of mental disorders such as schizophrenia, depression and anxiety disorders.
- *Cognitive psychology* is the study of all aspects of thinking, memory, problem-solving, pattern-recognition and attentional processes.
- *Developmental psychology* investigates developmental processes from conception, through the life course to the time of death.
- *Social psychology* is concerned with how people interact and how behaviour and beliefs can change as a result of the influence of others.
- *Occupational psychology* investigates how people interact at work, the optimal working conditions to promote health and well-being at work, and employer–employee relationships.
- *Forensic psychology* is the study of factors involved in criminality.
- *Clinical psychology* deals with the assessment and treatment of abnormal or maladaptive behaviour.

No one area of psychology can be separated from others as we are all social beings with brain activity and **cognitive** functions. Each person is shaped by a particular developmental history, but equally each person is influenced by his or her genetic inheritance. Applied disciplines of psychology, such as occupational, forensic and clinical psychology, draw on research from other areas to gain a full understanding of why people behave, think and feel as they do.

> **Cognitive** – aspects of mental activity that involve the manipulation of material in an abstract way. This includes thinking, memory, perception and problem solving.

Whereas it was once believed that the mind and body were separate, with disconnected influences and pathways, there is a large body of research which recognises that a person's psychological history and functioning has a large influence on his or her physical state. The placebo effect (described below) is an excellent example of this.

Health, stress and illness

A very clear example of how a person's thoughts and feelings can directly influence the body is the way the body reacts with the fight or flight response. To understand this, it is necessary for a little biological explanation.

The flight or fight response

When something potentially stressful happens, for example, taking a driving test or an important exam, the breakdown of a long-term relationship or a close relative being injured in a car accident, you make a judgement as to whether you find the situation stressful or not. If you perceive the event to be stressful, an important part of the brain, called the hypothalamus, is immediately activated. The hypothalamus has the role, among other things, of regulating eating behaviours and controlling **homeostasis**. It also sends messages to the **autonomic nervous system**, through a complex set of nerve fibres, and to the endocrine system, the part of the body which governs the secretion of **hormones**. A chain of events then follows, as summarised in Figure 4.01.

> **Fight or flight response**
> A sequence of physiological responses triggered by the perception of a danger. They prepare the body for running away from danger (flight) or defending or attacking (fight).

> **Homeostasis** – the processes by which the body maintains a constant internal physiological environment. For example, shivering to restore a drop in body temperature.
>
> **Autonomic nervous system** – a division of the nervous system consisting of the sympathetic and parasympathetic branches. Many of its functions occur without conscious awareness.
>
> **Hormones** – chemicals secreted by the endocrine system which have both behavioural and physiological functions. For example, the sex hormone testosterone causes hair growth and increased aggression.

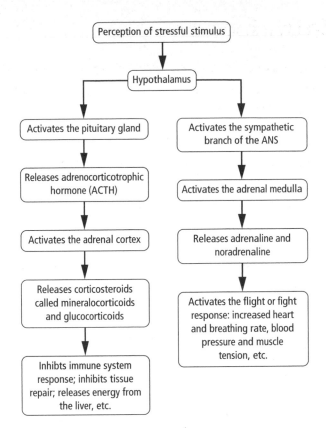

Figure 4.01 The stress response

The hypothalamus acts as a 'messenger', sending signals to the sympathetic branch of the autonomic nervous system. These messages result in the secretion of two neurotransmitters, adrenaline and noradrenaline, from the inner part of the adrenal gland (the adrenal medulla), which is located just above the kidneys. These two stress hormones are responsible for setting into action the fight or flight response.

> Did you know?
>
> *The fight or flight response is thought to have its evolutionary beginnings in dangerous situations where either running away or staying and fighting would increase the chances of survival. So, for example, if our human ancestors were faced with a sabre-toothed tiger, the ability to run away quickly would be an adaptive response that ensured survival. If, on the other hand, our ancestors were hungry and needed to hunt down wild boar, the ability to fight would also encourage survival.*

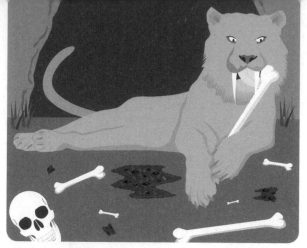

Figure 4.02 Those who developed a strong fight or flight response were most likely to survive!

The physical changes that occur when the fight or flight response is activated are:

- the pupils dilate (to increase the amount of light available)
- the heart rate and strength increases (so the maximum amount of oxygenated blood is available to the lungs and muscles)
- lung function is increased (to maximise the supply of oxygenated blood)
- blood supply is diverted from the stomach and skin to the muscles of the limbs (to enable faster and stronger movements)
- sugar is released from the liver to the muscles (to enable faster and stronger movements).

A second message sent by the hypothalamus is to the endocrine system. This message activates the pituitary gland (a part of the brain situated just below the hypothalamus) which then secretes a special hormone known as adrenocorticotropic hormone (or ACTH). This in turn activates the outer part of the adrenal gland known as the adrenal cortex, which then releases stress hormones known as glucocorticoids, such as cortisol. These hormones help increase the body's energy and also act directly to suppress immune system functioning. The reason is that, at times of stress, the body needs to direct all its energy and resources into dealing with the immediate emergency. As the immune system takes up a lot of energy in repairing and recharging the body, the functioning of this system is temporarily put on hold in order to deal effectively with the threat.

The role of control in health and illness

You may have wondered why some people seem amazingly resilient to life's ups and downs. People all around them succumb to colds and other infections, but they stay healthy. Similarly, one person may feel that life has come to an end if he or she is made redundant whereas another sees it as a challenge and sets off enthusiastically in a new direction to make the best of the situation. These latter type of people have what is known as a 'hardy' personality. Research by Kobassa (1979) has shown that hardy people have three personality traits, sometimes known as the three Cs. They see potentially stressful events as a challenge rather than a threat, they have a high sense of personal control, and they are highly committed to everything they do. As a consequence of this personality type, they tend to be resilient to stress and to make the most of their lives, taking set-backs in their stride and turning potential disasters into successes. This resilience to stress means the immune system is not compromised by constant activation of the stress response, and a diagnosis of illness tends to be met with a fighting response rather than one of giving up.

Christopher Reeve

Christopher Reeve was paralysed in a horse riding accident in 1995. After his accident, he and his wife opened the first centre in the United States devoted to teaching paralysed people to live more independently. Known as the Christopher and Dana Reeve Paralysis

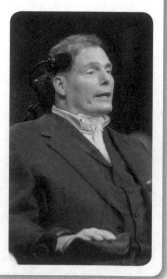

Over to you

Christopher Reeve turned his own personal disaster into an opportunity to improve life for others. Find out more about Christopher Reeve, in particular the interviews he gave. What does he say that indicates he approached life in a 'hardy' manner? Why do you think this might be?

Control as a modifier of stress and an indicator of improved health outcomes

Loss of control can be a major difficulty for some individuals, causing severe psychological responses. Elderly people admitted to residential nursing homes may find it quite a shock to experience loss of control over their lives after years of independent living, and this can be accompanied by quite negative psychological and physiological outcomes. An experiment by Langer and Rodin (1976) gave one set of residents in a nursing home a degree of control over their environment, which included responsibility for looking after house plants, choices about whether to take part in activities and freedom to rearrange furniture. Other residents were given plants but told the nursing staff would take care of them; they were assigned to activities rather than choosing them and were given no control

over how the furniture was arranged. These residents were all followed up for a period of 18 months and it was found that those with control were healthier, more active and alert than those without control. Even more important was the finding that the rate of mortality was halved among this group.

Type A and Type B personality types

Somewhat similar to the hardy personality is what is known as a Type B personality. This personality type was described by two cardiologists, Friedman and Rosenman, who were investigating cholesterol levels in groups of males who presented with heart disease. They found that those at high risk of heart disease also tended to be more stressed. By analysing behavioural characteristics of a large group of men, they identified certain typical kinds of behaviour which they named Type A and Type B. A summary of these is given in Table 4.01.

In a clinical setting, a range of behaviours, attitudes and beliefs is assessed to determine what personality type an individual has. There are, however, several short forms of this test.

Over to you

To do an online test to assess whether you are a Type A or Type B personality, go to www.heinemann.co.uk/ hotlinks and enter the express code 4256P. This test has been specially adapted for students.

While some studies have found that people with a Type A personality are at higher risk of asthma attacks, indigestion and nausea, the link is not consistent or strong. However, a much higher

Table 4.01 Summary of Type A and Type B behaviours

Type A	Type B
• Self-critical • Strives towards goals but without feeling pleasure in achievements • A sense of time urgency – working against the clock; taking on too much • Easily aroused to anger and tending to feel hostile (although this may not be expressed)	• Easy-going • Philosophical about life • Low levels of competitiveness • Little sense of time urgency • Low hostility • Able to take time to 'stop and smell the roses'

association has been found between Type A personality and risk for **coronary heart disease** (CHD). For example, a study in 1974 investigating 3000 men aged 39–59 years found that after 8½ years, Type A men were twice as likely than Type B participants to have developed and died of CHD (cited in Rice and Haralambos, 2000).

> **Coronary heart disease** – A number of illnesses that are a consequence of narrowing or blocking of the coronary arteries which supply blood to the heart muscle; they include angina, arteriosclerosis and myocardial infarction (heart attack).

The physical explanation for this links to the fight or flight response described earlier. The actions of the sympathetic nervous system during this response cause blood to be pumped at higher rates, due to the secretion of adrenaline and noradrenaline. At points in the cardiovascular system where the blood vessels branch, these become worn and thinner. Glucose released during the stress response is normally reabsorbed by the body when the stress passes, in which case no harm is done. For those who are constantly stressed, however, glucose builds up and can settle in the worn parts of the arteries and form a clot, thus leading to CHD.

There is also a behavioural component to the link between CHD and personality type. Type A personalities are significantly more likely than their Type B counterparts to drink frequently and excessively, to take up smoking and find difficulty in giving up smoking.

Both of these are risk factors in themselves for CHD. Finally, Type A personalities are more likely to try to struggle on despite being tired, or push themselves to the limit when injured.

Finally, a psychological factor that seems to be involved is the tendency to be hostile, cynical and suspicious. This may lead the Type A personality to treat potentially neutral situations as full of conflict, the individual thereby provoking others who in turn become less supportive. This leads to the loss of a socially supportive network and worsening of relationships, which in turn encourages feelings of hostility and suspicion.

Fighting spirit

A similar concept to control is the importance of what has been called 'fighting spirit', both in the development of illness and the response to a diagnosis. For example, it has been suggested that there might be a cancer-prone personality type. This is described as individuals who avoid conflict, suppress emotions, are passive, appeasing and helpless, and tend to be focused on others at the expense of their own needs. An examination of medical students over 30 years old found that those who were more likely to develop cancer were individuals who had low self-awareness, were self-sacrificing, inclined to blame themselves and unable to express emotions. These individuals were sixteen times more likely to develop cancer than individuals who did not show such personality characteristics.

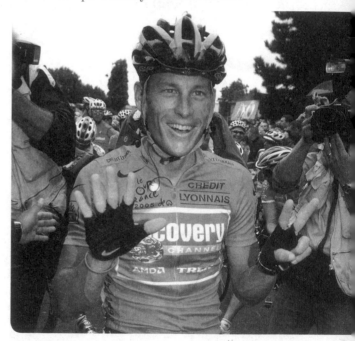

Lance Armstrong miraculously overcame testicular cancer to become a three-time Olympian champion and six-time winner of the Tour De France. He is an inspiration for millions

When it comes to dealing with illness, it has been found that those who displayed a 'fighting spirit' tended to be less anxious than more passive individuals. Similarly, individuals with cardiac disease tend to experience higher than normal levels of anxiety and depression during the first weeks or months after a heart attack. If very high levels continue for more than a few months, those individuals tend to show decreased compliance in their treatment regime. They are also more likely to suffer subsequent cardiac problems or to die in the next several months. Clearly, then, reduced anxiety and a pro-active and positive approach to recovery has major implications for recovery and mortality rates.

Explanations for feelings of control or lack of control

Learned helplessness

When people experience a high level of stress over a long time caused by events which they are unable to control, they may lapse into apathy and lose the capacity to take action to alter events which are controllable. This is known as learned helplessness. However, not all people who are exposed to uncontrollable events develop learned helplessness.

An experiment carried out by Hiroto and Seligman (1975) demonstrated how a sense of helplessness and a low sense of personal control can arise. They allocated healthy participants to one of two groups. All groups were subjected to an unpleasant noise, but there were variations in the degree to which participants could exert control by doing something to make the noise stop. The experiment was divided into two phases, as described in Table 4.02.

The findings of the experiment were that, during Phase 2, the uncontrollable-noise group (Group 2) performed much more poorly than the other two groups. The explanation for this is that they had learned, during Phase 1, that whatever they did made no difference. They had thus learned to become helpless and to believe they had no control.

Attributional style

Based on Hiroto and Seligman's (1975) experiment and many other similar experiments, a theory was developed known as attribution theory. Attributions refer to the explanations people give for the causes of events. For example, an individual who develops Type II diabetes after many years of smoking, drinking and following a high fat, high sugar diet with little exercise, may attribute (explain) the cause of the development of diabetes to his own lifestyle.

Table 4.02 Phases of Hiroto and Seligman's learned helplessness experiment (1975)

Phase 1		
Group 1: Controllable-noise group	**Group 2: Uncontrollable-noise group**	**Group 3: Comparison group**
Participants were told that a noise would occur from time to time and 'There is something you can do to stop it' (subjects were able to locate a button on the apparatus which turned off the noise).	The same instructions and apparatus were used as for Group 1, but whatever actions were taken by the participants, they were unable to turn off the noise.	The participants were told 'From time to time a noise will come on and off. Please sit and listen to it'.
Phase 2		
Instructions for all three groups were the same in this phase. Each group was told: 'A noise will come on and off and there is something you can do to stop it.' However, new apparatus (a sliding knob) was provided which would stop the noise in all three conditions.		

Attribution theory is used extensively to explain how people make sense of uncontrollable negative events. According to the theory, individuals consider possible causes by assessing three dimensions of the situation:

- *Internal–external:* the individual assesses whether an uncontrollable negative event arises because of his or her own personal inability to control outcomes or whether it is due to external causes beyond his or her control.
- *Stable–unstable:* here the situation is assessed as resulting from a cause that is long-lasting (stable) or temporary (unstable).
- *Global–specific:* here the assessment is made as to whether an event has resulted from factors that have wide-ranging effects or specific effects.

Attributions of negative life events to stable and global causes are likely to lead to helplessness and depression. Internal attributions also can lead to loss of self-esteem. A person's typical way of making attributions is known as his or her attributional style. The implications to health of attributional style can be summarised as follows:

- *Internal–external:* An internal attribution is likely to lead to loss of self-esteem. For example, if an individual receiving physical therapy for a limb injury cannot meet the goals set each week by his or her physiotherapist, the individual may feel either that he or she is not good enough (internal attribution) or that the regime is not suitable (external attribution).
- *Stable–unstable:* A stable attribution is likely to follow diagnosis of a chronic or disabling illness (which is long-lasting). This leads to a greater risk of depression and helplessness than if the condition is seen as temporary.
- *Global–specific:* A global attribution is more likely to lead to helplessness than a specific attribution. For example, the failure to stop smoking and adhere to a dietary regime may be attributed to a lack of will power and

general worthlessness (global attribution) or to acceptable and limited human failings – 'I am good at controlling many aspects of my healthy lifestyle with the exception of this' (specific attribution).

Locus of control

Locus of control refers to the extent to which an individual believes that he or she:

- is in charge of his or her own destiny
- is able to influence own behaviours and those of others.

In general, people with an internal locus of control are more likely to have a hardy personality, be resistant to stress, have a fighting spirit when diagnosed with illness, to adhere to medical guidance and be proactive in regaining health or dealing with illness. By contrast, those with an external locus of control feel they have little control over events and are more likely to be anxious and depressed.

Did you know?

Attributional style and locus of control can be measured online using an inventory. To access this inventory, go to www.heinemann.co.uk/hotlinks and enter the express code 4256P.

A questionnaire used to measure whether someone has a high or low sense of personal control is the Multidimensional Health Locus of Control Scale developed by Wallston, Wallston and DeVellis in 1978. This is reproduced below as Forms A and B (Tables 4.03 and 4.04). The Multidimensional Health Locus of Control Scale can also be found on the Heinemann website; visit www.heinemann.co.uk/hotlinks and enter the express code 4256P.

Table 4.03 Multidimensional Health Locus of Control Scale: Form A

Instructions: Each item below is a belief statement about your medical condition with which you may agree or disagree. Beside each statement is a scale which ranges from strongly disagree (1) to strongly agree (6). For each item, circle the number that represents the extent to which you agree or disagree with that statement. The more you agree with a statement, the higher will be the number you circle. The more you disagree with a statement, the lower will be the number you circle. Please make sure that you answer EVERY ITEM and that you circle ONLY ONE number per item. This is a measure of your personal beliefs; obviously, there are no right or wrong answers.

1 = STRONGLY DISAGREE (**SD**)	4 = SLIGHTLY AGREE (**A**)
2 = MODERATELY DISAGREE (**MD**)	5 = MODERATELY AGREE (**MA**)
3 = SLIGHTLY DISAGREE (**D**)	6 = STRONGLY AGREE (**SA**)

		SD	MD	D	A	MA	SA
1	If I get sick, it is my own behaviour which determines how soon I get well again.	1	2	3	4	5	6
2	No matter what I do, if I am going to get sick, I will get sick.	1	2	3	4	5	6
3	Having regular contact with my physician is the best way for me to avoid illness.	1	2	3	4	5	6
4	Most things that affect my health happen to me by accident.	1	2	3	4	5	6
5	Whenever I don't feel well, I should consult a medically-trained professional.	1	2	3	4	5	6
6	I am in control of my health.	1	2	3	4	5	6
7	My family has a lot to do with my becoming sick or staying healthy.	1	2	3	4	5	6
8	When I get sick, I am to blame.	1	2	3	4	5	6
9	Luck plays a big part in determining how soon I will recover from an illness.	1	2	3	4	5	6
10	Health professionals control my health.	1	2	3	4	5	6
11	My good health is largely a matter of good fortune.	1	2	3	4	5	6
12	The main thing which affects my health is what I myself do.	1	2	3	4	5	6
13	If I take care of myself, I can avoid illness.	1	2	3	4	5	6
14	Whenever I recover from an illness, it is usually because other people (for example, doctors, nurses, family, friends) have been taking good care of me.	1	2	3	4	5	6
15	No matter what I do, I am likely to get sick.	1	2	3	4	5	6
16	If it is meant to be, I will stay healthy.	1	2	3	4	5	6
17	If I take the right actions, I can stay healthy.	1	2	3	4	5	6
18	Regarding my health, I can only do what my doctor tells me to do.	1	2	3	4	5	6

Table 4.04 Multidimensional Health Locus of Control Scale: Form B

Instructions: Each item below is a belief statement about your medical condition with which you may agree or disagree. Beside each statement is a scale which ranges from strongly disagree (1) to strongly agree (6). For each item, circle the number that represents the extent to which you agree or disagree with that statement. The more you agree with a statement, the higher will be the number you circle. The more you disagree with a statement, the lower will be the number you circle. Please make sure that you answer EVERY ITEM and that you circle ONLY ONE number per item. This is a measure of your personal beliefs; obviously, there are no right or wrong answers.

1 = STRONGLY DISAGREE (**SD**)
2 = MODERATELY DISAGREE (**MD**)
3 = SLIGHTLY DISAGREE (**D**)

4 = SLIGHTLY AGREE (**A**)
5 = MODERATELY AGREE (**MA**)
6 = STRONGLY AGREE (**SA**)

		SD	MD	D	A	MA	SA
1	If I become sick, I have the power to make myself well again.	1	2	3	4	5	6
2	Often I feel that no matter what I do, if I am going to get sick, I will get sick.	1	2	3	4	5	6
3	If I see an excellent doctor regularly, I am less likely to have health problems.	1	2	3	4	5	6
4	It seems that my health is greatly influenced by accidental happenings.	1	2	3	4	5	6
5	I can only maintain my health by consulting health professionals.	1	2	3	4	5	6
6	I am directly responsible for my health.	1	2	3	4	5	6
7	Other people play a big part in whether I stay healthy or become sick.	1	2	3	4	5	6
8	Whatever goes wrong with my health is my own fault.	1	2	3	4	5	6
9	When I am sick, I just have to let nature run its course.	1	2	3	4	5	6
10	Health professionals keep me healthy.	1	2	3	4	5	6
11	When I stay healthy, I'm just plain lucky.	1	2	3	4	5	6
12	My physical well-being depends on how well I take care of myself.	1	2	3	4	5	6
13	When I feel ill, I know it is because I have not been taking care of myself properly.	1	2	3	4	5	6
14	The type of care I receive from other people determines how well I recover from an illness.	1	2	3	4	5	6
15	Even when I take care of myself, it is easy to get sick.	1	2	3	4	5	6
16	When I become ill is a matter of fate.	1	2	3	4	5	6
17	I can pretty much stay healthy by taking good care of myself.	1	2	3	4	5	6
18	Following doctor's orders to the letter is the best way for me to stay healthy.	1	2	3	4	5	6

Using findings from this questionnaire and similar others, the following conclusions have been drawn about the role of a sense of control in health and illness:

- People with a strong sense of personal control may be more likely or able to maintain their health and prevent illness than those with a weak sense of personal control.
- Those who have a strong sense of control adapt better to serious illnesses and promote their own recovery more effectively than those with a weak sense of control (particularly if such individuals see their illness as being severe).
- Individuals with illnesses such as kidney failure or cancer who have an internal locus of control suffer less depression than those with an external locus of control. The individual's belief that he or she or someone else can influence the course of the illness allows the individual to be more hopeful about the future.
- Individuals with strong internal locus of control beliefs probably realise that they have effective ways for controlling their stress.
- Those who have a low sense of control have poorer health habits, more illnesses and are less likely to take active steps to treat their illness than people with a greater sense of control.

Sheila

I am a care worker in a small local authority children's home. I have been allocated responsibility for a new eight-year-old child, Safraz, who has been taken into care because his mother, a single parent with three other children, has multiple sclerosis and is unable to look after him. Safraz is very quiet and reserved, doesn't make eye contact and doesn't interact with others. He has recently started attending a new school in the area and the staff there think he may be being bullied.

1 Work in small groups to discuss reasons for Safraz's shyness in terms of the dimension of control.

2 What could Sheila do to help Safraz increase his sense of control? How would this help him in life?

Promoting health and well-being

Adopting and maintaining a healthy lifestyle

With advances in knowledge and understanding of the mind-body link, there has been an increasing interest in health promotion. In 1977 the American physician John Knowles wrote that most people:

are born healthy and made sick as a result of personal misbehaviour and environmental conditions. The solution to the problems of ill health in modern American society involves individual responsibility ... and social responsibility through public legislation and private volunteer efforts. (Cited in Sarafino, 1998: 10)

Increasingly, the focus in medical and health initiatives is on the promotion of health protective behaviours and prevention of illness through a variety of measures, rather than living in a carefree manner and then accessing medical services when damage has occurred.

> **Health promotion**
> Initiatives designed to help people prevent becoming ill in the first place by adopting healthy lifestyles.

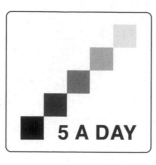

Just Eat More
(fruit & veg)

Image used as part of the government's 'five-a-day' health campaign, which encourages people in the UK to eat five portions of fresh fruit and vegetables daily

Types of health protective behaviours

There are three major types of actions taken to promote well-being and prevent illness, collectively known as health protective behaviours.

Primary prevention

This consists of actions taken to avoid illness, disease or injury. Examples include wearing a seat-belt, getting vaccinations, using sun screen and adopting healthy lifestyle behaviours.

Secondary prevention

This refers to actions and behaviours adopted to identify and treat an illness early on in order to stop the problem worsening or even reversing the problem. Sometimes referred to as 'illness behaviour' this includes seeking medical care, having regular screening or check-ups, breast and testicular self-examination, blood pressure and blood cholesterol level checks, physiotherapy for an injury, etc.

Tertiary prevention

Tertiary prevention takes place when a serious injury occurs or an illness progresses beyond the early stages. It involves actions taken to prevent disability and enhance rehabilitation. For example, a individual with arthritis will adopt tertiary prevention measures by taking prescribed medication and engaging in programmes designed to maintain mobility (such as physical therapy). For an individual with a serious injury such as a limb amputation, tertiary prevention may consist of the use of prosthetic limbs, physical therapy to adapt to activities in the absence of the amputated limb, and adopting new lifestyle behaviours to allow for continued independent living.

Understanding problems associated with adopting health protective behaviours

> **Over to you**
>
> *Discuss among yourselves what lifestyle factors and behaviours you think could contribute to illness. Decide which of them are due to the individual's behaviour (e.g. smoking) and which are due to the environment (e.g. ingesting industrial pollutants). Create a list of these and research one of them by looking up official statistics (e.g. deaths due to alcohol abuse or smoking). You may want to draw up a short questionnaire to hand out to fellow students asking them how much they are aware of the risks of various lifestyle behaviours (e.g. smoking, not taking enough exercise, etc).*

In the activity above you have probably come up with a long list of behaviours known to contribute to illness, two of the most obvious being smoking and eating an unhealthy diet. However, knowing that certain behaviour puts you at risk of later illness is not always sufficient to prevent you from doing it, as anyone who has tried to lose weight or give up smoking will acknowledge! For some behaviour, there is a genetic link. For example, people with an alcoholic parent are more likely to become alcoholic themselves than those without. Some people have a tendency to become obese more easily than others. But genes do not determine health behaviours. You can choose, for example, not to drink or to limit your food intake to prevent obesity. So what is it that encourages individuals to take up healthy or unhealthy behaviours?

Operant conditioning

One answer to this is learning. A particular type of learning called operant conditioning has been heavily researched and sheds much light on how people acquire, maintain and stop various behaviours. According to this theory, when a person does something that results in a desired consequence (e.g. eating a bar of chocolate), he or she is positively reinforced for that behaviour by the feelings of comfort and pleasure gained. Any behaviour that is reinforced is likely to be repeated. The person is thus more likely to eat a bar of chocolate in the future. If, on the other hand, a person is praised for eating some fruit instead of a bar of chocolate and the praise is perceived as desirable, he or she may learn to snack on fruit instead of chocolate. The praise has become a positive reinforcer.

Positive reinforcement
This occurs when a particular behaviour is followed by a consequence that is experienced as satisfying to the individual. There is more likelihood of the behaviour occurring again due to this process. For example, if spending five minutes meditating (behaviour) leads to an individual feeling relaxed and calm (consequence), he or she is more likely to repeat the behaviour in future (i.e. meditate more often).

Individuals can also be encouraged to adopt behaviours if they provide negative reinforcement. This occurs when the action of an individual removes an unpleasant feeling or event. An example of this would be drinking a glass of wine at the end of a stressful day. The sense of relaxation and relief obtained by drinking the wine takes away the negative sensation of stress

and anxiety. Once again, you will be more likely to drink a glass of wine the next time a similar situation crops up. An example of healthy behaviour as a result of negative reinforcement might be if you have a painful ankle due an injury and spend time swimming, which relieves the pain. You will thus be more likely to continue swimming because it is negatively reinforcing.

Negative reinforcement
This occurs when a particular behaviour is followed by the removal of an unpleasant event or stimulus. For example, if massaging the temples (behaviour) leads to pain relief (removal of the unpleasant event or stimulus), the behaviour of massaging the temples is likely to increase.

The principles of positive and negative reinforcement explain how behaviour can be acquired. It may not, however, be maintained if the reinforcement does not continue. The concept of extinction is relevant here; this refers to the weakening of learnt behaviour until it stops altogether. For example, a child may be given a star on a star chart as positive reinforcement every time he or she cleans his or her teeth. If, after a period of time, the parent or carer stops giving stars and doesn't supervise teeth cleaning, the child's tooth-cleaning behaviour may well be extinguished as the reinforcement is no longer being offered. Similarly, the person whose ankle has healed may give up swimming as it is no longer reinforcing for him or her.

The final principle that is relevant to operant conditioning is that of punishment. If an individual is punished for smoking (for example, by being grounded by a parent or carer), this may stop him or her repeating the behaviour. Punishment, however, is much less effective than reinforcement. Take the example of the child who is punished for hitting his little sister. It is very likely he will learn not to hit his sister in the presence of the person who punished him, but he may well continue the behaviour when that person is out of sight. In terms of encouraging people to give up unhealthy behaviours such as smoking, punishment from others is often not effective and so it is necessary to look at what is going on inside the individual to determine a better method.

Social learning theory

A second form of learning, which leads to the acquisition of healthy or unhealthy behaviours, is called social learning theory. According to this theory, people learn behaviours by observing others; for example, it is possible to learn dance steps by watching a pop video. Simply learning is not enough, however, to make a person actually perform the behaviours. The individual needs to be motivated to perform the behaviour, and this is influenced by many factors. In terms of health behaviour, if a young adolescent sees a highly popular individual at the school drinking vodka and receiving admiration from others for doing so, he or she may be motivated to copy this behaviour and thus gain admiration for him- or herself. If, on the other hand, the individual being observed is unpopular and his or her vodka drinking is seen as pathetic, there will be much less motivation to copy the behaviour. In general, people's motivation to imitate others is increased if they are high status (e.g. film stars, models or people known to us whom we admire), attractive or similar (e.g. similar age, race and gender).

Models of health behaviour

For a long time it was assumed that encouraging people to adopt a healthy lifestyle required nothing more than giving them information about what to do and what to avoid.

Health belief model

The relationship between knowledge and behaviour is quite a complex one. To understand this, psychologists have come up with what is known as the health belief model, which takes a more complex view to understanding healthy behaviours. According to this model, people make two assessments about potentially risky behaviour. They evaluate the perceived threat and then evaluate the advantages and disadvantages of taking action to reduce the threat. In doing this, people ask themselves a series of questions, as shown in Figure 4.03.

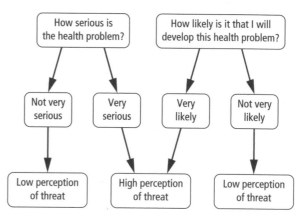

Figure 4.03 Health belief model: assessment of potential threat (Stage 1)

Factors that influence this first stage of appraisal comprise what are known as **demographic variables**; these include age, gender, race and ethnic background. Also relevant are social and psychological factors, including personality type, social class and knowledge about, or prior contact with, the health problem. Thus, a female with a family history of breast cancer will have knowledge about this disease through personal contact with the affected family member(s). She may be concerned about the age of onset and, if she leads a stressful lifestyle and has a vulnerable personality type, she may be highly likely to assess breast cancer as a very serious problem to which she is highly susceptible.

> **Demographic variables** – aspects of the population surveyed; for example, age, gender, ethnicity, social class, level of education, type of occupation, level of wealth and any other factors relevant to the research question.

The second step in this model involves an appraisal of the benefits and disadvantages of taking preventive action. These are referred to as the perceived costs or barriers and perceived benefits.

- Perceived benefits include better health, longer life, an improved lifestyle, staying well to watch one's children grow up, etc.
- Perceived costs or barriers could include the difficulty (financial or practical) and the inconvenience or discomfort of visiting a health professional or service to receive medical care.

If the costs or barriers exceed the benefits, the model predicts that the individual will not take action. For example, a cervical smear test is, to many people, an unpleasant procedure. This discomfort may act as a barrier to an individual having the test; in this instance, the barrier is greater than the perceived benefits of this preventative health measure.

Putting together all the aspects of the model, therefore, the following possible outcomes are identified (see Figure 4.04).

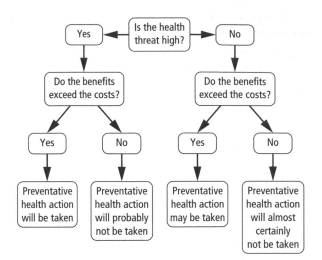

Figure 4.04 Health belief model: assessment of benefits and disadvantages of taking preventative action (Stage 2)

As mentioned briefly above, there are other variables which may influence both the appraisal of threat and the cost-benefit analysis. An individual with a hardy personality, for example, may be more likely to want to take control over his or her health and so, despite appraising a potential threat as low and the costs to taking action as high, continue to take the action required to ensure health. On the other hand, barriers to attending clinics, doctors' surgeries, etc., for preventative health measures are more likely to exist for people on a low income or the elderly or disabled. Poor transport facilities, the difficulties involved with looking after children whilst attending clinics, etc., may prove to be significant barriers, resulting in health promotion behaviours not being followed.

Research has supported this model. For example, it has been found that people who believe themselves to be susceptible to a particular health-related problem and believe that the benefits of taking action outweigh the costs, are more likely to visit the dentist regularly, take up vaccination programmes, get regular breast and cervical cancer tests and take part in exercise programmes when compared to those who do not perceive these to be health threats and/or feel that the costs outweigh the benefits.

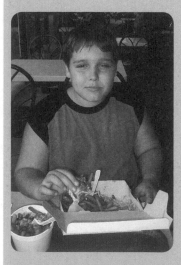

Despite the growing problem of obesity, many children continue to eat high-fat diets with little nutritional content

The health belief model suggests that to tackle a problem such as obesity, it is not enough to simply give information about healthy eating and exercise; many more factors seem to be involved. Work through the following activities to investigate this in more depth.

Understanding pain and individual responses to pain

Types of pain

Chronic pain is different from acute pain.

- Acute pain refers to pain experienced by temporary conditions that last less than six months or so; for example, migraines, toothache, the pain resulting from injuries or surgery. Acute pain induces high levels of anxiety in individuals but is accompanied by a reduction in distress and anxiety as the condition improves and the pain lessens.
- Chronic pain describes pain that continues over a period of many months or years.

It is associated with continuing high levels of anxiety and distress and accompanying feelings of hopelessness as attempts to alleviate the pain fail.

Living with chronic back pain

Sue Clayton is 56 years old and has suffered from chronic back pain for the last 23 years following surgery. Her pain is so chronic that sometimes she is incapable of moving. 'I get pain from my waist to my toes. It is like a burning pain and I feel like I am walking on glass. The only thing that really works for me is lying flat on my back.' Sue has tried all sorts of pain relief, from medication to complementary therapies, but little has worked and her life has been very severely limited. 'It has been very difficult to cope. I was in my early 30s when the back pain first started with sciatica. I had to give up work and had difficulty looking after my children. I had to put one child in boarding school and I had to import a lot of help to help me look after my two children.'

Did you know?

Research carried out in Scotland suggests that almost half of the population of Scotland is thought to be suffering from some kind of chronic pain. The two-year study questioned more than 5000 people in the north-east of Scotland. Details of the study can be accessed via the Heinemann website; go to www.heinemann.co.uk/hotlinks and enter the express code 4256P.

Classification of chronic pain

Psychologists Turk, Meichenbaum and Genest (1983) have identified three different types of chronic pain, classified with reference to both the cause and the frequency of pain.

Chronic recurrent pain

This type of pain has a **benign** cause, i.e. it isn't a sign of a serious and worsening illness or disease. Pain occurs on a temporary basis: pain-free periods are interspersed with painful episodes. A classic example of this is migraine or tension headache – the cause is benign (it is not a symptom of a brain tumour or other serious underlying cause) and when the headache or migraine is over, the associated pain is no longer present until the next episode (hence recurrent).

Benign – any condition which, untreated or with symptomatic therapy, will not become life-threatening. The term is used in particular in relation to tumours, which may be benign or malignant. Benign tumours do not invade surrounding tissues and do not metastasize to other parts of the body. (The word is slightly imprecise, as some benign tumours can, due to mass effect, cause life-threatening complications. The term therefore applies mainly to their biological behaviour.)

Chronic intractable benign pain

This refers to pain that is also benign. However, it tends to be present all of the time, sometimes being more intense than at other periods. As with chronic recurrent pain, this type of pain isn't related to an underlying malignant condition such as cancer or arthritis. A good example of this type of pain is chronic low back pain.

Chronic progressive pain

This type of pain is associated with a **malignant** condition and is likely to become worse as the condition progresses. Cancer is a very typical example of this type of pain, as is rheumatoid arthritis.

Malignant – in medicine, the term describes a clinical course that progresses rapidly to death. It is typically applied to neoplasms that show aggressive behaviour, characterised by local invasion or distant metastasis.

The influence of psychological factors in the perception of pain

It has been consistently found that treatments for pain involving medical intervention such as drugs or surgery have an effect on acute pain but lose their efficacy when treating chronic pain. This suggests that pain is not perceived in the same way at all times.

Individual tolerance for pain also seems to vary quite considerably. During the Second World War (1939–45), a physician called Beecher noticed that requests for pain relief from soldiers were much less frequent than those from civilians, despite a similar degree of injury. For example, 80 per cent of civilians asked for medication for pain relief compared with only 20 per cent of soldiers. The explanation for this was that the experience of pain by soldiers was associated with something positive – for them, the war was over and they would not be sent back to their units. For civilians, on the other hand, the experience of pain meant that their lives became worse.

Did you know?

Further evidence for psychological factors in the perception of pain comes from the puzzling phenomenon of phantom limb pain. This occurs following amputation when a individual continues to report pain in the limb that has been amputated. This is clearly a medical impossibility since there cannot be any nerve receptors to detect pain. An explanation clearly needs to be sought by looking at the psychological factors associated with the experience of pain.

Physiological responses to pain

In order to understand the experience of pain, and the methods of managing it, it is necessary to look at one of the most influential psychological theories of pain. This is known as the Gate-Control theory of pain and was introduced by Ronald Melzack and Patrick Wall in 1965 (later updated in 1982).

The Gate-Control theory of pain

This theory suggests that a 'gate' exists in the spinal cord (part of the central nervous system) which receives information from three sources:

1. A-delta and C fibres
2. peripheral nerve (A-beta) fibres
3. the brain.

Figure 4.05 The Gate-Control theory of pain

A-delta and C fibres

When an injury occurs, strong pain signals are sent from two types of small-diameter pain fibres known as A-delta and C fibres. A-delta fibres transmit messages very quickly and with intense pain; C fibres transmit messages more slowly and are responsible for longer-term throbbing and chronic pain.

Peripheral nerve fibres

Peripheral nerve fibres from the site of the injury (known as A-beta fibres) also send signals to this gate. These are large-diameter fibres which do not transmit pain stimuli but carry information about harmless stimuli or mild irritation (e.g. touching, rubbing and scratching the skin) at the site of the injury.

The brain

The brain sends signals to this gate about the psychological state of the individual. This includes information such as:

- behavioural factors, for example, focusing on the pain or diverting attention away
- emotional factors, including the degree of anxiety, fear or depression experienced
- previous experience of pain or injury; for example, a migraine sufferer who has experienced the pain before will be able to identify it and know that it passes in time; he or she will also know of strategies to ease it until the pain goes away.

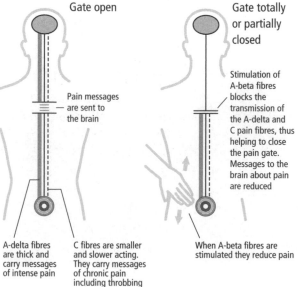

Experience of pain can be described in physiological terms by looking at the activity of nerve fibres. Activity in A-beta fibres tends to stop the action of the A-delta and C fibres, thus inhibiting the perception of pain. This can be demonstrated by massaging the back of the neck during a headache (stimulating the activity of the A-beta fibres) to bring temporary pain relief, or applying heat to a sore muscle to decrease the pain.

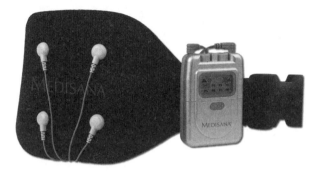

A portable TENS machine. This device can be attached to parts of the body using the four gel pads shown. It sends gentle pulses of electricity which serve to shut the pain gate, thus relieving pain. It is used by many women during labour (see Figure 4.06)

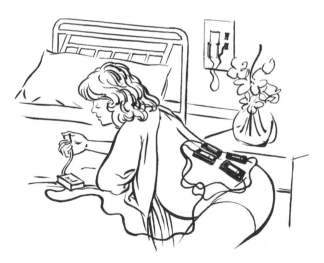

Figure 4.06 The attachment of a TENS machine to four areas of the back of a woman in labour. The positioning of the gel pads will depend on the most appropriate area where pain relief is needed

Psychological explanations of different types of responses to pain

Psychological factors have been shown to increase or decrease the sensation of pain. Imagine that you are suffering from intolerable toothache; the phone rings, and when you answer it the caller tells you that you have won £500,000. It is very likely that, in the excitement of the moment, you will not be conscious of the pain of the toothache. This is clearly not to do with stimulation of receptor nerve cells, but has a psychological origin.

Psychological factors that have been found to increase the sensation of pain include:

- anxiety, fear and tension
- depression
- focus on the pain itself, or anticipation of pain
- boredom, with little involvement in life's activities.

Psychological factors associated with closure of the pain gate and reduced pain sensation include:

- relaxation, **visualisation** techniques and **meditation**
- positive emotions such as happiness or optimism
- previous experience of mastery over pain.

Visualisation – concentrating on or imagining something very strongly as a visual image. A visualisation technique is often used to treat disease by inducing relaxation in the individual, who actually wills away his or her disease. It is also known as guided imagery.

Meditation – suspending the stream of thoughts that normally occupy the mind to induce mental calmness and physical relaxation. This form of alternative medicine is generally performed once or twice a day for approximately 20 minutes at a time. It is used to reduce stress, alter hormone levels and elevate mood.

Dealing with illness

Response to a diagnosis of illness

Illness frequently involves disruption to the individual's lifestyle, a high degree of dependency on others, unpleasant and maybe time-consuming procedures, and pain. If hospitalised or moved to a new environment there may also be a lack of privacy, the need to adapt to an unfamiliar, strange environment, and strict time schedules and rules.

If there is no diagnosis yet the individual may be anxious about the exact nature of the problem. Other questions may include: What will the outcome be? How will the illness influence my life? If the problem is known, this raises a new set of questions, such as: What will the treatment be like? Will it be successful? Uncertainties can be compounded by lack of information, perhaps because tests have not been performed yet or because information has not been communicated properly.

Shontz's stages of response

Shontz (1975) identified a sequence of reactions experienced by individuals following the news that they have a debilitating illness. The stages of response are as follows:

- *Shock* – the individual may feel stunned or bewildered; he or she may behave in an automatic fashion or may feel a sense of detachment. The feeling of shock could wear off quickly or last a long time. It is likely to be most severe when the diagnosis occurs without warning.
- *Encounter* – the individual experiences disorganised thinking and feelings of loss, grief, helplessness and despair. He or she feels overwhelmed by reality.
- *Retreat* –the individual uses avoidance strategies, prehaps by denying the existence of the health problem or its implications. This gradually wears off when either a second diagnosis confirms the original one

or symptoms worsen and retreat is no longer possible.

However, not all individuals react in this way. Some, instead of feeling shock, feel cool and collected; others may feel paralysed with anxiety. Some feel helpless and overwhelmed after the initial diagnosis, but others don't. When people feel they are powerless to change their situation they may respond with denial and other avoidance strategies (Lazarus, 1983). Those who use avoidance strategies may not absorb information given to help them deal with their illness; they may not take practical steps, nor follow up with adaptive strategies to manage the illness.

Coping behaviours associated with a diagnosis of illness

Short-term and long-term health problems can have similar consequences for the individual's initial emotional state. But long-term problems require different adjustments: individuals and families have to make permanent behavioural, social and emotional changes, and the way the individual views his or her life will alter.

People diagnosed with a long-term illness tend to cope in the following ways; these skills can be used selectively or in combination:

- Denying or minimising the seriousness of the situation. This can be helpful in the early stages of adjustment. Benefits include putting emotions aside for a while so as not to feel overwhelmed and allowing time to organise other coping resources.
- Seeking information about the health problem and treatment procedures. This will help the individual to deal with the symptoms of the illness.
- Learning to provide own medical care; for example, insulin shots, etc. This helps the individual to gain a sense of control and personal effectiveness with respect to the condition.
- Setting concrete, limited goals such as exercising, going to shows or social

gatherings, meeting friends and maintaining regular routines. These provide individuals (and their families) with opportunities to achieve goals they consider meaningful and events to look forward to. They may also encourage the individual to exercise and reduce his or her incapacitation.

- Recruiting instrumental and emotional support from family, friends and practitioners by expressing needs and feelings.
- Considering possible future events and stressful circumstances in order to know what lies ahead and to be prepared for unexpected difficulties.
- Gaining a manageable perspective on the health problem and its treatment by finding a long-term purpose or meaning for the experience. Individuals often do this by applying religious beliefs or by recognising how they have been changed in positive ways by the experience.

As you read on page 136, a sense of control can benefit people's health and help them adjust to becoming seriously ill. Loss of control is an inevitable result of hospitalisation. For example, an individual may not be able to walk because of a leg injury; may not be allowed to watch TV late at night because it disturbs others; may not be allowed to have visitors at certain times. Angry responses to such restrictions result from feeling controlled or believing that personal freedom is threatened.

The role of information in adapting to illness

Individuals can react in a number of different ways to a diagnosis of illness or impending surgery. Some want to find out all they can about their illness, the various treatments offered, rates of recovery, etc. Others find that information simply weighs them down – causes them to worry more and feel more distressed and helpless. Interestingly, the degree of fear experienced seems related both to the desire to obtain information and the amount of distress experienced following surgery. However, it seems

that if information is given in a situation where the patient experiences low levels of anxiety, it may be beneficial.

Research carried out by Beddows in 1997 involved extensive information-giving to one group of pre-operative patients (the experimental group) and comparing their levels of anxiety post-operatively to a group of similar patients who didn't receive this information (the control group). The researcher visited participants in their own home, where they were more at ease and better able to ask questions and fully absorb the information they were given. It was found that although both groups experienced anxiety when admitted to hospital, the experimental group experienced less anxiety post-operatively than the control group.

It has been found that different types of information can actually aid recovery as well as reducing distress.

- Sensory information is information about what comes in through the senses; for example, smells, tastes, touch, hearing and sight. Individuals who are given such information are much better aware of why things are happening (e.g. a nasty taste in the mouth after an anaesthetic; how it will feel when a needle is inserted, etc.) and this helps them to deal with or reflect upon feelings associated with such sensations. For example, individuals about to undergo an endoscopy were given sensory information and suffered less distress afterwards.
- Procedural information helps the individual learn how the procedure will be carried out.
- Coping skills information takes the individual through possible strategies for dealing with his or her illness.

Benefits of pre-operative information

The benefits of pre-operative information for the individual include the following:

- Reduced length of hospitalisation: individuals given coping skills plus sensory information before having abdominal surgery were able to leave hospital up to three days earlier than those not given such information.

- Reduced need for painkillers and a reduction in pain rating: individuals given coping skills and sensory information pre-operatively needed less pain-killing medication following the operation.
- Reduction in anxiety. This may be explained by the information helping individuals to rehearse worries, fears and changes following the operation, so that changes become more predictable and thus less distressing.

These findings all link to the role of control, as outlined above, and suggest that an increased sense of control gained through a variety of information-giving strategies can be beneficial to some, if not all, individuals.

Being ill: adopting the sick role

Sick role behaviour

The concept of the sick role was first identified by the sociologist Talcott Parsons. He saw illness as a deviant act which disrupts the smooth running of the social order; by falling sick, individuals are exempt from fulfilling their social role. The sick role also brings with it certain rights and obligations. The individual is:

- prevented from performing his or her social role
- exempted from personal responsibility for the illness (a temporary state)
- obligated to get well as soon as possible and to consult with medical experts.

The aim of the sick role is to reduce the disruptive effect of illness on the social system. Medicine exists to promote social cohesion and speed up the individual's return to his or her role in society; the role of doctors is to sanction ill health.

The three personal accounts below illustrate the consequences of adopting or rejecting sick role behaviour.

Clay

The day I left hospital after my stroke was a glorious day. I started planning all the things I could do with the incredible amount of free time I was going to have. Chores I had put off, museums and galleries I wanted to visit, friends I could meet for lunch. It was not until several days later that I realised I simply couldn't do these things. I didn't have the mental or physical strength and I sank into depression.

Clay's wife

As time went on and Clay was gradually improving at home, I occasionally was concerned about his dependency on me, which seemed unnecessary. It can easily become a habit after the need no longer exists. Gradually, I asked him to do certain things, leaving things undone which were previously his domain, acting indecisively and leaving decisions up to him. At first he was surprised, and then he did what was needed. He gradually took over more and more, giving up his 'stroke personality'.

Monika

If the doctor tells you that you cannot walk upstairs, he is telling you that you are weak, that you are no longer strong. He has taken something away from you – ah, your pride. You suddenly want to do what you are not supposed to do, what you have been doing all your life.

Sick role behaviour in hospital

Hospitalised individuals sometimes respond angrily to restrictions, feeling controlled or believing their freedom is being threatened. Brehm (1966) calls this 'reactance'. Shelley Taylor (cited in Sarafino, 1998: 309) has described how hospitalised individuals may sometimes show reactions in their:

petty acts of mutiny such as making passes at

nurses, drinking in one's room, smoking against medical advice, and wandering up and down the halls. Such minor incidents tend to irritate nursing and custodial staff, but rarely do any damage. However, petty acts of mutiny can turn into self-sabotage, such as failing to take medications which are essential to recovery or engaging in acts which have potentially fatal consequences. Coupled with these mutinous acts against the hospital routine and treatment regime are frequent demands upon the staff for attention, treatment and medication, and numerous complaints regarding the quality of same.

Sick-role behaviour is influenced by individuals' ideas about how they should behave and their reactions to restricted freedoms. Social interactions will also affect sick role behaviour. For example, individuals respond differently to medical personnel who are cheerful and friendly compared with those who are unpleasant or surly. Sick role behaviour also depends on how well individuals cope with their medical conditions and the medical treatment procedures they receive in the hospital.

Beliefs about appropriate sick role behaviour are shared by medical personnel. Lorber (1975) investigated the beliefs and behaviour of 100 individuals admitted to hospital for elective surgery. All participants were over 40 years of age and had been admitted for a range of complaints from routine to very serious. They were asked to agree or disagree with statements such as:

- The best thing to do in the hospital is to keep quiet and do what you're told.
- I cooperate best as an individual when I know the reason for what I have to do.
- When I'm sick I expect to be pampered and catered to.

Responses to such statements gave an indication of whether individuals believed the expected behaviour they should show was passive or active. Medical staff were then asked to rate individuals as either a 'good individual', an 'average individual' or a 'problem individual',

giving reasons for their choice. Those rated as 'good' were generally passive, cooperative, uncomplaining, stoical and unemotional. Those rated as 'problem' individuals were seen as uncooperative, constantly complaining, overemotional and dependent. Staff tended to overlook difficult behaviour from seriously ill individuals.

However, over-compliance is not necessarily beneficial for individuals. Taylor (1979) found that individuals who are too passive in hospital may not take an active role in their recovery.

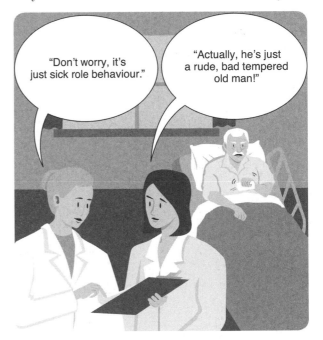

Figure 4.07 Beliefs about appropriate sick role behaviour are shared by medical personnel

Methods of reducing anxiety

Medical benefits of relaxation and anxiety relief

Stress and anxiety can aggravate some chronic conditions. For example, diabetics' ability to metabolise glucose can be reduced, asthma attacks can be triggered or made worse, and depression is strongly associated with anxiety and can exacerbate physical illness. Anxiety management techniques include:

- relaxation training
- visualisation or guided imagery
- biofeedback.

Relaxation training

Relaxation techniques directly counter the physiological arousal of stress. They help maximise energy and enhance coping mechanisms. Relaxation can help individuals deal with some of the distress their symptoms bring, as well as with the emotions that may be triggering or exacerbating their symptoms. Relaxation techniques have been found to be useful in helping diabetics manage stress and maintain blood glucose levels. They are also successful in some chronic diseases, such as arthritis, asthma, gastrointestinal disorders and chronic pain. Epileptics can be taught to recognise sensations and events associated with attacks and to use relaxation techniques when these occur.

Did you know?

It has been shown in individuals with cardiovascular disease that a low-fat diet as well as relaxation techniques can reverse the build-up of artery-clogging plaque.

Over to you

Below, a typical relaxation method is described. Read it through then try it for yourself.

- *Sit quietly in a comfortable position.*
- *Close your eyes.*
- *Deeply relax all of your muscles, beginning at the feet and progressing up to the face. Keep the muscles relaxed.*
- *Breathe through your nose. Become aware of your breathing. As you breathe out, say the word 'one' silently to yourself. Breathe easily and naturally.*
- *Continue for 10 to 20 minutes. You may open your eyes to check the time, but do not use an alarm.*
- *When you finish, sit quietly for several minutes, at first with eyes closed and later with eyes open. Do not stand for a few minutes.*
- *Do not worry about whether you are successful in achieving a deep state of relaxation. Maintain a passive attitude and permit relaxation to occur at its own pace. When distracting thoughts occur, try to ignore them by not dwelling upon them and return to repeating 'one.' With practice, relaxation should come with little effort.*

Visualisation or guided imagery

Similar to relaxation training, visualisation (guided imagery) involves using the mind to imagine a pleasant place where the person feels relaxed, peaceful and free of stress.

Over to you

Have a go at the following visualisation method:

- *Begin by breathing slowly and deeply.*
- *Think of yourself in a place where you feel relaxed and at ease, such as your favourite holiday spot, a beautiful garden on a sunny day or a snug room with a fireplace.*
- *Create all the details in your mind such as the sights, sounds, smells and colours of this special place. The more details from all your senses you can include in your visualisation, the more powerful and effective it will be.*
- *Focus on feelings of being relaxed and at peace in this place.*
- *In situations in everyday life when you feel yourself getting tense, anxious or upset, try to go somewhere quiet, take a deep breath and visualise yourself in this special place again. In this way you will be able to recapture the feeling of calm and relaxation you experience when doing the visualisation exercise.*

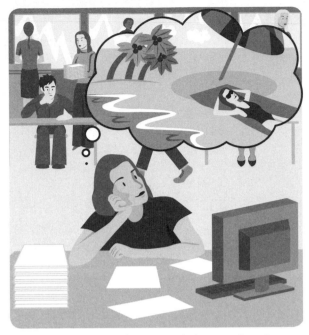

Figure 4.08 Use visualisation techniques to imagine a pleasant place and induce calm when feeling tense, anxious or upset

Biofeedback

Individuals who use biofeedback find they can not only alter their physiology, but can gain a sense of control over their lives. Biofeedback is a technique which involves feedback about physiological aspects of the person's state, such as heart rate, blood pressure and temperature, which manifest as visual or auditory signals on a monitor. Adrenaline produced by the body causes sweating, which can be measured by placing electrodes on the skin. This shows changes in skin resistance (known as the galvanic skin response) which then register as a visual signal or tone. If the signal or tone is high, the level of arousal is similarly high. Initially, by a process of trial and error, the individual attempts various relaxation techniques (deep breathing, visualisation, etc.) to reduce the level of signal or tone. As relaxation deepens, blood pressure and heart rate slow down and this is shown (the feedback part of the process) by a lowering of the signal or tone on the monitor. Over time, the individual learns to recognise signs of tension and finds it easier to control physiological functions.

A typical biofeedback monitor. This portable machine's

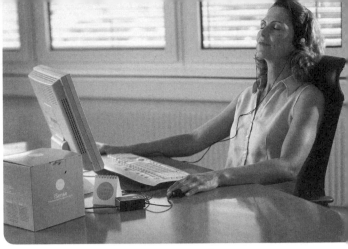

sensors are attached to the individual's fingers

Figure 4.09 Relationship between feedback from a

As the feedback signals deeper relaxation, the individual knows that what s/he has just been doing is producing relaxation, so does this more (e.g. visualisation, deep-breathing), thus increasing the feedback indicating relaxation.

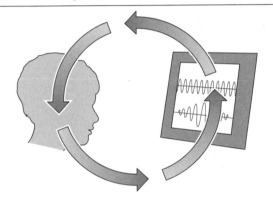

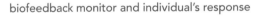

biofeedback monitor and individual's response

Some effective uses of the biofeedback technique are described below:

- *Migraine headaches* – the pain of this type of headache is caused by constriction of the blood vessels in the head. In the early stages of a migraine there is constriction of the arteries resulting in cold hands. By attaching a monitor to a finger, the individual can receive feedback (signals) on finger temperature. Learning to relax the muscular walls of the blood vessels in the finger causes an increase in temperature and also allows the blood vessels in the head to relax, thus easing the headache.

- *High blood pressure* – biofeedback can be used to lower blood pressure.
- *Urinary and faecal incontinence* –individuals can now use readouts of tension from their urethral and anal sphincters to control urinary and faecal incontinence, conditions that often resist all other medical and surgical interventions.
- *Epilepsy* – some epileptics use biofeedback from electroencephalograms to calm the irritable brain tissue that produces their seizures.
- *Asthma* – the monitor gives feedback regarding airflow in breathing, so an individual can learn to control the diameter of the bronchial airways.

Further benefits of biofeedback extend beyond merely physiological improvements. The individual learns to feel in control of his or her physiological state and thus gains a sense of mastery which can often be transferred to other life situations. It is a powerful technique for achieving relaxation when encountering stressful situations, as the individual can learn to recognise signs of stress and tension and use the power of the mind to induce the same physiological changes produced when using the monitor.

Understanding addictions

There are probably many among you who find it hard to start the morning without a strong cup of coffee. You may have commented at times, 'I'm addicted to caffeine'. So, what is addiction?

Addiction
'A condition, produced by repeated consumption of a natural or synthetic substance, in which the person has become physically and psychologically dependent on the substance' (cited in Sarafino, 1998).

You will have noticed from the definition of addiction that there are two aspects involved: physical and psychological. Physical dependence includes tolerance and withdrawal.

Tolerance
When a person's body adapts to intake of a particular substance and needs more of it to reach the same stage of pleasure or relief. For example, you may find that if you take a strong painkiller it has a powerful effect the first time, but if taken regularly, the effect reduces.

Withdrawal
When a person experiences unpleasant effects after stopping taking the substance to which he or she has become addicted. Depending on the extent of the addiction and the type of substance, the following withdrawal symptoms may occur: headaches, anxiety, irritability, hallucinations, nausea, tremors and a craving for the substance itself.

The psychological component of addiction usually comes before the physiological effects of tolerance. This is concerned with the need felt by the person to use a substance because it makes him or her feel good in some way or helps him or her to cope. For example, many young people begin drinking alcohol or smoking cigarettes because it gives them some sort of social status or helps them fit in with their peer group. At an early stage they will not be physically dependent on these substances, but with repeated use the body will adapt and withdrawal will be difficult.

When use of the substance becomes something that seems out of control of the individual, this is termed substance abuse. Not everyone who drinks alcohol or caffeine or smokes cigarettes would be diagnosed as suffering from substance abuse, however.

Addiction to smoking

While use of alcohol or recreational drugs such as heroin, cocaine, ecstasy and LSD may fit the 'problem' criteria for substance abuse outlined above, cigarette smoking appears to be a different kind of addiction. Smoking is problematic not so much for its effects on lifestyle (losing a job, gaining a criminal record, etc.) but because of the high risk it brings of developing serious illnesses such as heart disease and cancer.

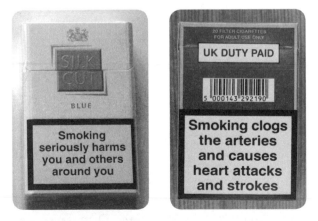

Health warnings on cigarette packets give a stark message about the health risks associated with smoking

There is widespread awareness of the dangers of smoking within society, and some specific outcomes of smoking are even printed on cigarette packets, as shown above. However, people continue to take up smoking despite these risks. To understand why, we need to look at both internal factors and situational influences associated with starting smoking. Since smoking usually starts during the teenage years, this outline will focus on adolescents.

Situational and environmental factors

These refer to the social environment in which young people grow up and the role models they are exposed to. Factors which make it more likely for teenagers to smoke include:

- having parents or friends who smoke
- smoking a first cigarette in the company of peers who encourage them
- belonging to a group of peers where smoking is associated with being glamorous, attractive to the opposite sex, looking mature, etc.
- being exposed to and influenced by admired **role models** who smoke.

Role model – a person who is admired for any reason and whose behaviour may be imitated by others. Role models can include celebrities such as sports players, film and pop stars, or people we know and look up to (e.g. a teacher, an older student at school).

Internal factors

Certain personality characteristics have been identified as increasing the likelihood of an adolescent beginning to smoke. These include:

- being rebellious
- being a risk-taker
- being unwilling or unable to meet the expectations of parents and/or other authority figures.

Thus, the picture that emerges is of an individual with a particular set of personality characteristics who belongs to (or joins) a peer group where smoking is valued. The attraction of taking up smoking lies in the image he or she can adopt of being 'cool', rebellious, individual, tough and independent of authority.

Alcohol addiction

The profile for addiction to alcohol is similar to that of smoking: there is an increased likelihood that those exposed to unhealthy drinking behaviours in their parents will adopt such behaviours themselves. Peer group use (and abuse) of alcohol is also highly influential. Internal personality factors such as risk-taking, sensation seeking and aggression are associated with a high likelihood of developing alcohol addiction. Finally, those with a history of getting into trouble with authority are also at risk.

Common disorders with a psychosomatic component

Asthma

Asthma is a chronic disease involving difficulty in breathing and coughing. When this occurs to a significant degree, it is called an asthma attack. The physiological cause of asthma is contraction of the bronchioles of the lungs. This reduces the amount of air that can be breathed in, causing the wheeziness so characteristic of this disorder.

There are a number of environmental causes of asthma, such as pollutants in the atmosphere, but there is also a psychological component. When an individual becomes highly stressed, asthma attacks may become more frequent and severe. As has already been described, psychological treatments such as biofeedback can be used to reduce symptoms and help the individual gain a sense of control.

Depression

Depression is a disorder characterised by the following psychological symptoms:

- emotional disturbances (feeling intensely unhappy, finding little or no pleasure in life)
- motivational symptoms (lack of drive, loss of enthusiasm for activities once enjoyed)
- behavioural disturbances (being markedly slowed down or agitated)
- cognitive symptoms (negative views of self, the world and the future; feelings of worthlessness).

Physical symptoms can include sleep disturbances, poor concentration, constant tiredness, changes in appetite and lack of sex drive.

Physiological explanations of depression

There is some evidence of a genetic basis in some cases of depression (i.e. a faulty gene is passed from one generation to the next). The strongest evidence for this comes from the study of identical twins. Since they share the same genetic make-up, it should logically follow that if depression is controlled by genes and one member of a twin pair has it, the second twin will also have the disorder. There is some evidence to support this explanation. McGuffin (1996) carried out a study of nearly 200 pairs of twins. The findings were as follows:

- For identical twins, if one twin had developed depression, there was a 46 per cent chance of the other twin sharing the disorder.

- For non-identical twins, who share only 50 per cent of their genetic material, the likelihood of both twins developing depression was reduced to 20 per cent.

McGuffin's research suggests that there may indeed be a genetic predisposition to depression, but other factors must be involved or the rates would be 100 per cent and 50 per cent respectively.

A second physiological explanation of depression suggests that there may be abnormally low levels of the **neurotransmitters serotonin** and **noradrenaline**, or an imbalance between these. Unfortunately, current understanding of the exact role of these neurotransmitters is not advanced. It has been found, for example, that anti-depressant medication which raises levels of serotonin or noradrenaline, or both, are effective in reducing depression; however, it does not follow that low levels of these neurotransmitters cause depression. (Similarly, a headache can be relieved by aspirin, but this does not mean that the pain was caused by the absence of the active ingredients of aspirin.)

Neurotransmitter – a chemical that is released by a neuron (a special nerve cell in the brain) and taken up by another neuron. In this way, chemicals can be transported around the brain.

Noradrenaline – a hormone secreted by the adrenal medulla as part of the 'fight or flight' response (see also page 135). It is also a neurotransmitter in the nervous system and affects parts of the human brain where attention and impulsivity are controlled.

Serotonin – a neurotransmitter found in the brain that affects mood and appetite. It is also thought to influence physical co-ordination, body temperature and sleep, and to play a role in the mechanism of migraine headaches.

Explanations of depression that account for physiological and psychological factors

A more realistic explanation of depression is that it results from a combination of factors, both physiological and psychological. For example, people with a hardy personality type and/or an internal locus of control show powerful resilience to stress; they tend to be optimistic and able to deal effectively with life's trials and tribulations. In comparison, those who lack hardiness and believe that most of what happens in life is out of their control may learn to see themselves, the world and their future in very negative terms.

A case of depression

Tanisha is a twenty-year-old student studying molecular biology at a prestigious university. She was referred to the student counselling service by her tutor who was concerned about her increasing withdrawal, apathy and dramatic weight loss. Over the course of the session, the counsellor found that Tanisha had always been the 'bright one' in the family and her parents had high expectations of her. Her father was a professor of law and was determined that Tanisha should follow his academic success by becoming a high-ranking academic in her subject. Throughout her school life her teachers had praised Tanisha for her successes, but her parents often criticised her for not doing perfectly in all subjects. When she achieved four A grades and one B grade at A level, her parents only commented on the B grade. She felt they were not only disappointed in her but felt her lack of perfection reflected on them and was a cause of disgrace to the family. The lifelong pattern of punishment for failure with no balancing recognition and praise for success led Tanisha to develop an extremely negative self-concept where she felt herself to be worthless and a failure.

Eczema

Eczema is a skin disorder characterised by itching and the scaling and thickening of the skin. It is usually located on the face, elbows, knees and arms, although eczema can affect any part of the body. Although the cause is unknown, one theory is that it may be related to malfunctioning of the immune system. The condition may be short-lived (acute) or long-term (chronic). One out of ten children develops eczema, but more than half of them lose it by the time they reach their teens. The mind-body link is apparent in some cases of eczema, with it worsening at times of stress or distress, as illustrated by the following case study.

Panic attacks

These consist of an intense and sudden feeling of fear and anxiety. When a panic attack occurs, the following physical symptoms are usually experienced:

- rapid heart beat
- trembling
- rapid shallow breathing
- pins and needles in the arms
- feeling faint.

Panic attacks can occur up to several times a day. Many people who have a panic attack fear that they will collapse or die. These attacks are not harmful and usually go away within 20 to 30 minutes.

Donna's therapist

For Donna, a forty-year-old mother of four teenagers, the problem seemed to be small, relentlessly itching bumps on her legs, buttocks, stomach and arms. Twelve years of dermatology, creams, lotions, baths and pills had occasionally helped but never resolved the problem. She was frustrated, angry and disappointed with herself and her doctors, and she was still tearing at her skin. In therapy, we quickly identified a key source of irritation in Donna's life: her husband. He was distant, withdrawn and sexually demanding – a combination that left her feeling used. She was caught between her anger and her inability to confront him. After several sessions, Donna came to see how her skin had been waving a red flag to express the frustrated feelings she couldn't feel directly: it was ceaselessly 'itching to change'. Her 'itchy' feelings started to move from her skin to a mix of anxiety, anger and sexual excitement as she began to take a more direct, even combative approach, with her husband.

(Extract taken from the Talk Eczema website with permission of Ted Grossbart.)

1   What physical effects does the fight or flight response have on the body?

2   Name two personality types that seem resistant to stressors and explain why this is so.

3   Why is control important in managing the negative effects of stress?

4   What methods could be used to help an individual gain a sense of control over his or her life?

5   What is meant by learned helplessness? Why does a sense of learned helplessness tend to be associated with negative outcomes for the individual?

6   How does the model of health behaviour explain why people do or do not take action to reduce (or deal with) a health threat?

7   What is meant by the pain gate theory?

8   Name one method of pain control that works to 'close' the pain gate and give examples of situations where it may be used.

9   List three types of information that can be given to an individual diagnosed with an illness and explain why these may be important.

10 What methods could be used to reduce anxiety in patients, either before or during an episode of illness? Explain how these work.

11 What is meant by the sick role?

12 List three methods of anxiety reduction and explain how they work.

13 Describe how learning theory can be used to understand why young people take up smoking and drinking.

14 What is meant by a psychosomatic disorder or illness?

References and further reading

Books

- Banyard, P. (1996) *Applying Psychology to Health*. London: Hodder & Stoughton
- Baum, A., Revenson, T.A. and Singer, J.E. (2001) *Handbook of Health Psychology*. New Jersey: Lawrence Erlbaum Associates
- Beddows, J. (1997) Alleviating pre-operative anxiety in patients: a study. *Nursing Standard* Vol. 11 Issue 37: 35–38
- Brehm (1966). Cited in Sarafino (1998), p309
- Hiroto and Seligman (1975). Cited in Sarafino (1998), p106
- Kobassa (1979). Cited in Sarafino (1998), p110
- Langer and Rodin (1976). Cited in Sarafino (1998), p109
- Lazarus (1983). Cited in Sarafino (1998), p388
- Lorber (1975). Cited in Sarafino (1998), p308
- McGuffin *et al.* (1996) cited in Comer, R.J. (2001) *Abnormal Psychology*. (4th ed.) New York: Worth Publishers, p198

- Melzack and Wall (1965). Cited in Ogden (1996), p223
- Ogden, J. (1996) *Health Psychology*. Buckingham: Open University Press
- Rice, D and Haralambos, M. (2000) *Psychology in focus: AS Level*. Ormskirk: Causeway Press, p106
- Sarafino, E.P. (1998) *Health Psychology – Biophysical Interactions*. (3rd ed.) New York: John Wiley & Sons
- Shontz (1975). Cited in Sarafino (1998), p388
- Taylor (1979). Cited in Sarafino (1998), p309
- Turk, Meichenbaum and Genest (1983). Cited in Sarafino (1998), p331
- Wallston, Wallston and DeVellis (1978) *Health Education Monographs* 6: 160–170

Useful websites

The following websites can be accessed via the Heinemann website.
Go to www.heinemann.co.uk/hotlinks and enter the express code 4256P.

- BBC Science and Nature's interactive human brain map.
- Stressfree – a system of healthcare professionals providing solutions to stress.
- Hardiness – provides stress management training for companies and organisations that aim to develop enduring qualities of hardiness.
- The Oxford Pain Internet Site, for anyone with a professional or personal interest in pain and analgesia.
- Keirsey – includes Keirsey Temperament Sorter questionnaire and descriptions of the personality temperaments.

Appendix

Table 4.05 Scoring instructions for the Multidimensional Health Locus of Control Scale

SUBSCALE	FORM(s)	POSSIBLE RANGE	ITEMS
Internal	A, B, C	6–36	1, 6, 8, 12, 13, 17
External	A, B, C	6–36	2, 4, 9, 11, 15, 16
Powerful others	A, B	6–36	3, 5, 7, 10, 14, 18
Doctors	C	3–18	3, 5, 14
Other people	C	3–18	7, 10, 18

The score on each subscale is the sum of the values circled for each item on the subscale (i.e. where 1 = Strongly disagree and 6 = Strongly agree). No items need to be reversed before summing. All of the subscales are independent of one another. *There is no such thing as a 'total' MHLC.*

CHAPTER 5

Health and safety at work including basic principles of first aid

Key points

- Hazards are anything that can cause injury to a person. It is important to identify hazards in the environment and take measures to prevent the risk of them occurring.

- Poor conditions of work will result in human illness, errors and an increase in the accident rate.

- UK laws put obligations on managers and owners to ensure the health and safety of employees.

- The Health and Safety at Work Act 1974 is the key legislation designed to protect people from harm while at work or in the workplace.

- Risk assessments are necessary to assess the risk from hazards in the workplace. These should be continually monitored and updated.

- Every workplace should have an accident report form as correct documentation of an accident, incident or near-miss.

- The Health and Safety (First Aid) Regulations 1981 require employers to provide adequate first aid cover for their employees.

Introduction

The aim of this chapter is to introduce you to health, safety and security in the health and social care environment. Health and safety is vital in the health and social care sector in order to protect individuals from harm. Through the exploration of health and safety legislation and guidelines, you will be able to develop an understanding as to how a safe working environment can be promoted. This chapter will also prepare you for the potential hazards that you may encounter in health and social care settings; these include waste materials, infectious diseases, chemicals, drugs, equipment and environmental factors. You will have the opportunity to explore hazards in various environments and consider the potential risks they present.

Hazards in health and social care

Hazards are anything that can cause injury to a person. There are hazards all around you all the time; for example, the chair you are sitting on, the flooring you walk on, the water you wash your hands in.

> ### Over to you
>
> *Think carefully about the room you are sitting in. List all the hazards you can see. Think how each hazard you have identified could cause injury to a person.*

Hazards and risks are not the same thing. A hazard is something which could possibly cause harm; risk is the likelihood of that hazard causing harm. For example, a wheelchair left in a corridor is a hazard to nursing staff but it poses a greater risk to someone who is visually impaired – most sighted people will notice it and walk around it.

Hazards in the working environment.

In the working environment it is necessary to first spot the hazards before being able to prevent injury. So, you need to ask yourself 'what could go wrong?' The trouble with trying to spot hazards in the workplace is that it is easy to become complacent – the common place can become familiar and hazards may blend into their surroundings. For example, if fire doors are always wedged open for visitors to access the building, this can easily become accepted practice. Remaining detached from the environment and looking critically at what is around you is the first step to correctly identifying potential hazards in the workplace.

> ### Over to you
>
> *Think about a working environment that you are familiar with. How is safety of the environment maintained?*

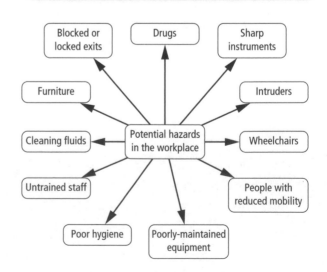

Figure 5.01 Hazards in the workplace

The Health and Safety at Work Act 1974 (see page 193) should be applied with regards to maintaining good working conditions. Poor conditions of work will result in human illness, errors and an increase in the accident rate.

- If an environment is too hot or too cold, staff will be uncomfortable in their work and may act in a way that could compromise their safety, for example putting on extra clothing to keep warm could restrict movement and make lifting and movement difficult.
- If staff work in an environment where there is poor lighting, it will be difficult for them to identify possible hazards, and accidents will be more likely to happen. Inadequate lighting in staff car parks may result in staff feeling unsafe and vulnerable to attack.
- Poorly maintained flooring may cause accidents, for example, people tripping on uneven surfaces. Cracks in flooring may harbour bacteria leading to the spread of disease.
- Lack of space could result in injury to staff as they try to manoeuvre around furniture or poorly stored equipment.
- Washing facilities should be easily accessible, well ventilated and located near toilets and changing areas; there should be soap and a method of drying provided. Inadequate washing facilities will result in cross-infection.
- A workplace smoking policy should outline the requirement for smoking safety. In some workplaces there may be a designated smoking room or area.

Over to you

Find out what the optimum room temperature is for a place of work.

Organisational premises

Hazards do not only occur within a building; they can also be the result of poor and inadequate building protection and maintenance. Buildings and their environments should be regularly checked and adequately maintained. Neglected buildings can lead to hazards occurring from loose brick work and dislodged building fittings.

Burglary can be prevented by all doors and windows being fitted with deadlocks; burglar alarms are also a deterrent. Some workplaces have fitted CCTV (close circuit television) which can monitor and record incidences.

Over to you

Closely examine the outside of the building you are currently using. How well has it been maintained?

Over to you

Draw a floor plan of a health and social care setting. Include in your plan details of potential hazards.

- *Explain why the hazards you have identified present a risk in your chosen setting.*
- *How could you reduce the risks to individuals and staff?*
- *What would be the effects of minimising the risks?*

Hazards in the home

Every object in the home is a potential hazard; the degree of danger (risk) will be different depending on who lives there (see Table 5.01). A home with young children will have different hazards than the home of two adults.

Hazard	What to check
Tables	Are tables a suitable height for the individual? Do they block any exits? Are they in a good state of repair? Are the corners sharp? Are they clean?
Chairs	Are the chairs at a suitable height for the individual? Are there too many chairs? Are all chairs stable? Are they in a good state of repair? Are they clean?
Furnishings	Are furnishings fire retardant? Are they clean? Are they in a good state of repair? Are they fit for the purpose?
Electrical appliances	Are electrical appliances maintained regularly? Are they stored safety? Are the plug sockets overloaded? Are there trailing leads? Are the leads frayed? Are electrical appliances placed on a suitable surface? Are they used away from water? Are they brought from a reputable manufacturer?
Bins for disposal of waste	Are the bins available for use? Are they kept clean? Are they kept away from food preparation areas? Are they emptied regularly?
Storage of chemicals	Are chemicals stored out of reach of children? Are they kept locked away? Do individuals know what to do if chemicals are accidentally swallowed? Are chemicals labelled with hazard symbols? Do chemicals have a use-by date? Are they stored in the correct container?

Table 5.01 Some of the more common hazards in the home

Hazards in the community

Hazards in the community include those from traffic and play areas (see Table 5.02). These can cause severe injury or even death if not taken seriously.

Hazard	What to check
Traffic	Is there a safe crossing area? Are there speed humps? Is there some form of speed control? Is the road well lit?
Play areas	Are play areas well maintained? Is the play equipment suitable for the age of the child? Is the playground flooring appropriate? Is the play area well lit? Are dogs allowed access? Are there any discarded, used syringes around? Is there any broken glass around? Has the bin been emptied?
Street lighting	Is the footpath adequately lit? Is there sufficient lighting for the area? Are the lights well maintained?
Animal faeces	Is there an appropriate bin to dispose of animal faeces? Are children expected to play in the same area in which dogs are exercised?
Street furniture	Are all signs, bollards, posts and railings well maintained? Is street furniture well lit? Is the furniture causing an obstruction to pedestrians or motorists?

Table 5.02 Hazards in the community

Children's play areas

Children's play areas and parks should be carefully constructed to meet the safety as well as the developmental needs of children. When examining the suitability of children's play areas, the following factors should be considered:

- soft floor coverings to prevent injuries from falls
- appropriate equipment for different age groups
- brightly coloured equipment for the visually impaired
- adequate lighting
- regular maintenance
- restricted access
- waste disposal and correct disposal of animal faeces.

Over to you

- *Draw a diagram of a children's play area marking on it all the health and safety features.*
- *Who is responsible for maintaining outdoor play areas?*

Dealing with intruders

In health and social care settings, we actively encourage strangers to come onto the premises. These 'strangers' are usually the friends and family members of individuals who are ill and distressed; their presence aids the recovery and support of those they come to visit. However, it is proving more and more difficult to ensure that strangers do not become intruders.

Staff should be actively encouraged to ask strangers who they are and why they are on the premises. Without good justification for their presence, strangers should be asked to leave. If a stranger is reluctant to leave then you should call security or the police as appropriate. Ensure all doors are locked and that the person cannot gain access to individuals or confidential information. Staff must also ensure that they wear appropriate identification and uniform where necessary.

By challenging people who do not possess identification, it is possible to maintain a degree of safety without locking too many doors, which can lead to a hostile restrictive environment. Locked doors, although keeping strangers out, also keep individuals in – this may sometimes be against their wishes. The freedom of choice of care makes it necessary to allow individuals the opportunity to exit buildings when they want to and not to be challenged about their reasons for leaving. Therefore, a fine balance must be obtained to ensure that safety is maintained and freedom of movement is not compromised.

Aggressive and dangerous encounters

Work-related violence is any incident in which a person is abused, threatened or assaulted in his or her workplace. This can include verbal abuse as well as physical harm. Physical violence and verbal threats have serious consequences for employees as they can cause distress, disability and even death. Today, one of the main causes of injury in the health and social care sector is assault and violence, and one of the main causes of staff sickness is work-related stress. The Health and Safety Executive (HSE) estimated the number of incidences of work-related violence in England and Wales in 2004–05 as 655,000. This is a reduction since 1995, when 1.3 million violent incidences were reported. The reason for this reduction may be the development of workplace policies to protect the work force.

Over to you

What other reasons do you think there may be for the reduction in the reporting of incidences of work-related violence?

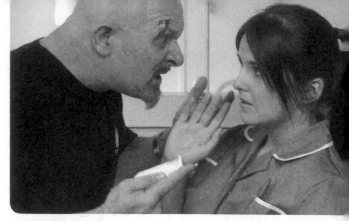

Work-related violence is a serious hazard for many people working in health and social care

Protecting lone workers

A high number of violent incidences happen to lone workers. For example, many social workers and care staff are required to work alone in the community visiting clients in their homes. Working hours can range from 7am to 10.30pm.

- Social workers are often required to deal with emotional situations such as removing children from their home; in these fraught circumstances, the social worker may be at risk of abuse by a distressed family member.
- Personal care staff may travel on foot and work set routines. These factors can put them at greater risk of assault from an abusive client or family member. Personal care staff have also been attacked because they have been mistaken as medical professionals carrying drugs.

Methods to reduce the risks of work-related violence

To ensure that staff are not put at risk from violent encounters whilst at work, a risk assessment should be carried out (see also pages 175–177). Some of the areas for assessment are considered in Table 5.03. Staff training is the most effective method of reducing risk of attack.

Risk assessment

Risk assessment involves carefully examining something that could cause harm and then deciding whether enough precautions have been taken to prevent injury.

Hazard	Precautions to minimise risks
Danger of attack whilst working in the community	• Carry a personal attack alarm. • Have access to a working mobile phone. • Attend self-defence lessons. • Attend training on appropriate responses to attack. • Ensure there is an appointed person available to respond to emergency phone calls. • Ensure facilities for staff to leave messages to indicate where they are working and when.
Danger of attack whilst working in healthcare settings	• Attend training on appropriate responses to attack. • Ensure staff are aware of how to access immediate help to defuse a potentially violent situation.

Table 5.03 Areas to consider when assessing the risks of work-related violence

Based on the risk assessment, a policy should be introduced to protect lone workers. The example of a lone working policy produced by Hampshire County Council is shown in Figure 5.02. Lone working policies help staff identify the risks associated with periods of solitary work. They offer advice as to how to carry out risk assessment and introduce appropriate preventative and protective measures.

Lone Working

Policy statement
Hampshire County Council is committed to reducing the risk to employees during periods of solitary working, and will provide proper monitoring, training and management of risks associated with lone working. The County Council accepts its responsibilities to reduce the risks to staff by carrying out risk assessments and introducing appropriate preventative and protective measures to reduce those risks so far as is reasonably practicable.

Policy standards
To comply with this policy the following standards must be met. Managers will ensure that:
• they identify any work situations where it is a legal requirement or local instruction that a person must not work alone, and ensure that the person is accompanied by a work colleague
• lone workers receive appropriate information about safe working practices, receive training as required and have access to equipment which is safe and well maintained
• persons who work alone receive adequate support, so far as is reasonably practicable, during their period of lone working
• persons who work alone have procedures in place for reporting their concerns about lone working to management
• persons who have to work alone are aware of their own respon-sibilities with regard to their health and safety, including the need to co-operate with management on health and safety matters
• they review their assessments on a regular basis and in any case after a serious accident or incident in which a person working alone is involved.

Figure 5.02 Hampshire County Council's lone working policy

The Health and Safety at Work Act 1974 and the Management of Health and Safety at Work Regulations 1999 state that it is a legal requirement that 'Employers must consider the risks to employees (including the risk of reasonably foreseeable violence); decide how significant these risks are; decide what to do to prevent or control the risks; and develop a clear management plan to achieve this.' This requirement can usually be fulfilled through a detailed risk assessment undertaken by workplace managers or health and safety officers.

Employees can reduce the risks of work-related violence by communicating with individuals in an appropriate manner using clear and concise language, and ensuring that the person fully understands the situation. Employees should have the skills necessary to enable effective communication to take place and to recognise when individuals begin to show signs of becoming agitated and aggressive. It is necessary to ensure that detailed records are kept when violent incidences occur, to allow for accurate recall of salient points which may be used at a later date.

Table 5.04 lists the responsibilities of employers and employees for reducing the risk of work-related violence.

Drunken assault

Lionne is working a night shift in a residential home for older people. She is catching up on some paper work alone in the office whilst the other members of staff are in the kitchen. At 1am in the morning the front doorbell rings. She opens it to find that one of the resident's sons is visiting. He appears to be drunk and starts shouting that he wants to visit his mother. Lionne, arms folded, begins to question him assertively, asking whether he has been drinking and why he wants to visit now. The son becomes more verbally abusive and aggressive and pushes Lionne against a door so he can get past. Lionne suffers grazing and bruising on her lower back and arms.

1 What should Lionne have done differently?
2 Describe the precautions that should be in place to protect staff from work-related violence.
3 Produce a risk assessment for night staff aimed at personal safety.

Bomb scares

Unidentified packages pose a risk due to the increased chance of terrorist activity. Suspicious packages can take many forms, for example, luggage, boxes and packages. The unknown nature of bomb threats makes taking the appropriate action very difficult. Any package that cannot be identified or accounted for must be treated with suspicion. A suspected bomb should not be touched, moved or opened. Most

Table 5.04 Responsibilities of employers and employees for reducing the risk of work-related violence

Responsibilities of employers	Responsibilities of employees
To carry out a risk assessment	To carry out a risk assessment
To provide access to safety equipment, e.g. personal alarms, mobile phones	To involve individuals in planning
To introduce a strategy for coping with violence in the workplace	To keep detailed records
To ensure appropriate staff training	To recognise and be alert to signs that an individual may become violent
To provide staff with a safe place to meet	Not to use jargon
To ensure appropriate safety procedures	
To share information with staff	

suspicious packages usually turn out to be harmless but it isn't worth taking the chance. If you find a package that you suspect may be harmful, treat it as you would a fire. Activate a fire alarm, ensure that the emergency services have been informed (fire brigade and police) and evacuate the building. The emergency services will alert the appropriate authorities and bomb disposal if necessary.

Care workers should not have to act alone but should inform their manager who will take responsibility for the situation. If a care worker is alone then he or she must consider the best action to be taken to protect individuals and staff. It is better to act than not to act and walk away.

Personal safety

To maintain safety and security, staff are usually given identity cards that help identify them from visitors and clients. Identity cards usually display a photograph of the individual and show his or her name and place of work. Personal identification helps limit access to strangers who should not be in the care setting.

Staff may also be identified by a uniform that indicates they work for the organisation. Remember, uniforms can be purchased or stolen so do not assume that a person in a white coat is a doctor; he or she could have bought it from a work wear shop in the high street.

> ### Did you know?
>
> *When attending a work experience placement, ensure that you wear a badge for identification at all times.*

> ### Reflection
>
> *What would you do if you saw someone in a restricted area who did not have an identity badge?*

Many healthcare settings have security procedures to prevent unauthorised people from entering the building. Staff enter a code on a keypad to open the door, while members of the general public use an intercom system where they have to identify themselves before gaining admission. Once inside, visitors may be asked to sign a register, which they sign again when they leave. With uniforms, identification cards, security locks and registers, it should be difficult for strangers to enter a care setting uninvited.

Personal safety should not stop there. People who work in health and care settings often work shifts. As care is offered 24 hours a day, it is necessary for staff to arrive for work at all times, including in the middle of the night. It is for these reasons that some establishments give their staff personal alarms or ensure that they are escorted to their cars. Staff may need to walk through dark alleyways and car parks, so it is important that these areas are well lit. Where possible, staff should walk together in high risk areas.

Risks and risk assessment

What is the difference between a hazard and a risk?

A hazard is anything that could potentially harm a person, for example, a wet floor. The risk is the likelihood of the hazard causing harm, for example, the likelihood that the person will slip on the wet floor and be hurt. When hazards have been identified it is necessary to consider the risks they present. The severity of risk may be rated as low, medium or high (see example of a risk assessment on page 177). Risks come in many forms, for example, the risk of infection or the risk of personal injury from damaged equipment or dangerous lifting practices.

This section looks carefully at how to identify risks and why it is important to abide by health and safety legislation. So that hazards and risks can be monitored, it is necessary that every workplace undertakes a detailed risk assessment and produces a plan of action to tackle health and safety issues.

Roles and responsibilities

Employers

UK laws put obligations on managers and owners to ensure the health and safety of employees. Managers have a role to show that safety matters within their organisation. Their attitudes to safety will ultimately affect the behaviour and attitudes of the employees.

Managers can influence safety by:

- setting appropriate health and safety policies to maintain a high standard
- ensuring that equipment and support is available to achieve aims
- holding local managers responsible for the health and safety of their workplace
- demonstrating a commitment to safety by giving the same value to health and safety concerns as to, for example, budgetary constraints and staff productivity
- being knowledgeable about health and safety
- getting personally involved.

Legal obligations placed on employers by the Health and Safety at Work Act 1974 are that they must ensure:

- arrangements are made to guarantee the health and safety of employees
- all equipment is safe and available for use by those that require it
- adequate health and safety training is provided to all members of staff to enable them to meet statutory safety requirements
- the working environment does not put anyone at risk
- a written safety policy which is understood by all staff
- safety policies are implemented correctly
- the establishment of a health and safety committee
- the workplace is kept in good condition
- there is no charge for use of personal protective equipment, e.g. gloves, overalls, uniforms
- the workplace does not emit toxic fumes or dusts.

The Health and Safety at Work Act 1974

The main piece of legislation that provides the legal framework for maintaining health and safety in the workplace. The Act requires all workplaces where there are five workers or more to have a written health and safety policy. It also places certain responsibilities on both employers and employees, who are jointly responsible for safeguarding the health and safety of anyone using the premises.

Employees

The Health and Safety at Work Act also places responsibility on employees, as follows:

- to take care of themselves and others that may be affected by their acts or omissions
- to co-operate with the employer in implementing health and safety regulations
- not to interfere with or misuse anything provided to meet health and safety requirements
- to report any dangerous situations to the manager
- to ensure that equipment is safe to use
- to maintain shared areas in a safe condition, including doorways, stairs, and lifts, etc.

View point

Viewpoint 1
It is the company's responsibility to protect me at work.

Viewpoint 2
It is my responsibility to keep myself safe at work.

Over to you

Think carefully about your job. What responsibilities does your employer have to protect you at work? Make a list, identifying the responsibilities regarding health and safety that are the employers' and those that are the employees'.

Risk assessment

You perform a risk assessment every time you cross the road. Is it safe to cross? Are there any cars coming? How fast are they travelling? Should I cross somewhere safer? Based on your assessment of the risks, you will either cross the road or not.

Risk assessment simply involves carefully examining something that could cause harm and then deciding whether enough precautions have been taken to prevent injury.

Risk assessment in the workplace

Every organisation must carry out a risk assessment – there is no choice, it is a legal requirement. The responsibility for completing risk assessments lies with employers; it is their responsibility to ensure the health and safety of employees is safeguarded.

The requirement to carry out a risk assessment is driven by three main reasons:

- *Moral reasons* – it is extremely upsetting for everyone concerned when a serious accident occurs. Nobody wants to see another person become ill, get injured or die as a result of activities at work.
- *Legal requirements* – the Health and Safety at Work Act 1974 requires that risk assessments are carried out as a fact of law (see above).
- *Economic reasons* – accidents carry a financial burden as well as a harming the workforce. Through poor health and safety management, money will be lost by:
  - staff absence due to illness and injury
  - loss of service to individuals
  - damage to the image of the care provider; this may cause individuals to change their health provider because of concerns about personal safety.

How to assess risks in the workplace

The Health and Safety Executive (HSE) suggests the following five-point process:

1 *Look for hazards*. Look carefully at your work environment and consider what could be a hazard. Make a note of your findings.
2 *Decide who might be at harm, and how*. Consider clients, staff, relatives, visitors and the general public.
3 *Evaluate the risks arising from the hazards and decide whether more should be done*. After identifying hazards, think carefully what risk they pose. Is it possible to reduce the risk? Or is it necessary to control the risk?

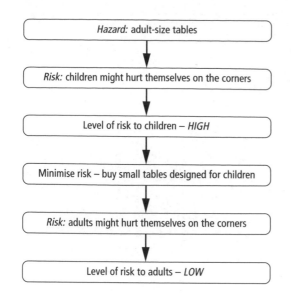

```
┌─────────────────────────────────────────┐
│      Hazard: adult-size tables          │
└─────────────────────────────────────────┘
                    │
                    ▼
┌─────────────────────────────────────────┐
│ Risk: children might hurt themselves on the corners │
└─────────────────────────────────────────┘
                    │
                    ▼
┌─────────────────────────────────────────┐
│      Level of risk to children – HIGH   │
└─────────────────────────────────────────┘
                    │
                    ▼
┌─────────────────────────────────────────┐
│ Minimise risk – buy small tables designed for children │
└─────────────────────────────────────────┘
                    │
                    ▼
┌─────────────────────────────────────────┐
│ Risk: adults might hurt themselves on the corners │
└─────────────────────────────────────────┘
                    │
                    ▼
┌─────────────────────────────────────────┐
│      Level of risk to adults – LOW      │
└─────────────────────────────────────────┘
```

Figure 5.03 Flowchart to show how the severity of risk is reduced in a nursery

Risks cannot always be totally removed, only the severity reduced (from high to medium or low). Figure 5.03 shows how the severity of risk is reduced in a nursery.

In Figure 5.03, the level of risk is reduced but not eliminated. It is important to consider that because children cannot control their environment and actions, they may put themselves at greater risk than adults in the nursery. For example, adults in the nursery are more likely to step out of the way of a small table and are unlikely to receive a head injury by running into a low table (young children would be at risk of such injury if adult-size tables were used in the nursery).

4 *Record your findings.* Workplaces should record their findings on a risk assessment form. This should show that:

● checks have been made
● hazards have been dealt with
● the number of people affected has been considered
● precautions have been taken to reduce the risk.

5 *Review your assessment from time to time and revise if necessary.* Hazards and associated risks do not go away once you have written them down on a form. Hazards need to be reassessed frequently, especially as technology changes and new equipment is used.

An alternative approach is to assess a risk and decide whether it falls into one of four categories:

● insignificant
● low
● medium
● high.

Table 5.05 contains an example of a risk assessment.

Table 5.05 Example of a risk assessment

Queen Elizabeth Day Unit, St Mary's Hospital							
RISK ASSESSMENT							
Hazard = task/ activity with potential to cause harm	Type of injury that could result if harm occurs	Type of people and number affected	Risk level (low, medium, high)	Current control measures in place	Further control measures required	Person responsible for implementation of further measures required and date to implement by	Date to review assessment (annual review unless task changes/alters)
Wheelchairs blocking fire exits	Unable to evacuate ward quickly – may result in people being trapped	All staff, clients and visitors to Day Centre	High	Storage provided away from fire exits	Folding wheelchairs for safer storage	Health and safety officer; Unit manager	
Meals kept aside on work sutface for clients absent from ward	Food poisoning	Clients	High	All meals should be sent back to the kitchens and fresh meals prepared when clients return to the ward	Fridge needed to store food safely	Health and safety officer; Unit manager	
Broken hoists	Lifting injuries	Staff	High		Maintenance book needed to ensure equipment is checked regularly	Staff in charge of each shift	

Health and safety survey

This in an on-going process which identifies what ought to be happening and compares it with what is happening. The survey should not be a one-off event because health and safety needs change with new equipment, new staff and new regulations.

The aim of a health and safety survey should be as follows:

1 *Identify what is required of the survey.* A survey may be performed for a particular reason, such as the arrival of a new piece of equipment or a change in the working environment. Sometimes it is necessary to undertake a survey because a pattern of incidences has been noted and there may be a serious risk of injury; for example, several staff noticing strangers hanging around the staff car park at night.

2 *Check what is really happening in the workplace.* This should be undertaken as a risk assessment. It is often assumed that health and safety is common sense, but more often than not this is not so. People have a tendency to assume that someone else will deal with a hazard or that it is there for a reason; for example, the wedged-open fire exit on a hot summer day.

3 *Specify the gaps in health and safety.* There may be gaps in health and safety needs that have not been identified, such as when new safety equipment is introduced into the working environment.

4 *Plan and take action to fill the gaps.* Following a risk assessment it is important to devise a plan of action so that recommendations are acted upon. A risk assessment is not a paper exercise but should be used appropriately to protect the workforce.

5 *Review what is required and start the process again.* A health and safety survey should be undertaken on a regular basis to ensure that the action plan has been implemented and that no further health and safety issues have arisen.

The health and safety needs of individuals

This section will look at different groups of individuals and the associated health and safety issues.

Children

Young children have not developed the ability to foresee the consequences of their actions. It is, therefore, the responsibility of adults to ensure that the child's environment is safe for him or her to play in.

Toys

Play is not risk free but, with a little thought, it is possible to control most of the dangers children will be exposed to. All toys bought in the UK must conform to the Toy Safety Regulations 1995, but how they are used and their appropriateness for the age of the child are also important factors in preventing accidents. Toys are involved in over 40,000 accidents each year (Royal Society for the Prevention of Accidents, 2005). Accidents do not always occur because toys are unsafe but because they have been left in the wrong place and people trip over them. Accidents may also happen when a toy intended for an older child is given to a younger child; for example, when a baby is given a toy with small, detachable parts designed for children aged 3 years and over, there is a risk of the baby choking.

Safety tips on toys

- Only buy toys from recognised suppliers or shops.
- Ensure children are supervised at play.
- Make sure that the toy is suitable for the age of the child. Children less than 3 years old should never be allowed to play with toys that are marked as unsuitable.
- Check the toy for loose hair, small parts and sharp edges.
- Check toys for signs of wear and throw away old and damaged toys.
- Keep the play area tidy.
- Follow any instructions or warnings that are supplied with the toy.

Before buying a toy or giving a toy to a child, look for the following safety symbols (shown in Figure 5.04):

- the European Community (CE) symbol is the manufacturer's statement that the toy meets European Union safety standards
- the Lion Mark is the British Toy and Hobby Association symbol of toy safety and quality
- a symbol or wording which indicates that the toy is not suitable for children under the age of three years.

A toy without any of the above has not been checked for safety.

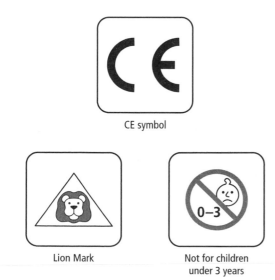

CE symbol

Lion Mark

Not for children under 3 years

Figure 5.04 Toy safety symbols

Toy safety

Belina has two children – Sarah aged 5 years and Jack aged 18 months. Sarah is playing with small beads and Jack has some toy cars. The phone rings and Belina leaves the children unattended to answer it. During the phone call, Sarah rushes in to say that Jack has swallowed some beads.

1 What emergency action should Belina take?
2 What should Belina have done when the phone rang?
3 Explain why toys are age specific?

School trips

During work placement visits you may have the opportunity, with a teacher, to take a group of children on a school trip or holiday. Before children can go anywhere it is necessary to perform a risk assessment to ensure that all hazards are carefully considered and minimised.

Over to you

The class you are working with is going swimming at the local leisure centre today. Produce a risk assessment looking at all the hazards that may occur during the trip.

As a result of several accidents during school trips, some fatal, the Health and Safety Executive has drawn up a list of questions to consider before taking children on trips, as follows:

1 What are the main objectives of the visit?
2 What is 'plan B' if the main objectives cannot be achieved?
3 What could go wrong? Does the risk assessment cover:
   - the main activity
   - 'plan B'
   - travel
   - emergencies
   - staff numbers
   - site-specific hazards, e.g. water sports, adventurous activities
   - variable hazards, e.g. weather and participant abilities.

4 What information could be provided for parents?

5 Is the leader competent?

6 What are the communication arrangements?

7 What are the arrangements for supervision, both during the visit and during free time – is there a code of conduct?

View point

Viewpoint 1

School trips are not worth the effort – too much work is required to meet health and safety legislation.

Viewpoint 2

School trips offer valuable experiences for children, and health and safety is very necessary to protect children whilst in your care.

A school trip

St Crispin's Junior School has arranged for Year 5 children to visit a local residential home to sing Christmas carols. As the home is only one mile away, the children are to walk there.

Immediately after break time, a teacher gathers together a group of children and starts walking to the home. No register is taken. It starts raining but the children have no coats. As they walk through the town centre, two children stop off at the sweet shop. Another child, who lives nearby, goes home to get his coat. On reaching the home they discover that they were not expected until tomorrow and the residents have gone Christmas shopping. The teacher turns the children around and starts heading back to the school.

- How could this trip have been made safer?
- What risk assessment should the teacher have undertaken before leaving?
- What could be the consequences of this trip?

Over to you

Complete the following risk assessment with reference to the scenario above.

Hazards	Actions to minimise risks
Supervision: • Is there enough staff to supervise the children during the visit?	
Road safety: • Where are the appropriate road crossing areas? • Are the children supervised whilst walking?	
Weather: • Are children and staff adequately dressed for changes in weather?	
Accidents: • Is there a trained first aider? • Is there a first aid kit? • Has parental consent been obtained? • Have children with health needs been considered?	
Preparations for the visit: • Is the home prepared for the visit? • Is there a suitable 'plan B'?	

Table 5.06 Risk assessment for a school trip

Older people

Older people are more vulnerable than adults. For example, as people grow older they have a reduced immune system which leaves them at greater risk of infection. Other reasons why the older population is more susceptible to injury from the environment include:

- reduced mobility
- reduced hearing
- failing eyesight
- fragility
- reduced reaction times.

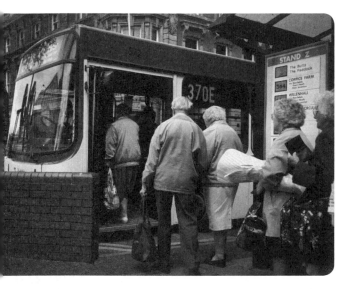

Escorting a client

Jessie is 89 years old. She is very mobile for her age but her eyesight has begun to deteriorate. You are working for an agency that provides domiciliary care, and Jessie has asked you to accompany her to the local supermarket on the bus.

You both arrive at the bus stop having just missed the bus and discover that there is a 30-minute wait for the next bus. During the wait, Jessie begins to get cold and tired as there are no seats available at the bus stop. When the bus arrives it is crowded with school children. Jessie needs help getting onto the bus as the step is high. The bus pulls away before Jessie has reached her seat, and she trips over a school bag falling to the floor.

1 How could you have been better prepared for the trip?

2 What changes should you have made to ensure a better trip?

3 What emergency first aid would you need to perform?

Over to you

Complete the following risk assessment with reference to the scenario above.

Hazards	Actions to minimise risks
Travel arrangements: • Which bus should you get to minimise waiting and overcrowding? • Is the bus suitable/equipped for older people? • What are the alternative travel arrangements?	
Weather: • Have variations in the weather been catered for?	
Accidents: • Is accompanying staff member qualified in first aid? • Are first aid provisions adequate or necessary?	
Preparations for the trip: • Is there a 'plan B'?	

Table 5.07 Risk assessment for escorting an older client by bus

People with disabilities

People with disabilities may be at risk from harm for many reasons, depending on the severity of their disability. These include:

- physical disability
- mobility difficulties
- lack of understanding of possible risks
- reduced intellect.

All healthcare workers have a duty of care towards clients with disabilities. Their role is to ensure that individuals do not put themselves at risk whilst supporting their efforts to achieve self-determination. In effect, this means that all those who manage or work with people with disabilities have a responsibility to:

- ensure a safe environment for staff and individuals
- safeguard the individual's interests
- protect individuals from danger, abuse or exploitation
- protect other people from any consequences arising from the provision of the service; for example, to protect the general public from a client who is unable to control his or her aggression.

People with disabilities have the same rights as everyone else – even the right to take risks

This does not mean that care workers should prevent people with disabilities from taking risks, but rather that these risks should be assessed and managed as part of planning for everyday care.

A walk in the park

Samira works in a day centre for young adults with disabilities. She has a close working relationship with James, a young adult with autism. Samira wishes to take James to the park to feed the ducks. Samira is very used to James and has thought carefully about the physical hazards that may be present in the short walk to the park. James' condition means that he expresses his emotions by hitting himself hard on the head. At the park James gets very excited and starts to hit himself. Samira has been trained to hold his arm to prevent James damaging himself. A member of the public witnesses James trying to hit himself and Samira restraining his arm and is convinced that Samira is abusing James. The bystander reports the incident to the police and Samira is suspended from work pending investigation.

1 How could Samira have prevented the incident from occurring?
2 What risk assessment would Samira have performed before going on the walk?
3 What actions could be taken in the future to prevent a repeat of this incident?

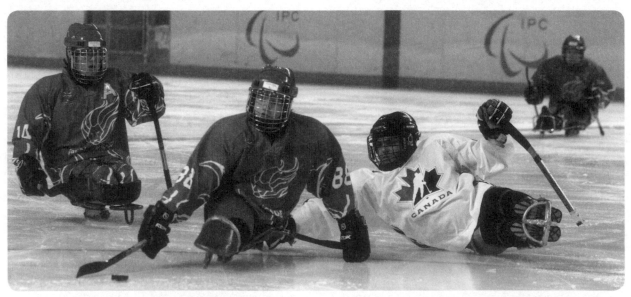

Complete the following risk assessment with reference to the scenario on page 182.

Hazards	Actions to minimise risks
Travel arrangements: • How will you get to the park? • If walking, where are the safest places to cross the road? • Does James understand the importance of good behaviour near traffic? • If taking a taxi, how will the client react to a new, confined space?	
Dangers near water: • What are the available precautions for water safety? • Who will you call in an emergency? • How deep is the water? • Is the water fast moving? • Are the weather conditions safe for being near water?	
Possibility of the client harming himself: • Does the accompanying staff member have the experience and training to care for the client? • How can help be sought, if necessary? • Is it appropriate for this client to have one-to-one care in the situation?	

Table 5.08 Risk assessment for escorting a client to the park

Viewpoint 1

People with disabilities should be encouraged to participate in the community, even if their actions may present some risk to the community.

Viewpoint 2

People with disabilities should stay in residential homes where the risks to the community are reduced.

Reporting and recording health and safety issues

Accidents

What do you understand by the word accident?

Although an accident may be unplanned, it is not unavoidable – the vast majority of accidents are predictable and preventable. Accidents may occur for obvious reasons, such as falls caused by cracks in a footpath or slipping on a wet floor.

Accidents can also be due to human factors; for example, illness, disability and fragility may increase the chance of accidents occurring.

Accidents

The Health and Safety Executive defines an accident as 'any undesired circumstances which give rise to ill health or injury, damage to property, plant products or the environment'. In others words, an accident is an unplanned event that may lead to harm or damage.

Accident report forms

Every workplace should have an accident report form as correct documentation of an accident, incident or near-miss. The person completing the form should make a detailed note of dates, times, witnesses and the treatment necessary. With a clear description of the event it may be possible to ensure that measures are taken to reduce the risk of a similar incident reoccurring.

When completing an accident report form it is very important that the correct information is gathered. To do this it is necessary to seek answers to six basic categories of questions, as shown in Table 5.09.

The only way that the questions listed in Table 5.09 can be answered after an accident is to ensure that a detailed record of events is taken in the form of an accident report. An example of a completed accident report form is given in Figure 5.05.

WHO?	Who was involved? Who was responsible? Who was the incident reported to? Who was notified?
WHEN?	When did the accident occur? When were people aware that the accident could occur? When did help arrive?
WHY?	Why did the accident happen? Why were safety measures not implemented? Why did safety measures fail?
WHAT?	What injuries occurred? What could have been done to avoid the accident?
WHERE?	Where did the accident happen?
HOW?	How did the accident happen? How could safety procedures be improved? How does the organisation learn from the accident?

Table 5.09 Categories of questions when completing an accident report form

Beeches Residential Home

Report of an Accident, Dangerous Occurrence or Near Miss

Date of incident *06/07/05* **Time of incident** *10:00*

Location of accident, etc. *Dayroom*

In the event of the casualty being absent from normal duties, please fill in the date of the first absence and date of return to work

Date off work *07/07/05* **Date return to work** *08/08/05*

Details of the person injured or involved in the accident, dangerous occurence or near miss

Full name, address and post code: *Daisy May, 39 Draft Street, Portsmouth PO1 1XX*

Age: *26*

Sex (M or F): *F*

Occupation of injured person or status if not an employee (e.g. Resident, Visitor) *Staff Nurse*

Nature of injury *Burn to hand*

Management of injury (Please tick appropriate box)

First aid only ✓ Advised to see doctor ☐

Casualty sent to hospital ✓ Admitted to hospital for more than 24 hours ☐

Account of accident, dangerous occurrence or near miss

Describe what happened and how. In the case of an accident, state what the injured person was doing at the time.

Daisy was handing out cups of tea to the residents when Mr Jones, who is blind, knocked in to her, causing her to spill tea on her left hand.

Witnesses (Please give names, address and occupation)

Health Care Support Worker, Kate Hill, 17 Beenthere Street, Portsmouth PO2 3ZY

Remedial action taken

(Note: All accidents, other than minor incidents, will require an accident investigation form to be completed.)

Kate Hill immersed Daisy's hand in cold water for ten minutes, wrapped it up in a towel and took her to A&E.

Signature of person making report *K. Hill* **Date** *06/07/05*

Signature of Safety Co-ordinator **Date**

On completion the residential home should retain a copy and send a copy to:
1. the Director of Environmental, Health and Safety Services (EHSS)
2. the Person(s) involved in the incidents

Figure 5.05
Accident report form

Incidents

Incidents are accidents that do not cause damage, harm or injury.

Incidents give you the opportunity to prevent accidents from occurring. For example, if it is realised that a client nearly received the wrong injection, this gives staff the opportunity to review their drug policy and prevent someone actually receiving the wrong drug in future. This is why it is important to record incidents (or 'near-misses'): the information gathered can prevent a major accident from occurring.

The importance of reporting incidents

Jean is 76 years old and lives on the second floor of a newly built small block of flats. Jean is visited daily by Jackie, a domiciliary worker. Jackie always uses the stairs after visiting Jean. On several occasions she nearly trips down the top step when leaving the flat, but thinks nothing of it. One day on visiting Jean, Jackie finds her at the bottom of the stairs following a fall. Jean is admitted to hospital with a broken neck of femur. Following an investigation by a health and safety officer it is found that when the building was built the stairs were fitted with a lip to accommodate a carpet. However, a carpet was never laid and, consequently, the lip of the step caused Jean to misjudge the step depth and fall. If Jackie had reported her 'near-misses' she may have prevented Jean's more serious accident.

The importance of reporting and recording health and safety issues

Every member of staff is responsible for reporting accidents, incidents and potential hazards. These should be recorded in an accident or incident book, as described previously. Failure to report may have serious consequences. If an accident or incident is not reported and the details accurately recorded then it becomes difficult to follow up.

Risk assessments are also needed to protect the employer, employee and individual. It is the employer's responsibility to ensure that all potential hazards have been assessed and that a risk assessment is in place. By law, all workplaces are required to carry out risk assessments. Accidents resulting from poor risk management may result in large fines and even imprisonment.

Poor risk management

Redbrook is a small maternity unit in a remote part of Scotland which employs six community midwives. The Healthcare Trust does not have a policy of ensuring that all staff members are vaccinated against Hepatitis B. Hepatitis B is carried in the blood and can be transferred from an infected individual to a healthcare worker. The long-term effects of Hepatitis B may include liver damage and liver failure.

1 If a midwife contracted Hepatitis B from an infected individual, who would be held responsible?
2 Find out how NHS Trusts usually ensure that all staff are protected against Hepatitis B.
3 Imagine that you are the insurance company representing the midwives at Redbrook maternity unit. Present your argument that the Healthcare Trust's lack of risk assessment has endangered the health and safety of its employees.

Infection control and disposal of waste

When assessing risk, it is not always the hazards you can see that you need to be careful about. **Micro-organisms** exist everywhere in the environment – in water, air, soil and blood, and even on your skin. They are invisible to the human eye. In the right circumstances, micro-organisms do not present a risk to human health. However, micro-organisms can also be disease-causing. The severity of the diseases they cause can range from mildly unpleasant, as in the common cold, to life-threatening, as in the case of AIDS resulting from HIV infection. Table 5.10 lists possible infections caused by micro-organisms in the workplace.

> **Micro-organisms** – life forms seen only under a microscope. They include bacteria, viruses, fungi and parasites.

Communicable diseases such as those in Table 5.10 are transmitted to a human host by a variety of different methods. Transmission may be through direct contact between two people or carried indirectly via a medium such as food or insects. Common routes of infection are shown in Figure 5.06.

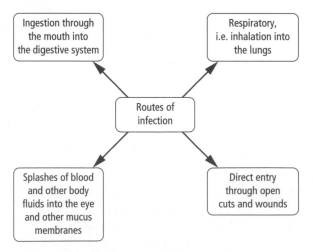

Figure 5.06 Common routes of infection

Things to remember: assessing the risks

The Health and Safety Executive gives the following advice about the spread of infection.

- Although micro-organisms can cause harm by infection, they can also cause allergies and/or be toxic.
- When considering direct contact with people or animals, you need to address risks from the living and the dead, as well as risks from handling material such as raw meat.
- You have a duty under health and safety law to consult with employees about health and safety matters. As well as giving employees information, you need to listen and take account of what they say before making any health and safety decisions. Ask your employees if they have come across any hazards you haven't identified, e.g. areas where dirty/used needles might be dumped.
- Make sure you identify all those who might be affected, not just employees – remember contractors, members of the public and others.
- There may be animals, including insects, in your workplace that you cannot see or that you have no direct control over: pests such as rats, pigeons, cockroaches, ticks, etc.
- If your work involves people or animals, they may appear healthy because infection may not be associated with obvious signs. But if you know they are suffering from an infection, or that there is an increased risk of infection because of behaviour, e.g. animals can be unpredictable and bite and scratch when unsettled, or background, e.g. recent immigrants may be from countries where there are diseases that are not usually found (or are only rare) in the UK, you should take this into account in your assessment.

(Source: Advisory Committee on Dangerous Pathogens – Infection at work: controlling the risks)

Organism	Type	Nature of infection
Bacteria	Legionella	Caused by the inhalation of infected airborne droplets; these can be spread via air conditioning systems. Potentially fatal.
	Salmonella	Usually found in poultry, eggs, unprocessed milk, meat and water. Attacks the stomach and intestines. Vomiting and diarrhoea are accompanied by painful abdominal cramps. Often spread from person to person through poor hygene. Associated foods include salads, raw vegetables, milk, dairy products, poultry and contaminated water. Symptoms include diarrhoea, fever, vomiting and abdominal pain.
	Streptococcus suis	There are several groups of streptococcal bacteria, causing a range of diseases. Group A streptococcus causes diseases ranging from mild infections of the throat and skin to more serious infections such as rheumatic fever. Group C and G streptococci under certain conditions can cause severe disease such as meningitis and septicaemia.
	Tuberculosis	Passed via airborne droplets when infected people sneeze or cough. Usually attacks the lungs but can attack any part of the body, such as the brain, spine and kidneys. Can be fatal.
	(MRSA) Methicillin Resistant Staphylococcus Aureus	There is no specific disease associated with this bacterium, but because it is resistant to antibiotics it causes a wide range of untreatable conditions from wound infections, ulcers, abscesses and lung infections to fatal septicaemia.
Virus	Hepatitis A	Transmitted via contaminated food and water, and from person to person where there is poor hygiene. Symptoms include loss of appetite, nausea, aching muscles and joints, and a mild fever.
	Hepatitis B	Highly infectious disease spread via the blood of an infected person. Healthcare workers are at risk of contracting the disease if accidentally pricked with a contaminated needle. Early symptoms include poor appetite, nausea, aching muscles and joints, and mild fever; in the long-term, Hepatitis B can result in liver failure.
	HIV (human immunodeficiency virus)	Most often transmitted through unprotected sex but can also be passed via blood transfusion and contaminated needles. HIV infection can lead to acquired immune deficiency syndrome (AIDS), a collection of diseases or illnesses caused by a weakened immune system that will eventually lead to death.
	Gastroenteritis	Common and highly infectious illness causing inflammation of the gut. Usually caused by a viral infection but also caused by bacteria and parasites. Symptoms include vomiting and diarrhoea.
Fungus	Ringworm	Common name given to a group of fungal infections of the skin, hair and nails. Usually causes reddened and scaly patches on the skin that may be itchy; the nails become thickened and discoloured.
Parasite	Roundworm	Parasites that live in the intestine. They have a long cylindrical body and are 20–30 cm long. Mild infestation often produces no symptoms; heavy infestation can result in vomiting, diarrhoea and abdominal pain.

Table 5.10 Possible infections caused by organisms in the workplace

Control of infectious diseases

Hand washing

Florence Nightingale once said 'Hospital should do no harm'. As a care worker, you will be responsible for the health of vulnerable and sick people. It is your duty to reduce their risk of contracting a disease by taking preventative action. Hand washing is one of the most important and easiest methods of preventing cross-infection from person to person.

Touch is a valuable tool for communicating compassion and understanding. In the healthcare professions, touching others can provide physical comfort and reassurance. However, one of the main ways that cross-infection occurs is through touch. As a care worker you must, therefore, constantly be vigilant in your hand washing to ensure that bacteria and viruses have as little chance as possible to spread.

You must always wash your hands:

- before starting work and when finishing work
- before and after eating
- after using the toilet
- before and after touching someone
- after handling dirty laundry or emptying waste bins
- after sneezing, coughing or blowing your nose.

Wearing gloves

Wearing disposable gloves will also offer a protective barrier against infection. Infection can travel in body products, especially blood. Cuts and grazes on hands that are not covered by gloves may allow someone else's blood to enter the body and cause an infection.

Gloves must be worn when:

- dealing with body products, e.g. blood, urine, mucus, sputum, vomit
- before and after eating
- changing soiled bed linen
- clearing up spillages
- dressing wounds and pressure sores
- changing nappies.

Protective clothing

As well as protecting your hands, it may be necessary to protect your clothing and others from the bacteria you carry. Disposable aprons should be worn and disposed of immediately before going to attend another person. In some situations, it is necessary to cover hair and shoes or to wear disposable gowns and masks.

Figure 5.07 Steps to good hand washing

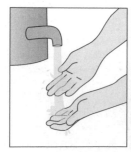
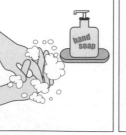
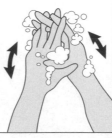
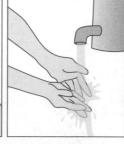
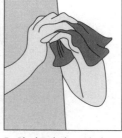

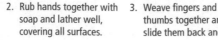

1. Wet hands with running water.
2. Rub hands together with soap and lather well, covering all surfaces.
3. Weave fingers and thumbs together and slide them back and forth.
4. Rinse hands under a stream of clean, running water until all soap is gone.
5. Blot hands dry with clean paper towel.

Protective clothing should be worn when:

- coming into contact with bodily fluids or wastes
- disposing of waste
- caring for someone who is being treated for an infection
- changing soiled linen.

Cleaning equipment

In addition to keeping yourself clean and carrying out precautions to prevent cross-infection, it is essential to ensure all equipment and work surfaces are clean. Many items are designed to be used only once and should be disposed of immediately after use. Large items such as mattresses and trolleys should be washed with antiseptic solutions and allowed to dry thoroughly before being used again. Smaller items such as instruments may come in packets and can be sterilised after use. Clean equipment before use on a new client, immediately after use and before putting it away.

Disposal of hazardous waste

In is important that hazardous waste is disposed of correctly, to ensure a safe working environment. Table 5.11 describes the method of disposal for each type of waste.

Preventing cross-infection

As a nurse on a busy geriatric ward, you are responsible for the care of Mrs Handley who has been incontinent of urine during the night. You and a new member of staff need to help Mrs Handley to wash and dress, and change her bedding and incontinence dressings.

1 How would you protect yourself and Mrs Handley from cross-infection?
2 Describe all the methods of waste disposal you would use to perform your duties in accordance with health and safety requirements.
3 Explain which two pieces of health and safety legislation you are using and who it is protecting.

Dealing with spillages

Spillages should be dealt with immediately using the appropriate disinfectant and the area cleaned thoroughly. Cleaning is one of the basic control measures that should be in place to reduce the risk of exposure to micro-organisms and other hazardous substances. In the health and care sector, it is necessary to remember that spillages may carry body products such as blood, urine, faeces, sputum and sweat, and consequently contain potentially harmful micro-organisms.

It is the responsibility of every employee to deal with spillages and hazardous waste.

Table 5.11 Waste disposal guidelines

Type of waste	Method of disposal
Clinical waste, e.g. used wound dressings, bandages, nappies, sanitary dressings, soiled gloves	Yellow bag – when the bag is full, carefully seal and tag it indicating where the waste has come from, e.g. labour ward, paediatrics, accident and emergency. The waste is burnt in an incinerator.
Sharps, e.g. needles, glass, syringes	Yellow sharps box – when the box is full, seal and tag it indicating location of box.
Body fluids, e.g. vomit, urine, faeces, blood, sputum	Wash down the sluice drain, and disinfect.
Dirty and soiled sheets and linen	Red bag – seal and send to the laundry (the bag will disintegrate in the wash).
Recyclable instruments and equipment for sterilisation	Blue bag – seal and return to central sterilisation services department (CSSD) for cleansing, sterilising and repackaging.
Waste paper	Black bag – seal and tag for incineration or shredding of confidential information.

Sometimes this responsibility requires that you find an appropriately trained person to deal with the incident.

When dealing with spillages you need to consider the following factors:

- Protect yourself and others around you.
- Do not tackle a spillage that you are not trained to handle – find someone who is.
- Use appropriate protective clothing for the job, i.e. gloves and aprons.
- Prevent others from contact with a spillage. This can be done by instructing somebody to remain with the spillage until it can be cleaned up and placing safety warnings around the infected area.
- Collect appropriate cleaning fluids and equipment to deal with the spillage.
- Use appropriate types of disinfectant for the spillage. Some disinfectants do not destroy viruses present in body fluids; for example, it would be no use cleaning a soiled mattress with washing-up liquid.
- Use the correct dilution of disinfectant for the task. If a disinfectant is not diluted correctly it may burn skin or be inhaled and damage the lining of airways.
- Some disinfectants require contact time with the spillage to work effectively. If mopped up too quickly they will not work sufficiently.

Inadequate cleaning

Teresa is a newly qualified physiotherapist. She is caring for a confused elderly gentleman, who suddenly takes out his false teeth and puts them on the table. Teresa hands him his teeth to put back in, which he does. She wipes saliva off the table with a paper towel and continues with her treatment.

1 Identify the ways in which infection can be spread in this scenario.
2 How should Teresa have dealt with the risk of cross-infection?
3 Analyse why Teresa acted as she did. What factors do you think prevented her from taking adequate measures to prevent the spread of infection?

Over to you

Dora and Jen are two cleaners on a medical ward. Jen has been to a study day to look at new changes in cleaning requirements. Dora hasn't. Dora continues to clean as she always did. Jen uses new improved chemicals and equipment in her work. Which member of staff presents the greater hazard to the working environment, and why?

Health and safety legislation and guidelines

Many of the hazards present in the workplace are covered by health and safety legislation. Table 5.12 will help you identify which legislation is relevant to particular hazards.

Fire Precautions (Workplace) Regulations 1997

The potential for fire is one of the main hazards in all healthcare settings. Yet, with a little thought and careful consideration, the chances of this dangerous hazard occurring can be drastically reduced and, in the event of a fire, its effects minimised.

The Fire Precautions (Workplace) Regulations 1997 state the following:

- All workplaces must have a fire risk assessment. These can be performed with the help and advice of the local fire brigade, who will inform employers how best to minimise the risk of fire.
- There must be a fire and evacuation procedure and at least one fire evacuation practice each year. Many workplaces opt for more frequent fire drills to ensure that every employee, trainee or temporary worker is aware how to act in an emergency.
- All staff, whether full-time, part-time or temporary, must take part in fire training and drills.
- All workplaces must have in place the appropriate fire fighting equipment, alarms

Hazard	Relevant legislation
Rooms and outdoor play areas that pose a risk	Health and Safety at Work Act 1974
Equipment in an unsafe condition	Health and Safety at Work Act 1974
Toys in an unsafe condition	Health and Safety at Work Act 1974
Incorrect storage of chemicals	Control of Substances Hazardous to Health (COSHH) Regulations 2002
Inadequate control of infectious diseases	Reporting of Injuries, Diseases and Dangerous Occurrences Regulations (RIDDOR) 1995
Fire	Fire Precautions (Workplace) Regulations 1997
Poor working conditions	Health and Safety at Work Act 1974
Unsafe furnishings	Health and Safety at Work Act 1974
Inappropriate furnishings for individuals	Health and Safety at Work Act 1974
Inappropriate use of equipment	Health and Safety at Work Act 1974
Inadequate equipment maintenance	Health and Safety at Work Act 1974
Poor staff training	Health and Safety at Work Act 1974
Lack of security measures	Manual Handling Operations Regulations 1992
Inadequate building maintenance	Health and Safety at Work Act 1974
Inadequate personal safety precautions	Health and Safety at Work Act 1974
Close proximity to radio transmissions	Health and Safety at Work Act 1974
Pollution of air and/or water	Control of Substances Hazardous to Health (COSHH) Regulations 2002

Table 5.12 Legislation covering particular hazards

and detectors. Staff should be trained in the use of available safety equipment.

- All safety equipment should be kept in a good state of repair.
- Emergency exits and all other exits must be kept clear at all times. Emergency exits must be kept locked, clearly labelled and lead directly to a place of safety.
- Emergency exits must open onto a direct means of escape which must be supplied with emergency lighting and well illuminated.

Evacuation in a care setting has additional problems, including moving people with mobility problems due to age, disability, immaturity or medical treatment.

What to do if you discover a fire

- Get everyone out of the building as quickly and calmly as possible, closing fire doors behind you.
- Ensure a member of staff calls the fire service.
- Take with you any registers of clients/individuals.
- If safe to do so, work in teams to evacuate wheelchair users and immobile individuals.
- Use equipment provided to move individuals.
- If unable to move an individual, leave him or her in a fire-free area, with all fire doors closed, and immediately inform fire fighters where the person is.
- Never put yourself or others at risk.
- Never return to a burning building.

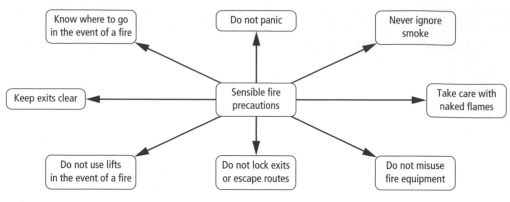

Figure 5.08 Sensible fire precautions

Safety equipment

Fire extinguishers

Fire extinguishers are designed for different purposes (see Table 5.13). Using the wrong fire extinguisher can make a situation worse.

Fire blankets

Fire blankets are usually located in kitchens or where there is a risk of coming into contact with flames. Fire blankets are flame retardant and are designed to place over a fire to smother the flames. They must be used in a calm and controlled manner, as flapping a blanket about will cause the flames to spread.

Table 5.13 Types of fire extinguisher

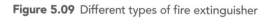

Extinguisher	Type	Colour	Uses	NOT to be used
Electrical fires	Dry powder	Blue marking	For burning liquid, electrical fires and flammable liquids	On flammable metal fires
	Carbon dioxide (CO_2)	Black marking	Safe on all voltages; used on burning liquid, electrical fires and flammable liquids	On flammable metal fires
Non-electrical fires	Water	Red marking	For wood, paper, textiles, fabric and similar materials	On burning liquid, electrical or flammable metal fires
	Foam	Cream/yellow markings	On burning liquid fires	On electrical or flammable metal fires

Figure 5.09 Different types of fire extinguisher

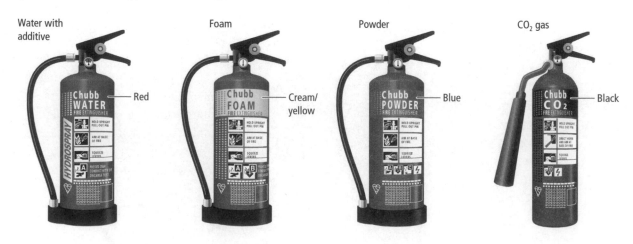

Water with additive — Red

Foam — Cream/yellow

Powder — Blue

CO_2 gas — Black

Health and Safety at Work Act 1974

The Health and Safety at Work Act (HASWA) applies to all work situations. It covers everyone at work or anyone, such as the general public, who may be visiting a workplace. HASWA covers all health and safety legislation, providing a safe environment for all employees and employers.

Employers

The Health and Safety at Work Act states that employers must ensure the workplace is safe and without risks to health. Employers must:

- provide a safe workplace
- ensure there is safe access to and from the workplace
- provide adequate and accessible information on health and safety
- have a written safety policy if employing more than five people
- maintain the workplace in good condition.
- ensure the safe use, handling, storage and transport of equipment and chemicals
- ensure the environment does not put anyone's health at risk
- provide information and supervision, where necessary, to protect the health and safety of their employees
- provide necessary health and safety training, e.g. manual handling training
- undertake risk assessments for all hazards.

Employees

Employees also have legal duties to comply with the Health and Safety at Work Act. Employees must:

- be responsible for their own safety and that of others

- co-operate with employers regarding health and safety
- not intentionally damage any health and safety equipment or materials provided by the employer
- correctly use any work items provided by the employer.
- report any dangerous situations to a manager.

Provision and Use of Work Equipment Regulations 1998

The Provision and Use of Work Equipment Regulations (PUWER) 1998 regulates the use of any equipment in the workplace. It is the responsibility of the employer and any person managing the use of equipment to ensure that all equipment:

- is suitable for the use to which it is put
- is used only for these purposes
- does not increase risks in the workplace
- is well maintained
- is inspected regularly, and records of inspection kept
- is used only by those trained to do so
- includes written operating instructions.

Manual Handling Operations Regulations 1992

More than a third of all injuries that require over three days off work are a result of a manual handling injury (Health and Safety Executive, 2002). Manual handling is the moving or supporting of loads by hand or by bodily force.

Manual handling injuries can occur wherever people are at work.

The Manual Handling Operations Regulations 1992 require employers to:

- avoid the need for manual handling as far as possible
- assess the risk of injury from any manual handling that cannot be avoided
- reduce the risk of injury as far as possible.

Employees must:

- follow systems of work laid down for their safety
- assess the risk of injury from any manual handling that cannot be avoided
- make proper use of the equipment provided
- co-operate with their employer
- inform their employer of any hazards to health they identify
- take care to ensure that their activities do not put others at risk.

Poor lifting techniques result in many thousands of lost working hours due to injury. As a result, the Health and Safety Executive (HSE) has set out guidelines to follow to avoid muscular and skeletal injury (see Figure 5.10).

> **Did you know?**
>
> *Always lift with a straight back and bent knees. Where possible, always seek help when lifting. If you are unsure, do not lift.*

Caring for frail and vulnerable people may occasionally involve different forms of lifting. It is very important that when you lift a person you do not put yourself or him or her at risk.

Before lifting, carefully consider if there is a safer alternative and what equipment is available to help you. **Lifting should be the last option when moving a person and should be done only in emergency and life-threatening situations.**

Tips for safe lifting in a care environment

- Practise lifting in a safe, controlled environment.
- All members of staff should be trained in manual handling.
- Assess the situation – do you really need to lift the client? Can he or she assist with the lift or move?
- Plan a lift carefully before starting.
- Make sure that you have enough room in which to lift.
- Inform the individual that you need to lift him or her. The individual's consent and co-operation will prevent any sudden movements.
- Adjust the bed to suit your height and check that the brakes work.
- Where possible, lift with another person.
- Decide who is going to lead the lift, giving clear instructions planned beforehand.
- Where possible, get the client to help move him- or herself.
- Staff that have undergone appropriate training should use the available equipment.
- Use rhythm and timing when moving; do not jerk.
- Never hurry a lift.

Figure 5.10 Safe lifting procedures must be observed

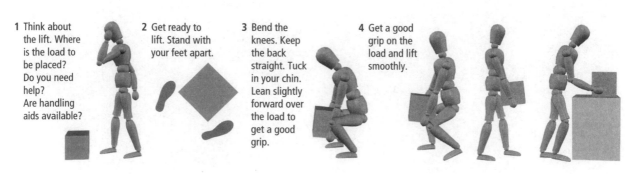

1 Think about the lift. Where is the load to be placed? Do you need help? Are handling aids available?

2 Get ready to lift. Stand with your feet apart.

3 Bend the knees. Keep the back straight. Tuck in your chin. Lean slightly forward over the load to get a good grip.

4 Get a good grip on the load and lift smoothly.

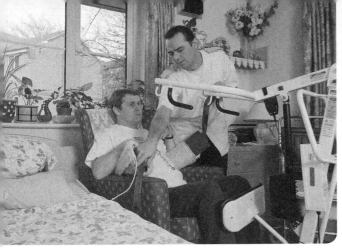

Equipment for moving and handling

Lifting technique

Renaye has run the Maple Residential Care Home for many years. She is working with a new member of staff, Tasha, when they are asked to help lift an obese patient into a bath. Renaye starts to manually lift the patient. Tasha questions her actions, suggesting they use the hoist provided. Renaye overrules Tasha saying that her method is quicker.

1 What could the consequences be if they decide to lift the client manually?
2 Who would be responsible if one of the staff received a back injury following the procedure?
3 Should Renaye have the personal choice to lift manually?

Reporting of Injuries, Diseases and Dangerous Occurrences Regulations (RIDDOR) 1995

The reporting and recording of injuries is a statutory obligation, i.e. it is required by law. This is necessary to help and assist with insurance claims as well as helping to prevent accidents from reoccurring. All records of accidents must be available for inspection and kept for a period of three years.

By law, employers must report the following to the Health and Safety Executive:

- *Death or major injury* – if an employee at work is killed or suffers a major injury; if a member of the public is killed or taken to hospital.

- *Over-three-day injury* – any injury that is not major but results in the employee being off work for more than three days, not counting the day of the injury itself.
- *Disease* – reportable diseases include:
  - poisoning
  - some skin diseases such as **dermatitis** and skin cancer
  - lung diseases including occupational asthma and those linked to **asbestos**
  - infections such as hepatitis, TB, anthrax and tetanus
  - conditions such as occupational cancers and musculo-skeletal disorders.

> **Dermatitis** – inflammation of the dermis, the outer layer of the skin, caused by contact with an external substance.
>
> **Asbestos** – fireproof material. Inhalation of asbestos fibres can lead to lung cancer and lung disease.

A dangerous occurrence is when something happens that did not result in a reportable injury but clearly could have done, for example, an explosion, the release of toxic gases or the collapse of a lift.

Data Protection Act 1998

The Data Protection Act 1998 governs the processing of personal information held on individuals (see also Chapter 2, page 53). The eight principles of the Act are that personal data should be:

- processed fairly and lawfully
- processed only for the purposes for which it was intended
- adequate and relevant but not excessive in relation to the purposes for which it is processed
- accurate and kept up-to-date; inaccurate data should be destroyed or corrected
- kept for no longer than is necessary
- processed in line with the rights of the individual (this includes the individual's right

to be informed about information held on him or her)

- secured against accidental loss, damage or unlawful processing
- not transferred to countries outside the European economic area unless that country ensures an adequate level of protection for the rights and freedoms of data subjects.

Management of Health and Safety at Work Regulations 1999

Much of the law regarding safety in the workplace can be found in the Health and Safety at Work Act 1974. However, any prospective employer setting up a new business should be aware of six important regulations which came about as a result of membership to the European Union and are now incorporated into UK law. The main one of these was the Management of Health and Safety at Work Regulations 1999, which merely adds specific detail to the Health and Safety at Work Act to allow for the safe management of health and safety.

Control of Substances Hazardous to Health (COSHH) Regulations 2002

COSHH regulations are intended to ensure control measures when employees are exposed to hazardous substances in the workplace. In health and social care settings, hazardous substances include cleaning materials, acids, disinfectants, as well as body products such as blood and urine.

Every workplace should have a member of staff who is responsible for implementing the guidelines set down by COSHH regulations.

COSHH regulations carefully consider how hazardous substances are used in the workplace:

- where they are kept
- how they are labelled
- their effects
- the maximum amount of time of safe exposure to a hazardous substance
- how to deal with an emergency involving a hazardous substance.

Correct storage of chemicals

- All substances should be stored in a safe place.
- Where there are children present, the storage area should be locked and out of reach.
- Chemicals must be kept in the appropriate containers supplied by the manufacturer.
- Where appropriate, containers must have safety lids and caps. (Some drugs are not stored in safety containers as they are needed for emergency use.)

Chemicals and solutions used in health and social care settings include drugs, cleaning fluids, antiseptics, solutions for cleaning wounds, replacement body fluids and blood.

Labelling

- Hazardous substances should be labelled with an appropriate symbol indicating the associated danger.
- The contents of the container should match the name on the outside. Never reuse a container designed for a different substance.
- The container should display a use-by date.
- Instructions on how to use the substance safely should be supplied with the chemical.
- There should be clear instructions on what to do in the case of a spillage.
- The length of storage time from opening should be given.

Dust

Toxic

Flammable

Irritant

Corrosive

Oxidising agent

Figure 5.11 Symbols showing types of hazardous substance

Health and safety policy

A health and safety policy is a document required by law to support health and safety legislation. A policy must be effective and worthwhile, not a meaningless jumble of words written down with no intention of ever being used. A good policy should come from the most senior members of an organisation to show a commitment to health and safety. It is no good writing a policy that is impossible to implement and has no relationship to the actual work taking place within an organisation.

When implementing a health and safety policy it is necessary to consider the following questions:

- Who is responsible for implementing the policy?
- Does the policy set achievable and measurable objectives?
- Are the resources available to implement the policy?
- How can the policy be explained in a way that every member of staff will understand?
- How will the policy be reviewed and improved?

Principles of first aid

> **First aid**
>
> First aid is the initial assistance or treatment given to a casualty for any injury or sudden illness before the arrival of an ambulance, doctor or any trained medical professional.

The Health and Safety (First Aid) Regulations 1981 require employers to provide adequate first aid cover for their employees. Every workplace must have enough first aid personnel and facilities to be able to:

- give immediate assistance to casualties
- summon an ambulance or other professional help.

This section will develop your knowledge of how to act in an emergency. All healthcare workers should have a detailed understanding of the principles of first aid; this is best developed by completing a recognised first aid course. First aid can mean the difference between life and death.

The role of the first aider

The aims of first aid are:

- to preserve life
- to limit worsening of condition
- to promote recovery.

The person offering first aid must act calmly and with confidence whilst continuing to reassure the casualty. The first aider should be:

- highly trained
- subject to regular examination
- up-to-date in his or her knowledge and skills.

Life-saving procedures

As well as dealing with minor injuries arising from accidents, first aiders must be able to perform life-saving techniques.

For life to continue there must be an adequate uptake of oxygen by the blood via the lungs (see Chapter 3, pages 68–73). Lack of oxygen in the

blood supply will result in organs such as the brain and heart failing, possibly resulting in death.

There are three important elements involved in getting oxygen to the brain, as shown in Figure 5.12.

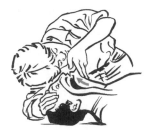

A–Airway

The casualty's airway must be open to allow air to pass into the lungs. To check that the casualty has an open airway, the first aider needs to gently tilt the casualty's head back and lift the chin.

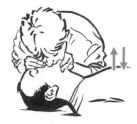

B–Breathing

If the casualty is not breathing, the first aider can breathe for him or her by exhaling into the casualty's lungs.

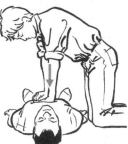

C–Circulation

If the heart stops, the first aider can use chest compressions to force the blood through the heart and around the body.

Figure 5.12 The ABC of resuscitation

When dealing with a collapsed casualty, following the resuscitation sequence will keep circulation going until help arrives. The casualty has a greater chance of surviving a life-threatening incident if the first aider can restore the oxygen to the brain by means of artificial ventilation and chest compressions, known as cardio-pulmonary resuscitation (CPR).

Step-by-step cardio-pulmonary resuscitation (CPR)

On finding a collapsed casualty you should carry out the following sequence:

- Check that you are safe to approach the casualty.

- Call for help. When someone comes to help, ask the person to phone for an ambulance. If you are alone and the casualty is not breathing, start the CPR sequence for one minute then call for an ambulance.
- Try to get a response from the casualty by asking him or her a question, gently shaking the casualty's shoulders or gently pinching the skin.
- If the casualty does not respond, open the airway by placing two fingers under the chin and lifting the jaw. Place your other hand on the casualty's forehead.
- Check breathing for 10 seconds:
  - put your cheek close to the casualty's mouth looking along the body
  - look for signs of the chest rising
  - listen for sounds of breathing
  - feel for breathing on your cheek.
- If the casualty is breathing, follow the procedure for treating an unconscious person (see below). If the casualty is not breathing, breathe for the casualty:
  - ensure the casualty is lying flat on his or her back
  - remove any obstructions from the mouth, leaving dentures in place
  - open airway as above
  - pinch the casualty's nose closed
  - take a full breath of air and place your lips over the casualty's, making a good seal
  - blow into the casualty's mouth until the chest rises
  - remove your lips allowing the chest to fall
  - repeat once.
- If breathing returns, follow instructions for treating an unconscious person (see below). If the casualty is not breathing, check for signs of circulation:
  - observe skin colour
  - observe for any movement
  - press your finger on the casualty's forehead; there should be a return of normal skin colour when you remove your finger.

- If there are signs of circulation but no signs of breathing, continue with mouth-to-mouth breathing until the person's breathing returns or an ambulance arrives. If there are signs of circulation and breathing returns, put the person in the recovery position, stay with them and monitor breathing and circulation until an ambulance arrives. If there are no signs of circulation, begin CPR:
  - with one finger, measure two finger-widths up from the point of the breastbone where the lower ribs start
  - place the heel of your hand on the breastbone
  - place your other hand over the lower hand, interlocking your fingers so that the fingers do not press on the casualty's chest
  - lean over the casualty
  - press down about 4–5 cm (1.5–2.0 inches)
  - complete 30 chest compressions quickly (aiming for 100 per minute)
  - give two mouth-to-mouth breaths
  - continue with 30 more compressions
  - alternate 30 compressions with 2 breaths.
- Continue with CPR until help arrives.

Treating an unconscious person

If a casualty is breathing but unconscious, he or she should be placed in the recovery position. This will prevent the tongue from blocking the throat and ensure the person does not inhale his or her own vomit. To place an unconscious person in the recovery position:

- Kneel beside the casualty and remove any bulky objects from their pockets.
- Open the airway by tilting the head back and lifting the chin.
- Straighten the legs and place the arm nearest to you at a right angle.
- Gently place the back of the hand furthest from you on the cheek nearest to you.

- Gently pull up the knee furthest from you so that the foot is on the ground. Keeping the hand on the cheek, pull carefully on the raised leg so that the body rolls towards you on its side.
- Arrange the bent leg at a comfortable right angle.
- Ensure the head is still tilted to keep the airway open and stay with the casualty until an ambulance arrives.

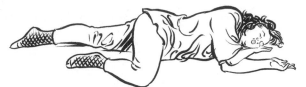

Figure 5.13 The recovery position

Over to you

List the hazards in a chosen workplace that could result in a life-threatening situation.

Fractures

A fracture is a break or crack in a bone caused by force. This force can be direct, as in a car accident of fall, or indirect, for example, a twist or wrench.

Fractures are generally described as being closed or open:

- A closed, or simple, fracture is when the bone is broken but the skin is not cut.
- An open, or compound, fracture is when the bone is broken and the skin is cut. The skin may have been cut by the bone or simply at the same time as the break occurred; the bone may or may not be visible in the wound.

Other types of fracture include:

- *transverse fracture* – the break is at right angles to the long axis of the bone
- *comminuted fracture* – the bone shatters into three or more pieces
- *greenstick fracture* – a partial split in a young (immature) bone, causing a bend on the other side of the bone.

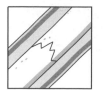
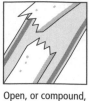
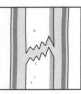
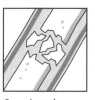

Closed, or simple, fracture

Open, or compound, fracture

Transverse fracture

Comminuted fracture

Greenstick fracture

Figure 5.14 Types of fracture

Fractures may be complicated by injury to adjoining nerves, blood vessels and organs. For example, a fractured rib may puncture a lung or an internal organ such as the spleen.

Treatment of fractures

- Check that you and the casualty are safe.
- Check ABC, during which time you should have called for help.
- Cover any open wounds to prevent blood loss and infection.
- Immobilise the injury by preventing movement of it.
- *Do not move* the casualty unless you have to.

Strains and sprains

Strains and sprains are both types of injuries to soft tissue. A strain is twisting, overstretching or tearing of a muscle, whilst a sprain is a stretching or tearing of a ligament (the tissue that holds two or more bones together). Both types of injury are usually caused by a sudden movement or wrenching of a joint. Symptoms of both a sprain and strain include pain, swelling, bruising and restriction of movement in the affected area. Strains and sprains are common injuries in many sports and usually occur in the ankles, shoulders and knees.

Treatment of strains and sprains

To treat a strain or sprain, you should follow the RICE procedure:

- *Rest* – support the injury in the most comfortable position for the casualty.
- *Ice* – apply an ice pack or cold compress to the area to reduce the swelling.
- *Compression* – apply pressure to the injured part by applying a thick layer of padding secured with a bandage.
- *Elevate* – raise the injured part to reduce the blood flow and minimise bruising.

Finally, send the casualty to hospital.

Bleeding

Bleeding is also known as haemorrhaging. Bleeding is classified depending on the type of blood vessel that has been damaged.

- *Arterial bleeding*
  Arteries are strong muscular vessels that carry blood rich in oxygen away from the heart (see also Chapter 3, pages 79–80). Blood from a damaged artery is bright red in colour. As arterial blood is under pressure, a damaged artery will rapidly spurt blood, resulting in severe loss of blood volume if not stopped.
- *Venous bleeding*
  Veins are thin-walled vessels which contain valves that help blood return to the heart (see also Chapter 3, pages 79–80). Blood from a vein is dark red in colour and will gush from a wound.
- *Capillary bleeding*
  Capillaries are very fine vessels within body tissue that link arteries with veins (see also Chapter 3, pages 79–80). Capillary bleeding is a gentle slight oozing that occurs at the site of the wound. Broken capillaries under the skin result in bleeding into the tissues, known as a bruise.

Treatment of bleeding

When dealing with bleeding, the aim of the first aider is to control the bleeding, minimise the effects of shock and infection, and then organise for the casualty to get to hospital.

> ### Did you know?
> *When dealing with blood, remember to protect yourself from cross-infection. Use disposable gloves where possible.*

When dealing with bleeding, the following procedure is required:

- Talk to the casualty at all times.
- Remove clothing from the wound, leaving in place any object protruding from the wound.
- Apply direct pressure over the wound or around any protruding object.
- Raise the bleeding wound above the level of the casualty's heart. This slows down the bleeding as the heart has to pump against gravity.
- Lay the casualty down to minimise the risk of shock.
- Place a pad over the bleeding area and bandage securely. Pad either side of a protruding object, do not remove the object.
- Keep checking for signs of shock. These include: pale, clammy skin; rapid pulse; sweating; feeling cold; shallow breathing; weakness; giddiness.

Burns

Burns are caused by dry heat, extreme cold, corrosive chemicals and radiation (including sun burn). Scalding is caused by wet heat (liquids and vapours).

Before treating a burn it is necessary to establish the extent and depth of the burn. By understanding the extent of the burn the first aider can assess the risk of the casualty developing shock as a result of loss of tissue fluid. Burns also destroy the body's natural barrier against infection: damaged skin will allow airborne bacteria to enter the body.

Treatment of burns

Most small, superficial burns can be treated by a first aider. The aim of treating burns is to stop the skin from burning further, to relieve pain and swelling, and to minimise the risk of infection.

When treating burns you should:

- check for danger
- check ABC
- lay the casualty down, protecting the burnt area
- flood the injured part with cold water for up to 10 minutes
- remove any jewellery or clothing from the injured area before it begins to swell
- cover the area with a sterile or clean dressing
- seek medical help as soon as possible.

Do not:

- remove any clothing that may be stuck to a burnt area
- touch the injured area
- burst blisters
- apply any lotions or creams to the injured area.

Treating a scald

Gerry is a resident in a centre for adults with learning difficulties. He has been practising making cups of tea for visitors. Today, it is his key worker's birthday and Gerry decides to make him a cup of tea, unsupervised. Unfortunately, Gerry pours boiling water over his hand.

1 As the centre's first aider, what is your immediate response to the situation?
2 In addition to pain, what other symptoms should you check for?
3 What is the role of the manager in this situation?

Asthma attacks

An asthma attack is a distressing and potentially life-threatening condition. It results from spasm of the respiratory muscles, causing the airways to narrow and breathing to become difficult (see also Chapter 3, page 74). Attacks may be triggered by smoking, having a cold or an allergic reaction; some attacks have no obvious trigger. Asthmatics are usually able to deal with attacks by using a reliever inhaler; these are usually blue. They may also carry a preventer inhaler which helps avert attacks; these are usually brown, red or white.

The signs of an asthma attack are:

- difficulty in breathing
- wheezing when the casualty exhales
- grey-blue tinge to the skin
- cough
- distress and anxiety
- difficulty in speaking.

Treatment of an asthma attack

When responding to an asthma attack you should:

- keep calm and reassure the casualty
- encourage the casualty to adopt a position that he or she feels comfortable in – usually sitting upright
- encourage the casualty to use his or her reliever inhaler (usually blue).

If the attack does not improve after five minutes, seek medical help.

Do not:

- force the casualty to lie down
- use a preventer inhaler (usually brown, red or white) to relieve an asthma attack.

Over to you

Research some of the reasons given for the rise in the incidence of childhood asthma.

Epilepsy

Epilepsy is a common condition characterised by convulsions. A convulsion, or fit, is the result of a neurological disturbance causing many of the body's muscles to contract simultaneously. Convulsions usually result in the individual losing consciousness.

Reflection

From experience, what do you know about how to deal with a person who is having an epileptic seizure?

There are a number of possible causes of epilepsy, including head injury, brain damage, lack of oxygen to the brain and the ingestion of poisons. There are two types of epilepsy: minor epilepsy, known as 'petit mal', and major epilepsy, known as 'grand mal'.

Minor epilepsy (petit mal)

It can be difficult to recognise a petit mal fit. Petit mal can present as a short blurring of consciousness similar to a daydream, the twitching of lips and eyelids, and odd movements such as lip-smacking and chewing. On recovery, the casualty may be confused or simply have lost his or her train of thought. It is important to be aware that a major fit can sometimes follow a minor fit.

If you think a person has suffered a petit mal fit, you should sit the person down and offer reassurance. Do not pester him or her with questions.

Major epilepsy (grand mal)

This condition is characterised by violent seizures and loss of consciousness. Epileptic fits can occur suddenly, without warning. Signs that a person is having a grand mal fit include:

- the casualty suddenly falls unconscious, sometimes letting out a cry
- the casualty becomes rigid, arching his or her back
- breathing may stop, resulting in a grey-blue tinge to the face
- convulsive movements begin
- the jaw may be clenched
- there may be a loss of bowel and bladder control
- the muscles finally relax and breathing becomes normal
- consciousness is regained
- the casualty may feel dazed
- a fit may be followed by a deep sleep.

If you see a person suffer a grand mal fit, you should aim to protect the person during the episode and provide care when he or she recovers.

- Try to protect the casualty from injury by easing his or her fall, if possible, and clearing the surrounding area.
- Protect the casualty's privacy by asking bystanders to move away.
- Loosen clothing around the casualty's neck.
- After the fit, place the casualty in the recovery position (see page 199), check breathing and pulse, and resuscitate if necessary.
- If the person is fitting for more than 5 minutes, call an ambulance.
- Note down for how long the fit has occurred.

Do not:

- lift or move the casualty
- place anything in his or her mouth
- use force to restrain him or her.

Diabetes

Diabetes is a medical condition caused by insufficient insulin, a hormone produced by the pancreas (see also Chapter 3, page 144). This means that the body is unable to regulate the concentration of sugar in the blood. Insufficient insulin leads to raised blood sugar levels which cause hyperglycaemia; too much insulin or low blood sugar levels result in hypoglycaemia.

Hyperglycaemia

Prolonged high blood sugar can result in unconsciousness followed by a diabetic coma. It is necessary to treat this condition quickly by giving the casualty insulin and intravenous (into the vein) fluids.

Signs of hyperglycaemia include:

- dry skin
- deep, laboured breathing
- a faint smell of acetone (similar to nail varnish remover) on the casualty's breath.

When responding to a person with hyperglycaemia, you should phone for an ambulance, follow the procedure for treating an unconscious person (see page 199) and monitor the casualty's condition carefully until help arrives.

Hypoglycaemia

Hypoglycaemia may occur in diabetics after binge drinking, heat exhaustion or hypothermia. A rapid fall in blood sugar levels may affect brain function and be accompanied by an epileptic fit. However, most diabetics know how to monitor their own blood sugar level, to ensure this remains within safe limits. If the hypoglycaemic attack is well advanced then the casualty may begin to lose consciousness.

Signs of hypoglycaemia include:

- weakness, hunger
- confusion
- possible violence
- sweating
- cold, clammy skin
- fast pulse
- shallow breathing.

When treating hypoglycaemia, the casualty may be unconscious or conscious. If the casualty is unconscious, treat as described on page 199. If the casualty is conscious, help him or her to sit down then give the casualty a sugary drink, sugar lumps, chocolate or any other sweet food. If the person's condition does not improve, seek medical assistance.

Bites and stings

Most animals and insects will not bite or sting unless injured or provoked. Bites and stings are usually minor injuries resulting in pain, swelling and discomfort. The aim of first aid should be to:

- make sure that no further injury occurs to you or the casualty
- treat any visible wound or pain
- obtain medical help if necessary
- note the time and cause of the injury, identifying the creature if possible.

See also Table 5.14.

Allergies

An allergy is sensitised reaction to a substance that is not generally thought to be harmful. These substances, known as allergens, may include pollen, foods, chemicals or drugs. Allergies can cause problems in one of three ways:

- respiratory allergies may result in asthma or hay fever
- intestinal allergies may result in vomiting or diarrhoea
- skin allergies may result in rashes.

Table 5.14 Treatment of bites and stings

Animal	Insect
<ul><li>Control bleeding by applying direct pressure and raising the injured part.</li><li>Cover the wound with a sterile dressing.</li><li>Take the casualty to an accident and emergency department.</li></ul>	<ul><li>If the casualty shows signs of anaphylactic shock (see below), dial 999 immediately and ask for an ambulance.</li><li>If possible, remove sting from wound with tweezers.</li><li>Apply a cold compress to the injury.</li><li>If the pain and swelling continue, advise the casualty to see a doctor.</li></ul>

Allergies very rarely result in a major medical emergency; generally, only minor treatment is required. This usually involves treating the symptoms with medication prescribed by a doctor. In very rare cases, however, an allergic reaction may result in anaphylactic shock.

Anaphylactic shock

Anaphylactic shock can be the result of a major allergic reaction to substances such as antibiotics, bee stings and peanuts. It is a very serious condition as death may occur within a few minutes. It causes the casualty's blood pressure to fall dramatically and makes breathing difficult. The face and neck may swell and the person may suffocate. A person suffering from anaphylactic shock urgently needs oxygen and a life-saving injection of adrenaline.

The signs of anaphylactic shock are:

- anxiety
- red blotchy skin
- swelling of the face and neck
- puffy eyes
- difficulty in breathing
- rapid pulse.

When responding to anaphylactic shock:

- dial 999 immediately and ask for an ambulance
- give as much information about the situation as you can
- help the casualty sit up to relieve breathing difficulties
- if the casualty become unconscious, put into the recovery position and prepare to resuscitate if necessary.

Did you know?

People who are at increased risk of anaphylactic shock, for example, because of a bee sting or peanut allergy, may carry adrenaline with them. When responding to anaphylactic shock, you should always check for medication and assist the casualty to use it.

Responding to an emergency

You are visiting an older client in his home. You walk in to find the client, who is known to have epilepsy, fitting on the wet, cramped, bathroom floor.

1 What are your immediate actions?

2 Describe in detail the symptoms of epilepsy.

The client stops fitting but does not regain consciousness and stops breathing.

3 Describe the life-saving techniques you would use on the client.

1   What is the difference between a risk and a hazard?

2   What is the name of the act responsible for maintaining health and safety in the workplace?

3   List the five steps you would take to assess risk in the workplace.

4   Who is responsible for implementing health and safety legislation?

5   Why is it necessary to record accidents?

6   Which regulations are concerned with the storage of chemicals hazardous to health?

7   Describe four things that you would check for on a bottle of prescription pills.

8   List three microorganisms that you may find in a healthcare setting.

9   How do microorganisms enter the body?

10   What colour extinguisher would be used to put out an electrical fire?

11   What does ABC stand for?

12   Define what is meant by a sprain.

13   How does arterial blood differ from venous blood?

14   What should you never do if someone is suffering an epileptic fit?

15   In the workplace, who should you inform if there has been an accident or injury?

References and further reading

References

● British Red Cross (2003) *New Practical First Aid*. London: Dorling Kindersley
● McGuiness, P. and Smith, L. (2004) *The Health and Safety Handbook*. London: Spiro Press
● Morris, S. and Willcocks, G. (1996) *Preventing Accidents and Illness at Work*. London: Pitman Publishing
● Ridley, J. (2004) *Health and Safety in Brief*. (3rd ed.) Oxford: Elsevier
● St Andrew's Ambulance Association, St John Ambulance Association and the British Red Cross (2006) *First Aid Manual*. London: Dorling Kindersley

Useful websites

The following websites can be accessed via the Heinemann website.
Go to www.heinemann.co.uk/hotlinks and enter the express code 4256P.

● BBC Health
● NHS Direct Online
● RoSPA (The Royal Society for the Prevention of Accidents)
● Health and Safety Executive – information on stress
● Department of Health
● The University of Edinburgh College of Medicine and Veterinary Medicine
● Business Link
● Food Standards Agency

CHAPTER 6

Research methods in health and social care

Key points

- All health and social care work is underpinned by good research.
- Research has to be planned and carried out systematically, and there are a number of key stages which must be completed, from planning through to evaluation.
- Primary research methods in health and social care include using questionnaires, interviews and observation.
- Primary research should be supported by secondary research.
- Data collected should be analysed and presented objectively and clearly.
- Good research methodology observes ethical principles and practice.

Introduction

The findings and outcomes from research underpin every aspect of health and social care. Worldwide, hundreds of journals, books and websites are devoted to reporting the findings of research projects relating to new developments in medicine and healthcare or the impact of new initiatives in social care. Almost every day, television and radio news bulletins report the outcomes of significant pieces of research relevant to the health and social care field. Health and social care practitioners need to be familiar with basic research methodology, whether in order to conduct their own small-scale research or to be able to evaluate work done by others.

Within this chapter you will learn about:

- why we should do research
- who does research
- key concepts in research
- primary and secondary research methods
- ethical issues in research
- the research process.

Chapter 6 is structured to allow you to follow the progress of a student, Jon, as he plans, implements, presents and evaluates a small-scale research project. You will consider Jon's choices at each stage, what he has done well, how he can learn from his mistakes and how he could have improved the project. Before you consider Jon's project, the wider context of the world of professional research, with particular reference to health and social care issues, will be described.

Why do research?

Figure 6.01 summarises the key purposes of research in health and social care.

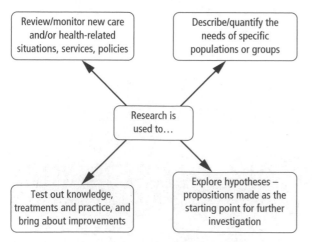

Figure 6.01 The purposes of research in health and social care

> **Research**
> The term research is used to denote a systematic enquiry designed to add to existing knowledge and/or solve a particular problem (Bell 1993: 2).

Over time, specific approaches and methods for carrying out such enquiries have developed, some of which are linked to particular disciplines. Laboratory experiments, for example, are often used when developing new drugs; clinical procedures might be set up in a controlled environment to assess, say, the impact of damage to the human brain after a stroke. Outside the laboratory environment, questionnaires may be used to find out how people respond to the provision of a new service, or the observation of behaviours might be employed to give an insight into the impact of a certain environment on how people interact.

Researchers will choose and adapt from a range of approaches and methods in order to seek answers to the questions or hypotheses they wish to test out. The important thing about all research is that whatever method is used, the findings should be reported systematically and scientifically, in as clear and honest a fashion as possible.

Who does research?

The short answer to this question is that anyone can do research. A brief trawl through the Yellow Pages to find out the names and addresses of all the local dentists is, in a sense, a piece of research. However, in this chapter you will consider some rather more elaborate research projects.

In the UK, there are a number of bodies that undertake research into health and social care issues. Some of these bodies are:

- universities
- hospitals
- the Medical Research Council
- the Research Council for Complementary Medicine
- the Prince of Wales' Foundation for Integrated Health
- private organisations such as large pharmaceutical companies.

In social care, there are a number of bodies in the UK that sponsor or promote research. The Joseph Rowntree Foundation, for example, sponsors research that impacts on the development of social policy, as does the Institute for Public Policy Research. These are only two of a number of bodies and organisations that promote social care related research.

Over to you

Using an Internet search engine, see how many organisations you can identify that conduct research into health or social care related issues. (The Joseph Rowntree Foundation publishes a list of useful websites.) Access one of these sites to find out what research is going on at the moment.

- *Who is paying for this work?*
- *What are the aims?*
- *What difference might it make when the findings are published?*

In the UK, the government initiates a great deal of research, sometimes in-house (within specific government departments) and sometimes commissioned from outside organisations and independent researchers. Such research is often concerned with establishing the cost-effectiveness of a particular government policy or initiative, ultimately aimed at enhancing the health and well-being of all sectors of the population. Each government department, such as the Department of Health, has its own website where details of ongoing and published research can be accessed easily. The Office for National Statistics (ONS) is the government department that deals with information from the National Census, the most recent of which was in 2001. The website for this department may be searched for easily accessible data on the population of England and Wales, with links to sources for Census data for Scotland and Northern Ireland (to access this site, go to www.heinemann.co.uk/hotlinks and enter the express code 4256P).

Demographic data provides an essential background to research studies of many kinds. It is fairly easy to access Census data, and the following exercise invites you to try this out for yourself.

Demography – the large-scale study of populations.

*Access the National Census data for your country of
residence. (For information on how to access this data,
go to www.heinemann.co.uk/hotlinks and enter the
express code 4256P.) Search the data for details of
your locality (this might be a town, city or small locality
such as one or two small **Output Areas**).*

See if you can identify:

- *the total population*
- *the population in terms of males and females (gender)*
- *how many people are aged over 75 years*
- *how many lone parent households there are*
- *how many people have a limiting long-term illness.*

Output Areas – the small local divisions within
which Census data is counted.

The study of populations can be very useful for
health and social care practitioners; the placing
of services is one obvious use of such data.

Dr John Snow and the Broad Street pump

Cholera is a highly infectious and potentially fatal
disease of the small intestine that causes severe
vomiting and diarrhoea. Until the late 1850s, it was
commonly believed that cholera was an airborne
disease. Matter such as rotting corpses or food
and the contents of sewers and cesspits were
considered to exude bad air, or 'miasma'. It was
thought that breathing in this miasma would result in
any number of diseases, including cholera.

Dr John Snow, a London anaesthetist, observed
incidents of cholera in the neighbourhood of
Soho, London, during the outbreak of August
and September 1854. He noticed that they were
clustered around a water pump in Broad Street.
He followed up his observations with a properly
documented study, including inspection of water
from the pump. He took a list of those who had died
of cholera from the General Register Office and then
made further enquiries about each of these people.

He found that nearly all the deaths were of people
living very close to this particular water pump. Five of
those who died lived closer to another water pump,

but on enquiry it was discovered that they always
sent for water from Broad Street. Nine people using
a local coffee shop which used the Broad Street
pump also died from cholera. A number of other
Broad Street residents, who worked for a local
brewery, always drank free beer provided by their
employer; none of these people were infected with
the disease.

Snow then persuaded the Board of Governors of St
James's parish to remove the handle of the Broad
Street pump to prevent its further use.

1 In what ways can Dr Snow's research be
considered properly scientific?
2 How does this story demonstrate the importance
of scientific research to maintaining public health?

Dr Snow supported his hypothesis with maps and
tables documenting the incidence of the disease.
He considered possible alternative explanations for
seeming anomalies (such as the apparent immunity
of the brewery workers). In 1857 he published a
paper in the *British Medical Journal* demonstrating
that customers of the Southwark water company
had a cholera death-rate that was six times higher
than customers of the Lambeth water company
(Halliday, 2001). Snow suggested that this was
because in Southwark, customers received water
drawn from a particularly polluted section of the
Thames. Initially, support for Snow's hypothesis was
limited, but after the 'Great Stink' of 1858, when
MPs were unable to enter the House of Commons
because of the smell from the Thames, the notion
that polluted water was the cause of diseases like
cholera was taken more seriously. Shortly after
this, the engineer Bazalgette was commissioned to
construct a new sewage system for London, and
this took much of the effluent away from the city.

Snow's **epidemiological** studies, in which he
rigorously tested his hypothesis about the spread
of cholera, led ultimately to improved sanitary
conditions in the City of London. His studies
provided a clear demonstration of the relationship of
disease and the environment, in this case between
cholera and polluted water.

Epidemiology – the study of the geographical
incidence of disease in order to demonstrate
potential causes (and cures).

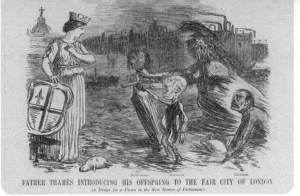

FATHER THAMES INTRODUCING HIS OFFSPRING TO THE FAIR CITY OF LONDON
(A Design for a Fresco in the New Houses of Parliament.)

The Great Stink of London, 1858. Before a proper sewage system was constructed, people in large cities suffered from diseases (including cholera) carried in polluted water

Demographic and epidemiological data is used constantly by politicians and service planners in order to explore the characteristics and needs of local populations, and to make informed decisions about new service developments or health interventions. An excellent example of the use of such data is provided by the Annual Report of the Chief Medical Officer (CMO), which can be accessed easily via the Department of Health website (to access the report, go to www.heinemann.co.uk/hotlinks and enter the express code 4256P). The report presents the recommendations of the CMO on a number of issues, based on research which is explained and fully referenced. Some of these recommendations are general to the whole population, such as the impact of smoking on skin ageing, the economic case for creating smoke-free workplaces, and the importance of early diagnosis of HIV (CMO's Report, Department of Health 2003). However, some recommendations are specific to local populations. For example, in 2003, the CMO's Report highlighted certain regional areas of concern for England, including that of the dental health of five-year-olds in the north-east. Using epidemiological data from dentists, the report notes a wide variation in the rates of decayed and filled teeth, from Hartlepool (average 0.86 per child) to South West Durham (average 2.82 per child). The report concludes that related factors are deprivation and the presence (or otherwise) of fluoridation, and notes that 'the provision of fluoridated water remains a priority in tackling inequality' (CMO Report 2003: 55).

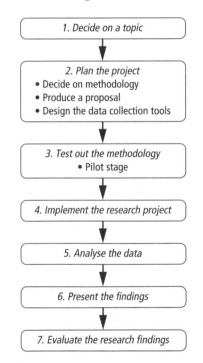

The process of research

Systematic research usually follows a series of steps, as shown in Figure 6.02.

1. Decide on a topic

2. Plan the project
• Decide on methodology
• Produce a proposal
• Design the data collection tools

3. Test out the methodology
• Pilot stage

4. Implement the research project

5. Analyse the data

6. Present the findings

7. Evaluate the research findings

Figure 6.02 Research usually follows a series of steps

In the rest of this chapter, you will track the progress of Jon, a mature student who is required to plan, implement and evaluate a piece of research on a topic of his choice, but which must be relevant to professional practice in health and social care.

Deciding on a topic

A starting point...

Jon is a care worker in a privately run residential establishment for older people. He is now working towards a care qualification, with a view to training as a social worker at some time in the future. He wants to broaden his knowledge of the care sector, so for his project he has chosen to study services for children and their families. He is also quite interested in the concept of community-based work, because so far his experience has been limited to residential care work.

As a starting point, Jon's tutor suggests that he should visit the local community-based social work team, to see what kinds of things are going on in his locality. He learns that there is a relatively new drop-in facility for mothers and toddlers based in a previously empty flat on a local council estate. This centre has been funded by Sure Start money. He visits the drop-in centre and talks to the manager. She suggests that Jon might like to evaluate the impact of the centre on the people who use it. This piece of work will be of interest not only to the manager, but also to planners at the Children's Services Authority who are responsible for the project.

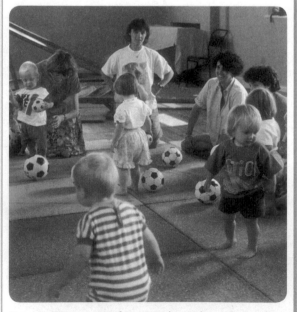

Drop-in centres are often popular with mothers who have young children

Did you know?

- Services for children are now being combined into new Children's Services Authorities. This means that the term Social Services will gradually be replaced. In some areas, Children's Trusts will be set up.

- Sure Start is a government-funded initiative that supports projects for young children and families. Local authorities can apply for funding to pay for schemes that will benefit this group of people.

Over to you

Find out what is happening to services for children in your local area. What existing services have been combined into the new Children's Services Authority? Is there a Children's Trust?

Finding the right place

When Jon discussed the Sure Start centre with the manager, he was curious to know why the local authority had decided to put it in this particular location. The manager explained that planners working for the council had used Census data to locate areas of potential need within the authority's boundaries.

The Census data had revealed a significant concentration of lone parent households with dependent children in two Output Areas. These two Output Areas were adjacent to each other. The council planners had then looked for suitable premises in both these areas, and the empty flat on this estate had been identified as being in a good place, close to bus routes and also shops.

Jon's research into the Sure Start centre will not be as far-ranging as some of the studies described in the previous paragraphs. However, he has to be just as clear about why he is doing it. Look back at Figure 6.01 on page 208, which sets out the key purposes of research. Jon's project comes into the category of reviewing a new care-related service in order to assess its impact on the people using it. In the next section, you will consider Jon's options in planning his project.

Planning a research project

> **Defining the research project**
>
> *Title:*
>
> **An investigation into the impact of the Fresh Start Centre in Crowdon, a new facility for parents and young children.**
>
> *Aims:*
>
> 1. To quantify service take up in this new facility in its first 12 months of operation.
> 2. To establish levels of user satisfaction by means of both quantitative and qualitative data.
> 3. To collect user views on future service developments.
> 4. To make recommendations to management about how current services could be improved and/or developed.

You will read more on what should be in a research proposal on page 231. Before Jon can actually write the proposal, he has to familiarise himself with a number of key concepts and a range of research methods. These are discussed in the following two sections.

Primary and secondary data

Researchers make a key distinction between primary and secondary data.

> **Primary data**
> The information collected by a researcher during the course of a study. Such information might include:
>
> - information from questionnaires
> - notes made during the observation of a person or group of people
> - notes/transcripts/recordings made during an interview
> - measurements and other data collected during experiments.

Jon's primary data will include the views of centre users collected by questionnaire and by a series of structured interviews. The following scenario describes the primary data collected by another researcher in a similar project.

You might have come up with the idea that Nas could take a video or tape recording of an actual reminiscence session. However, he would have to keep certain ethical issues in mind, as would anyone else about to embark on a research project involving information about people. Ethical issues are discussed more fully on pages 232–233, but it is important to stress that all data should be collected with permission and that everyone involved should be given full details of the project (how information will be collected and used). Nobody should be coerced into taking part, and if someone refuses to do so, this should be respected.

Did you know?

*A piece of primary research becomes secondary when it is **cited** by someone else in another study.*

Citation – the act of making reference to another piece of research.

Over to you

Working from the research that you identified in the activity on page 209, find out what secondary data might be available to you if you wanted to investigate further. For example, if you are interested in a particular medical or pharmacological treatment, where might you look for other instances of similar experimental or clinical work?

A specific use of secondary data is known as triangulation. Sometimes, particularly in large-scale studies, researchers will cross-check their findings by collecting data from a number of different sources and informants. A case study of group behaviours in a mental health day centre, for example, may be compared with data from a different centre elsewhere. Such a comparison will allow a more balanced account to be made of observed behaviours.

Jon's secondary data includes statistics produced by the council's own research department. These statistics show how many mothers have been using the centre, where they live, their age and the ages of their children. These figures show the times at which the centre is most heavily used. Jon also looks at the Census data collected and used by the council researchers, showing why this location was chosen for the new service. All these figures have been published by the council in a report on the centre.

The data also reveal a puzzle. Although the original Census data showed three Output Areas with a high number of lone-parent households (Upton, Crowdon and Snaresley), centre users come mainly from only two of these areas; hardly anybody using the centre lives in Snaresley. This has been pointed out in the council report and Jon thinks this is worth investigating.

Setting research aims

Setting clear goals and aims for a study is critical. The aims dictate the methodology and the kind of data collected. Clarity at an early stage is vital in order to avoid bad practice such as collection of irrelevant data or time wasting (both of data subjects and the researcher).

Quantitative and qualitative data

Quantifiable data is useful to a researcher because it allows conclusions or inferences to be drawn. (The interpretation of data will be discussed more fully on page 235). The production of quantitative data is an important element of scientific enquiry. For example, it would be unscientific to say 'most of' the participants in a study responded well to a certain treatment; this means little in scientific terms. It is more meaningful to quantify this and to state that, for example, 80 per cent of participants in a clinical trial of 3000 people responded well to the same treatment. Note, too, that in a well-conducted research study, both the results of the treatment and the total number of people in the sample are quantified (see page 218 for sampling methods).

Even in studies whose primary aim is to collect quantitative data, researchers will often collect qualitative information to supplement the hard facts. A real-life study that skilfully combines both quantitative and qualitative data is the University of York's study of Hartrigg Oaks (see below).

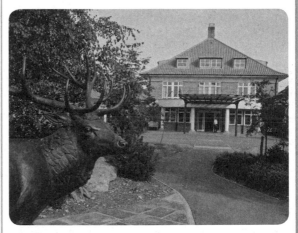

The University of York study used a range of data collection methods to provide both qualitative and quantitative data. The first report, published in 2003, provides quantitative data in the form of tables and bar charts, giving basic statistical information (numbers of residents, age profiles, short-term use of the facility, etc.) and information about satisfaction levels. Some of the latter is expressed quantitatively (for example, a bar chart showing satisfaction levels), whilst qualitative data is given in the form of direct quotations of residents' observations and comments. Researchers used two postal surveys, face-to-face interviews and discussion groups with both staff and residents to gather the evaluative data. The full report is available from the Joseph Rowntree Foundation.

To find out more about the Joseph Rowntree Foundation and Hartrigg Oaks, go to www.heinemann.co.uk/hotlinks and enter the express code 4256P.

Structured and unstructured data

These two terms refer to methods of data collection. Broadly speaking, data that is collected in a structured way can be quantified, whereas unstructured data cannot.

First steps

Jon is starting his enquiries into the use of the centre with an open mind. He doesn't ask people to fill in questionnaires at this point; although he does have some questions of his own, he is prepared simply to listen to centre users talking about their experiences. Jon hopes this will give him clues about what will be worth researching in a more structured way.

The centre manager invites Jon along to a morning session at the Sure Start centre. The centre users have been told that Jon is coming to talk to them, and he arrives at about coffee time.

Jon uses **open questions** such as 'What do you think about the new centre?' and 'Who do you think I need to talk to?' Jon is happy to let the centre users talk about what is important to them, and the discussion moves naturally to the issue of transport. Getting to and from the centre is a problem for some people. Some of the group also state they would like to have a greater say in how the centre is run.

Jon makes notes after the session, which he discusses with the manager to make sure he hasn't left out anything important.

Open question – a question that cannot be answered with 'yes' or 'no'; it requires a response to be made in the person's own words.

Although Jon did ask some questions, the data was collected in an unstructured way because he allowed people to respond in their own words and to raise whatever topics they wanted to. During the next stage of his project, Jon will be collecting some more structured data by means of questionnaires. Structured data is standardised in that **respondents** are required to decide between a number of options. (There is much more on structured data in the sections on primary research methods, pages 218–231, and analysing results, pages 235–241.)

Respondent – a person who takes part in a survey and who responds to the questions (either by self-completion of a questionnaire or during interview).

Both structured and unstructured data can be equally valuable to any research project. Figure 6.03 shows a specimen questionnaire designed to collect both structured and unstructured data.

The first two questions on the form in Figure 6.03 collect structured data. This can be analysed numerically: the researcher can add up the responses to each question and then express the results in terms of numbers or percentages. For example, the results might show that 40 per cent of respondents considered the community centre to offer a good service, 40 per cent considered the service to be average and 20 per cent thought the service to be poor.

In contrast, the second part of the questionnaire makes no attempt to structure what people want to say and, in theory, any responses are possible here. Of course, it is always possible that the researcher can classify these 'free-ranging' responses into broad areas. He or she might be

COMMUNITY CENTRE: USER SATISFACTION SURVEY

How many times a week do you visit the centre?
(Please enter number in the box)

Do you consider the service provided to be:
(Please tick the relevant box)

Good

Average

Poor

Use this space to make any comments you wish about the community centre.

_____

_____

_____

_____

_____

Figure 6.03 Specimen questionnaire designed to collect both structured and unstructured data

able to say, from such an analysis, that about 30 per cent of respondents indicated they would like to see different opening hours to the ones currently operating, or that 23 per cent found the centre difficult to access due to mobility problems. However, because of the unstructured way this information is collected, any conclusions drawn will have to be cautious and may need further investigation.

Over to you

Design a very short questionnaire for self-completion by a group of people aged over 75 years. The aim is to find out either what medication or what services respondents are receiving.

Some specialised terminology

Jon is now familiar with the terms qualitative and quantitative. He can also distinguish between structured and unstructured methods of data collection, and between primary and secondary research. There are two more terms that he needs to be able to use appropriately, and these are

subject and population. Jon is familiar with the term subject to refer to a topic for study, such as English or Science. Similarly, he has been familiar with the term population with respect to the people who live in a specified locality, such as Glasgow or Australia. However, in research, these words have different meanings.

Subject
In research, this word refers to the person or people who are being studied. The centre users are thus the subjects of Jon's study.

Population
In research terminology, the population is the total number of people being studied. In Jon's study, all the centre users are potentially part of the survey population.

Armed with these new concepts, and the information from his secondary research, Jon can now move forward to consider what primary research methods he will use.

Primary research methods

Sampling

One of the first tasks of any researcher is to define the population that will be studied. In a small-scale study, the choice of population may be relatively straightforward. In the Hartrigg Oaks study (see page 215), all the residents of this community formed the population targeted by postal questionnaire. In the scenario on page 213, Nas is studying the impact of reminiscence sessions on older people in a residential unit. His main population for study is thus all those residents who attended the sessions. Similarly, as there are at present about 50 parents using the Sure Start centre, in theory Jon can include all of these people in his study.

However, sometimes it is not possible to include all relevant subjects within the scope of a piece of research. It would be very difficult, for example, to measure the physiological changes resulting from smoking by studying every single smoker in the UK. This would involve testing possibly hundreds of thousands of individuals, and the logistical problems would be immense. For larger-scale studies such as this, a procedure known as sampling is necessary in order to reduce the population to a manageable size.

> **Sampling**
> Sampling is the selection of a representative cross-section of the population being studied.

Opportunity sampling

Sometimes, even when a population is well-defined, the researcher may have to be content with whoever is available to form the subject group. Not everyone may be prepared to take part in a survey, for example, and some people may be willing but not able to attend. Similarly, members of a group that is being observed may not all be present at the time the observation is made. This is very likely to be the case in a small-scale study where time and human resources are limited.

Who is available?

The total population of Jon's study is comprised of everyone who uses the centre, and these people will be invited to answer general questions by means of a questionnaire. However, Jon plans to collect some more detailed information, and it will not be possible to interview everybody in such depth. Opportunity sampling will result in interviews with those people who have the time and are willing to help Jon in this way.

Random sampling

Researchers may use a number of different sampling methods to arrive at the population of a study. One such method is known as random sampling. Before this can be done, a sampling frame has to be drawn up. This is basically a comprehensive list of potential subjects.

If, for example, researchers want to monitor the effectiveness of a new diagnostic technique designed to pick up early signs of cancer in older women, the total population may be defined as all women living in a certain area aged 50 years plus. One way to make a random sample would be firstly to ask all GP surgeries in that area to print out lists of all female patients of that age. This list would then be the sampling frame. The next stage would be to select names from that list, perhaps every tenth one, in order to give a smaller scale list of subjects for study. A better way to ensure a truly random sample would be to generate a random list of numbers by computer, and then to ask GPs to produce those names corresponding to the numbered places on the sampling frame list.

Stratified random sampling

Sometimes, researchers will want to use a different sampling technique, especially if it is important to make sure that key sub-groups within a given population are properly represented.

Suppose, for example, that the objective is to establish satisfaction levels among people using a new community outreach scheme. An initial survey of everyone using the scheme might be done easily by using a very simple questionnaire, but there may be too many users to do in-depth interviews with everyone. The sampling frame would be the list of all people known to use the service. However, if the list showed that there were far more women than men using the scheme (for example, 70 per cent of users were women), researchers would need to make sure that the sample chosen for the in-depth interviews represented this 70:30 gender split. This means that if 100 people were selected for interview, 70 must be women and only 30 should be men. This technique is known as proportionate stratified sampling.

There is yet another kind of stratified random sampling known as disproportionate random sampling. Suppose, for example, that a very small number of people using the outreach scheme are from a particular ethnic community. Perhaps only five people are from this cultural group and they represent less than 1 per cent of the total population of the study. If proportionate stratified sampling were to be used, only 1 out of 100 people selected for interview would be from this group. However, if cultural issues were felt to be important then researchers might want to ensure that the views of all five people in this cultural group were recorded. There might be important reasons why people from this group were not using the outreach facility, and interviewing all five people might provide important information for service planners.

Quota sampling

Yet another sampling technique is known as quota sampling. This is often used by market researchers, who might be instructed to stop a specified number of, for example, men of a certain age in the street, and then to ask questions, perhaps about a particular product or service. Suppose a council wanted to assess reactions to a new one-stop shop facility in a shopping centre, then the quota sampling method might involve interviewers stopping 100 men and 100 women as they left the premises, in order to get their views on the service.

It may not be necessary for you to show that you can use these more sophisticated sampling techniques. However, awareness of these techniques may help you to evaluate the research of others.

Questionnaires

Jon is going to collect the structured data for his study by means of questionnaires. Questionnaires can be issued to respondents for them to complete by themselves or they can be completed by the researcher during an interview. Jon will be using both methods to obtain his data. Self-completion questionnaires will be posted to all centre users (the centre administrator will do this for him), and later Jon will hold interviews with ten centre users. His analysis of the ethnicity of centre users leads him to target five centre users in particular (see below), but the remaining five are made up of people who are able and willing to take part. (The advice in this section applies mainly to the self-completion situation.)

When questionnaires are self-completed, clear instructions must be given and the form must be user-friendly and easy to complete. Short, simple forms are more likely to be completed fully than long, complicated ones.

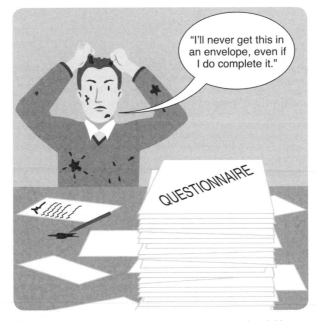

Figure 6.04 Self-completed questionnaires should be short, simple forms, not long, complicated ones

The distinction between structured and unstructured data was discussed on pages 216–217, and a mini-questionnaire was shown giving examples of questions designed to collect both types of data (Figure 6.03). To recap: structured data is that which can be expressed numerically, whilst unstructured data is less easy to quantify.

Questions to collect unstructured data

Unstructured data is usually collected by means of the verbal or open question. Open questions cannot be answered simply with 'yes' or 'no', so a respondent has to find his or her own words to give an answer. Open questions usually begin with the words 'what', 'why' and 'how'. For example:

- What are your views about the meals on wheels service in your locality?
- What differences have you observed as a result of taking this drug?
- Why did you choose to use this service?
- How are you feeling as a result of having acupuncture?

Open questions are useful in questionnaires for collecting qualitative data, such as respondents' views or opinions, or where researchers are interested in exploring all angles of an issue. This may be in addition to quantitative data collected in the structured part of the form. Sometimes, such qualitative data can be analysed and expressed numerically, especially if the researcher can detect a trend in the responses. However, you need to be very experienced in order to do this well, particularly if there are a lot of questionnaires to analyse.

Questions to collect structured data

There are a number of different options when seeking to collect structured data by questionnaire, six of which are set out in Table 6.01 below (following Bell 1993: 76–77).

The *list* (Table 6.01) is useful when you want to establish which of several options applies to each of your subjects. A respondent can tick as many items in the list as are applicable. You may also want to pre-code items in the list for ease of analysis (analysing and presenting data is discussed further on page 241).

With the *category* type of question, a respondent will tick only one of a number of boxes and, again, you may wish to pre-code each item for future analysis. As with lists, it is often useful to add the category 'Other' to allow for options that you may not have anticipated.

The *ranking* type of question is normally used to establish the relative importance that a respondent attaches to specific characteristics, qualities or even services. For example, you might use this method to find out which activities potential users of leisure services might value and use.

The *scale* has a similar use to the ranking type of question, and can be employed to ask respondents to attach values to specific characteristics or services. In the example in Table 6.01, people have been asked to rate the service provided at the local GP surgery. Here, respondents have been allowed a choice of five scores, allowing them to select a mid-point score if they feel ambivalent about an issue. Some researchers would offer only a four-point scale (e.g. Excellent, Good, Fair, Poor), as it is claimed that a five-point scale allows people to sit on the fence and leads to meaningless scores of 'average'. However, others criticise the four-point scale on the grounds that it can polarise scores artificially; people may be genuinely ambivalent about certain issues and should have the opportunity to express this. Forcing respondents to choose between 'better' and 'worse' ends of a scale may not necessarily lead to meaningful scores.

The *grid* can be used to express more than one parameter at the same time, and does the job of collating the data into more than one category. An example is shown in Table 6.02. Using this example would mean that the researcher could produce tables to show the total number of people using types of service and the number using each type of supplier. Preferences towards

Type	Example
List	Which of the following services do you use? (Please tick those that apply to you.) • Home care • Meals service • Residential care • Other (please specify)
Category	Which of the following age groups do you belong to? (Please tick one category only.) • 19 years or under • 20–25 years • 26–30 years • 31 years or over
Ranking	Place the following leisure activities in order of their importance to you by giving a number to each (1 = least important, 5 = most important): • swimming • movement and music • art classes • drama group • craft activities.
Quantity	How many times have you visited your GP in the last six months? (Please enter the number of times in the box.)
Scale	The service given at my local GP surgery is: Excellent Good Average Fair Poor 1 2 3 4 5 (Please circle the number that most closely corresponds to your opinion.)
Grid	(An example of a grid to collect data is given in Table 6.02).

Table 6.01 Question types: structured data collection

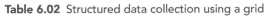

Please indicate by ticking the appropriate boxes which services you receive and who provides them.

	Council	Age Concern	NHS	Private company	Don't use this service
Day facilities					
Meals service					
Chiropody					
Community nurse					

Table 6.02 Structured data collection using a grid

particular types of supplier would show up, for example, if the people in the sample preferred the Age Concern day facilities over and above those provided by the council.

Using one or more of these types of structured questions will provide you with data that can be analysed numerically, even if it concerns people's views and opinions of something. In practice, researchers often use a number of different types of question on the same questionnaire, although they keep it simple by grouping question types together. Structured questions can be supplemented by unstructured data collection on the same form.

The closed question can also be used on a self-completion questionnaire. A closed question can be answered with a 'yes' or 'no', and can be useful in determining which categories a respondent falls into. For example:

- Do you use medication to control your condition?
- Does your child need physiotherapy?
- Do you need help getting in and out of bed?

The closed question can also be used in conjunction with a technique known as routing. If a respondent answers in a certain way to a closed question, then he or she can be redirected on to a different part of the form. For example:

- Question 3: Do you use medication to control your condition? If your answer is 'no', please go straight to question 7.

In the above example, questions 4, 5 and 6 would then deal with aspects of taking medication. (The person who answered 'no' at this point would not need to answer these particular questions.)

Questionnaire design and layout

It is important to give careful consideration to the design of a questionnaire, which should be neither too complex nor too long. Points to consider regarding questionnaire design include:

- type the questionnaire
- consider the font size and design – will any of your respondents have visual problems?
- use plenty of white space: this aids clarity
- make instructions clear
- explain abbreviations, acronyms and specialised terms (jargon)
- if using tick-boxes, align to the right-hand side of the sheet
- leave complex questions to the end
- avoid 'leading' questions
- avoid ambiguity.

Over to you

Go back to the questionnaire you designed earlier (page 217). In light of what you have studied in this section, consider whether you might revise this questionnaire to include other types of question. Would you alter the layout or change the number of questions? Redesign the questionnaire accordingly.

Interviews

Interviews can be structured, unstructured or semi-structured in the way they are designed and carried out. In practice, an interviewer may opt to use a combination of these techniques. Whichever method you use, an important pre-consideration is to value and respect your interview subjects.

Planning an interview

Thorough planning is essential to conducting successful interviews. There are a number of practical considerations to bear in mind, and these are set out in Table 6.03.

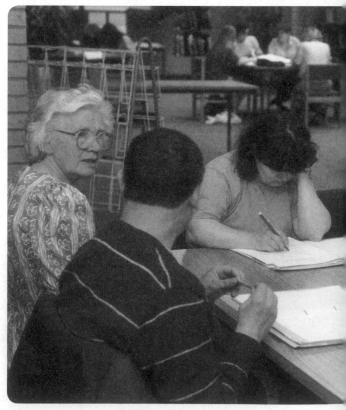

Facilitated sessions are often used to empower people with learning disabilities to express themselves

Time	Choose times that are mutually convenient for both interviewees and yourself. Make sure that your interview sessions don't clash with something else that people would normally be doing.
Pacing	Don't take on too many interviews at one time. Conducting even one interview can be very tiring, depending on its length and content.
Venue	Choose a venue that is convenient for everybody who is going to be involved. It should be suitable for holding private, quiet conversations. The room needs to be comfortable, neither too hot nor too cold, and well-ventilated.
Furniture	Furniture should be comfortable, but not so comfortable as to cause drowsiness. Consider whether you will need a table to lean on (to take notes) or whether you will have your papers on a clip-board.
Accessibility	This is another factor to consider with respect to the venue. If you or your respondents have mobility problems for example, you will need to make sure that everyone has easy access to the building/room you have chosen.
Additional help	Consider whether you will need a signer (for deaf people) or an interpreter. You may have your own sensory or language needs. In either case, you will need to check whether the venue is adequate to accommodate yourself, your subjects and any helper who is present. Similarly, people with learning disabilities may require the presence of an advocate or care worker.
Recording unstructured data	Consider whether you will use a tape recorder, take notes yourself or have a second person to take notes. (Note: the interviewee must be quite comfortable with whatever method of recording you choose.)

Table 6.03 Checklist for preparing to conduct an interview session

Structured and semi-structured interviews

In the structured interview, the researcher uses a schedule which might be very similar to the self-completion questionnaire. The interviewer will read out each question, completing or ticking the boxes and circling the relevant responses as required. If the respondent doesn't understand something, the interviewer can explain further.

When conducting a structured interview, the researcher aims to ask the questions in the same way for each respondent. This is to make sure that the data collected is standardised, and to minimise **bias**.

> **Bias** – distortion of the results of a piece of research, due to the undue influence of a specific factor.

Some advantages of structured interviews are:

- all or most of the questions are likely to be answered (respondents may leave unanswered questions in a self-completed questionnaire)
- the risk of misunderstanding of questions is minimised
- the risk of collusion between respondents is avoided
- the interviewer can dictate the pace of the interview
- additional responses/reactions may be observed by the interviewer
- problems of reading, writing and comprehension can be overcome
- quantitative data will be produced in a standardised way
- sensory and physical problems can be overcome.

The interviewer may also have a list of prompts or probes to help respondents provide further detail in specific areas.

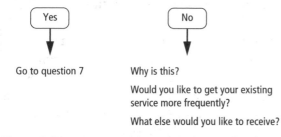

6. Do you consider that you receive enough practical support?

Yes → Go to question 7

No → Why is this?

Would you like to get your existing service more frequently?

What else would you like to receive?

Figure 6.05 Using prompts to obtain more detail

In Figure 6.05, the technique of routing is also used. If the respondent answers 'Yes' to question 6, then the interviewer moves straight on to question 7. If the answer is 'no', then the interviewer moves to a series of prompts to elicit some further data from the respondent.

This use of a combination of question types is also known as semi-structured interviewing. This method involves starting from a list of prepared questions, but then allowing the respondent to answer these in his or her own words. In the example above, the respondent is steered towards a number of aspects of service delivery. The technique can also be used to allow interview subjects to introduce their own themes within a given topic.

Unstructured interviewing

Unstructured data collection occurs when interviewees are allowed to talk about anything they want to, without any further prompting on the part of the interviewer. Although the interviewer will probably initiate the topic, there will subsequently be little attempt to control what the subject wants to disclose. This method is also known as in-depth interviewing, as it often allows a respondent to say what he or she really thinks about something.

An example of an opening prompt for an unstructured (in-depth) interview with a young person is 'Hi, how are you doing?' In this example, which is from a research study into the attitudes of young people, the researcher wants to know what is important to her subjects and doesn't want to be prescriptive about the topics to be discussed. There is no pre-designed schedule, and although the researcher might be interested in some specific topics (like drug use, for example) the course of the interview will actually be led by the young person. The original interview may be tape-recorded, and a technique known as **discourse analysis** then used to analyse what happened, so the interviewer can establish the key issues and concerns for each subject. Subsequently, the researcher may want to conduct further interviews which are more structured in design.

> **Discourse analysis** – a research technique in which speech or conversation is recorded and then analysed to determine how someone uses and structures language.

In practice, and in the context of specific research, it is likely that the researcher will want to retain ultimate control of the interview, whether or not it is structured, semi-structured or unstructured.

Table 6.04 Collecting semi-structured data

Topic	Open questions/prompts
Social circumstances	Tell me about yourself. What's it like where you live?
Health	Tell me about your current state of health. What's your state of health like at the moment?
Service use	Why do you come to this drop-in centre? Tell me about the things you do here.

Observation

Another method of data collection is observation. Observation is often used when making case studies (for example, observing aspects of service use in a mental health drop-in centre) or ethnographic studies (for example, watching the interaction of a group of young children and adults). It can also be used in conjunction with the experimental method. An example of this might be when two groups are observed separately, one of which is subject to certain conditions and the other is not. The objective in this case is to see if there are noticeable behavioural differences between the two groups.

Observation can be by a participant observer (someone who takes part in the activities with the subjects of the study) or a non-participant observer. Table 6.05 describes the key differences in techniques used for each of these observational research methods (for more on this see Bell 1993: 109–21).

One of the problems with the participant method of observation is that subjects will often modify their behaviour simply because of the presence of a stranger (the researcher). This is sometimes referred to as the observer's paradox.

When using the observational method, it is extremely important to decide exactly what is being measured or recorded. Bell (1993: 111) notes that the focus of observation is usually one or more of the following:

- content (what happens)
- process (the way in which something happened)

Figure 6.06 Specimen observation sheet

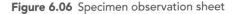

Observing social interaction in individuals using a day unit for people with a learning disability

Group: _____
Number in group: _____
Date: _____
Time from: _____ To: _____

Aim:

Activity during observation:

Are there any 'friendship groups' evident within the group as a whole?
_____

Are there any individuals who appear not to get involved with the activity?
_____

Are there any obvious group leaders?
_____

Are there any individuals who seek more attention from the session tutor than the others?
_____

Do people share equipment with each other?
_____

Do people help each other?
_____

Are there any individuals who appear to be actively avoiding interaction with the others?
_____

Candidate's Signature: _____
Supervisor's Signature: _____

Notes:

Type of observation	Techniques used
Participant	• Researcher works/lives alongside the subjects of the study. • Data collection is often unstructured. • The researcher records significant behaviour, situations and events.
Non-participant	• Researcher watches events whilst remaining as unobtrusive as possible. • May use grids or charts to record what goes on (e.g. interaction between individuals in a group). • The process may be video-recorded or tape-recorded.

Table 6.05 Observational research methods

- interaction (how participants respond or react to each other)
- the way in which participants contribute to what is going on
- specific aspects of behaviour (e.g. violence, concentration span).

There are some very sophisticated classification systems for describing behaviour which are too complex for inclusion here. These are discussed and documented in Bell (1993: 112–14).

Experiments and trials

Experiments and trials involve the setting up of specific situations in order to test the validity of particular theories or hypotheses. Experiments are often concerned with establishing causal relationships, for example, that music therapy helps control post-operative pain. In principle, the researcher is in control of all the variables and parameters within an experiment, which should provide quantitative data for analysis. A good experiment is capable of replication, that is, it can be repeated using exactly the same conditions in order for several sets of results to be compared. If results are similar over a number of experiments, firm conclusions may be made from the data.

Some experiments are relatively straightforward to design and control, such as the testing of pharmaceutical products. Currently, the gold-standard for the testing of medical knowledge and treatments is the randomised clinical controlled trial (RCCT). A sampling frame will be set up according to certain pre-defined criteria (for example, age, medical condition) and a population selected at random from this sampling frame. This group will receive the new drug. A second, or control, group (which satisfies the same criteria as the first group) will either receive no treatment, a **placebo** or the existing standard treatment. Experiments can also be used to compare and contrast the impact of different kinds of treatment on people with the same medical condition.

Placebo – something that looks like a medical intervention, but which is in fact inactive.

When a large number of such trials have taken place, researchers can then take a look at all the results by means of a systematic review. Such a review will be able to assemble the evidence for a particular intervention in a range of settings and patient groups. This kind of research activity is called meta-analysis, and it can sometimes reveal a common 'global' outcome from specific research.

Systematic reviews are extremely important in the production of guidance for practitioners. The National Institute for Health and Clinical Excellence (NICE) provides national guidance (in England and Wales) on the promotion of health and the prevention and treatment of ill-health. NICE's guidelines are based on reviews of clinical and economic evidence. NICE also invites interested parties such as manufacturers, patients, carers and health professionals to give evidence on the use and effectiveness of specific interventions and treatments. The resulting guidelines are then publicly available to patients, professionals and carers. You can access the NICE website by going to www.heinemann.co.uk/hotlinks and entering the express code 4256P.

Early intervention in Multiple Sclerosis: a longitudinal study

Multiple Sclerosis (MS) is a condition in which the immune system goes into overdrive, and the body's immune cells actually start to attack the myelin sheath in the white matter of the spinal cord.

Researchers want to test out the hypothesis that early intervention with people who have MS has a greater impact on the progression of this disease than treatment which is given at a later stage. The scientists have recruited 180 patients known to be in the early stages of MS, two-thirds of whom will receive a new drug, Campath-1H. The remaining third of the sample will receive Beta Interferon, which is currently quite commonly used to treat this disease. Subjects in both groups will be monitored regularly for five years, and the final results will not be available for seven years. (Coles and Cox, 2002)

1 In an experimental study, how can researchers avoid influencing results?
2 In this trial, the participants will not know which drug they have been given and the scientists will not know who has received each drug. This is known as a 'double-blind' technique. How relevant is this technique to experimental research?

This kind of project is known as a **longitudinal study** because it lasts for a significant period of time. This particular study contrasts two groups, one receiving a new treatment and the other a conventional, existing treatment. Researchers can avoid prejudicing the outcome of an experiment by not telling subjects which group they belong to. This eliminates any possible psychological bias. This is considered to be even more effective when researchers themselves do not know which group subjects have been allocated to. This 'double-blind' technique is often used when the control group receives a placebo rather than another pharmaceutical product.

> **Longitudinal study** – a research study that lasts for a significant period of time, allowing the impact of a number of variables to be taken into account.

Sometimes, the results of research are inconclusive or even controversial. The current debate on the safety of the combined MMR (Measles, Mumps and Rubella) vaccine is an interesting example of this.

In the late 1990s, Dr Andrew Wakefield published research suggesting a possible link between the MMR vaccine and the condition known as autism, together with associated bowel and gut abnormalities (Wakefield 1998). As a result of subsequent media coverage, many parents stopped having their children vaccinated with the combined drug, despite advice to the contrary from the government and health officials.

The debate on the safety of the MMR vaccine has continued since 1998. There are still researchers who dispute the official Department of Health conclusions and advice, and the debate continues within the scientific community. The government's position on this, together with a list of research articles, can be accessed via the Department of Health website. A conflicting view can be explored via the What Doctors Don't Tell You website. (To access both of these sites, go to www.heinemann.co.uk/hotlinks and enter the express code 4256P.)

1 What are your views on this particular issue?
2 Would you let your child be vaccinated with the combined MMR vaccine?
3 What are the advantages and risks of this procedure?

Experiments to measure or predict human behaviour are harder to set up and control. Nevertheless, researchers, especially psychologists, do use the experimental method to investigate aspects of human behaviour. They often combine the setting up of an experimental situation with aspects of the observational method of data collection. (See pages 232–233 for the ethical implications of such research.)

Action research

Action research is a method that focuses on a particular task or problem. The project is conducted by a number of people (often a group of colleagues) who regularly review and monitor aspects of an issue in order to make decisions about how it should be tackled.

The term 'action research' derives from the fact that the actions of practitioners are the focus of study; it is categorised as research because whatever happens during a project is recorded just as systematically as for an observation or an experiment. The practitioner-researcher involved in such a study will also engage in reflection on his or her own practice, in order to evaluate what happens, to draw conclusions, and to make recommendations for the benefit of other practitioners.

An example might be that of a group of health staff who want to make improvements in the way that individuals are assessed and then admitted to a treatment programme. Staff keep diaries of what is going on, interview individuals and analyse service data. They also analyse their own responses and reactions to situations as these develop. As time goes by, they will introduce changes to the system and then monitor the impact of those changes. In a sense, therefore, the practitioner engaging in action research is both the subject and object of the study, and this method also provides a means by which a health or social care professional can further his or her own professional development.

As this method usually involves the collaboration of a group of people over time in the context of an ongoing work situation, it is unlikely to be relevant to a small-scale project. However, the findings of other action research projects may provide useful secondary information.

Case studies

Case studies involve the in-depth observation, description and analysis of a particular situation. A case study might involve just one person or it might encompass a total situation, such as a group of people in a therapy group or an early years' class.

The case study method involves several techniques and might combine observation with, for example, interviews, surveys, the keeping of logs and diaries and, in particular, the recording of 'critical incidents' which may have a bearing on what is being studied.

Critical details

Researchers want to assess the usefulness of a new piece of equipment designed for assisting people with disabilities to move between the bed and a chair. They ask care assistants in a residential unit to try out the equipment when appropriate, keeping diaries of what they do. In particular, they want care assistants to note any difficulties and record any specific incidents – good or bad – relating to the new device. They also ask the individuals who have been assisted to keep similar diaries.

After a six-week period, researchers study the diaries and accounts of the critical incidents. They also interview care assistants and residents to obtain further qualitative data. The number of occasions on which difficulties were experienced (and the types of difficulty encountered) can be expressed quantitatively.

1 Can you see any potential difficulties with the diary technique of data collection?

2 How objective might such data be? Does this matter?

You might want to combine the use of questionnaires with one or more of these research techniques, depending on the topic.

Research methods: some advantages and disadvantages

There are advantages and disadvantages to the major methods of data collection – questionnaire, interview and observation, and research methods should always be chosen keeping these in mind. By doing this, you can use one or more methods to best advantage whilst avoiding the potential for error and bias which is inherent in each. Tables 6.06–6.10 list the advantages and disadvantages of different research methods, for you to consider.

Table 6.06 Self-completion questionnaires

Advantages	Disadvantages
• Relatively cheap. • Can include a large number of participants. • Some respondents may prefer this to being interviewed. • No danger that interviewer can influence the answers.	• Questions may be misunderstood. • Respondents may collude in answering the questions. • Some questionnaires may not be returned (especially if being sent by post). • Some questions may be left unanswered. • Some responses may be hard to understand. • Questions may be wrongly completed (e.g. two boxes ticked instead of one).

Table 6.07 Using questionnaires in interviews

Advantages	Disadvantages
• All questions will be answered. • All questionnaires will be completed. • Interviewer can ask extra questions (via probes). • Data will be uniform if researcher uses same format each time. • Interviewer may also collect extra (unstructured) data.	• Requires more researcher time (and, therefore, usually involves a smaller sample). • Respondents may be hard to contact/convenient times may be hard to arrange. • Respondent may give answers he or she thinks the researcher wants (bias). • Respondent may take a dislike to the interviewer (bias). • Questionnaire format may restrict responses.

Table 6.08 Unstructured interviews

Advantages	Disadvantages
• Much qualitative data will be collected. • Respondents can say exactly what they think and feel. • Interviewer can probe/follow through on any topic of interest. • Useful at the planning stages of a research project.	• Very time consuming, so sample may need to be smaller. • Interviewer needs very good communication skills. • Potential for bias because of personality of interviewer. • Applicability of results may be limited. • Very hard to produce quantitative data. • Findings may be limited to sample group.

Table 6.09 Non-participant observation

Advantages	Disadvantages
• Observer can watch subjects in their own environment. • Observer may see behaviours that subjects are not aware of. • Useful for non-literate subjects, e.g. young children. • Both interpersonal interactions and group behaviours can be observed. • May be recorded to view again.	• Some ethical problems – especially if the observation is secret. • Observer may misinterpret behaviour. • Some behaviour may be missed if note-taking is recording method. • What happens may not be relevant to the aim of the research. • Behaviours may be affected if the observer is visible to the group.

Table 6.10 Participant observation

Advantages	Disadvantages
• Observer gains in-depth and accurate knowledge of group behaviours. • Valid data is produced. • Can give access to hard-to-reach or closed groups (e.g. homeless people).	• Presence of observer will inevitably affect behaviours to some extent ('observer's paradox'). • Ethical problems if observer does not disclose true identity. • Time consuming. • Advanced social skills needed. • Observer may lose sense of objectivity. • Non-acceptance by group may limit value of data.

It takes courage, time and dedication to become a participant-observer, and there are also ethical issues involved if the researcher's true identity is withheld. Recording and publishing details of people's behaviour without their permission is arguably bad practice. However, it should be possible to gain permission before engaging in an observation exercise. Spending time with a group to allow them to become accustomed to your presence before data collection starts is not only courteous to the subjects but also increases the chances of natural behaviours being observed.

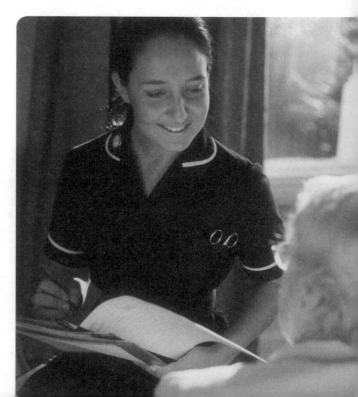

The semi-structured interview combines the advantages of both the structured and unstructured approaches

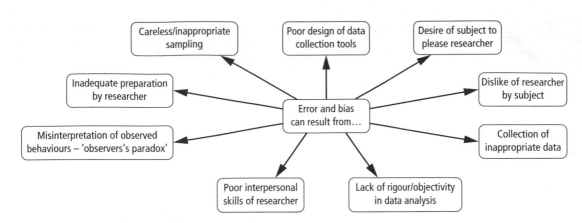

Figure 6.07 Sources of error and bias in research: a summary

Drawing up a research proposal

Once Jon has familiarised himself with the key concepts in research, together with the range of data collection methods available, he can write a research proposal to give to his own manager, the day unit manager, and any other interested parties.

A good research proposal will include:

- the aims of the study
- the rationale for the study (i.e. why you are doing it)
- the methodology to be used
- details of any piloting or preliminary activity
- an explanation of the ethical considerations and how these will be addressed (see pages 232–233)
- specimen data collection tools
- a timescale for the project.

Testing out the methodology

An essential part of any research study is to test out the data collection method. Sometimes, a full-scale pilot project is carried out, in which the methodology is tested on a relatively restricted group of subjects in order to identify any potential errors or snags.

Even in a small-scale study, it can be useful to have a 'dry-run' to test out the questionnaire before moving on to the collection of 'real' data.

Asking other people to complete prototype forms may throw up some unforeseen ambiguities or problems.

Piloting the questionnaire

After the unstructured interviews he held with centre users, Jon wants to include data collection on transport use. In particular, he wants to find out about the frequency of public transport use.

In his first attempt at questionnaire design, the relevant question is:

- How much do you use public transport to get to the centre?
  (Please tick) Very often / Sometimes / Not very often

1 What problems might be anticipated if this wording is used?

2 How might the questions be improved?

A pilot exercise involving the centre manager, a staff member and a centre user reveals that Jon's questions are too vague and won't give him reliable data. Each of the three choices is open to personal interpretation. For example, 'Very often' to one person might mean every week, whilst to another person it might mean every day. On reflection, Jon therefore opts for a quantity-type question, which limits respondents to specific choices which can be counted. Jon's revised question is:

- How many times a week do you use public transport to get to the centre? (Please enter a number in the box. If you do not use public transport, please enter a zero.)

Implementing the research plan

Ethics in research

When conducting research, it is important to keep ethical considerations in mind.

Considering the participants' rights

The British Psychological Society (BPS) Code of Ethical Principles sets out some guidelines for conducting research with people, in order to guide psychologists. These principles are set out in Figure 6.08. The BPS Code is actually intended for use by chartered psychologists, but it represents good practice and provides a point of reference for the ethics of interview (and other) research.

Over time, a number of principles have developed as a matter of good practice. These are the result of some unfortunate experiences arising from the conduct of a number of psychological studies. The following scenario describes a controversial controlled observational study conducted in the 1960s by Professor Stanley Milgram of Yale University (Milgram, 1963). The study has become famous for the ethical issues it raises as much as for the subject matter itself; a more detailed description of Milgram's study can be found in Gross, 2003 (pages 103–23).

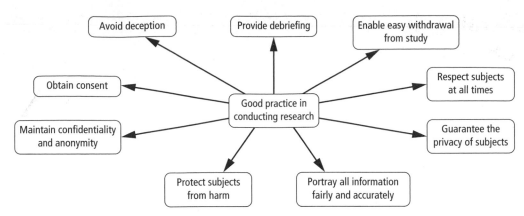

Figure 6.08 Guidelines for research set out in the BPS Code of Ethical Principles

All of the volunteers were debriefed afterwards and told that they had not harmed anyone. A year later, they were sent questionnaires to check for any longer-term emotional damage.

1 Does the deception involved in Milgram's experiment breach ethical principles, or could it be acceptable?

2 How important is it for people taking part in any study to be fully informed about what is going on?

3 How might such information affect people's behaviour during the course of the study?

4 Is deception ever justified as part of a research project?

Proceeding with consent

Before the questionnaires are sent out, Jon prepares some very short leaflets (based on his research proposal) explaining the aims of his research study and how he intends to proceed. Every centre user is sent one of these leaflets, which also invites co-operation.

It is made clear that all information given during interviews will be treated as confidential and the questionnaires will be anonymous. Volunteers are invited to take part in the interviews. Jon makes himself available at the centre before he starts his data collection, just in case anyone wants to ask him any further questions about the study.

Practical considerations

Postal questionnaires

When using postal questionnaires, it is essential to make sure that there is enough funding to pay for paper, cost of printing and production, envelopes and postage. In Jon's case, because the centre manager wants to see the results of this project, the Children's Services Authority will fund all administrative costs.

It is vital to allow enough time for respondents to complete and return their questionnaires, with plenty of time for their subsequent analysis. Jon has allowed two weeks for completion of the initial questionnaires, a further two weeks for analysis, and then one month to schedule in the individual interviews. He calculates he will then need a further three or four weeks to process all the data he has collected. He negotiates this with the centre manager and administrator, to make sure that the additional work doesn't clash with any other demands within the unit.

Jon's timings are based on his personal workload and that of the Sure Start centre. They are relative to this particular project. If you are doing research of your own, you will need to customise the project timetable to suit you and those you are working with. Some other practical considerations are set out in Table 6.11 on page 234.

Task	Notes
1. Give advanced notification of the study.	Notify everyone concerned, giving full information about the nature of the study and what is involved. A good research proposal might be used at this stage to give information to key individuals.
2. Ask permission where appropriate.	Permission will be needed from the subject population (if personal information is sought). Managers and/or staff in health or social services facilities should also give their assent.
3. Give assurances of confidentiality and anonymity.	Consider yourself bound by the BPS Code of Ethics as much as any professional researcher.
4. Keep appointments, be punctual and courteous.	
5. Collect data using tools as designed.	Make sure that a supervisor is present, particularly if working with children or people in a social services or health care facility.
6. Record data carefully onto questionnaires, observation sheets, etc.; use video or tape-recording as appropriate.	Anonymise your notes and questionnaires. Store all data securely.

Table 6.11 Checklist for conducting a research project

Conducting interviews

Thorough planning is essential to conducting successful interviews. There are a number of practical considerations to bear in mind; a checklist for preparing to conduct an interview session is given in Table 6.03 on page 223.

A quiet place

For the individual interviews, the centre manager allows Jon to use his own office. This is a quiet and pleasant room that is adequately ventilated and warm. In the room are two easy chairs and a coffee table, so Jon and his interview subjects can be relatively relaxed. There is no need for Jon to sit behind a desk to conduct his interviews, since this might intimidate his subjects and inhibit disclosure of information.

Jon has to make sure that he schedules interviews for times when the room is not required by the manager. Interview times also need to be convenient for his respondents.

Analysing the data

Bell (1993: 127) advises that in working through data, you should be 'constantly looking for similarities and differences, for groupings, patterns and items of particular significance'. A good way to see these patterns emerging is to begin to arrange the data into tables, bar charts and/or graphs from quite an early stage. In this way, these data presentation methods also become data analysis methods.

The reliability and validity of research data

Key concepts in assessing the value of data are reliability and validity.

Reliability

This relates to the extent to which a set of results can be replicated by repetition of a test, experiment or survey. For example, if a response to a medical treatment is replicated by researchers in different places and at different times, then the accumulated data might be said to be more reliable.

Analysing quantitative data

It is advisable to query the data in as many ways as possible. Are there, for example, differences between men and women in the sample population? Are there age differences or anything particularly significant about one group of people within the sample (e.g. disabled people)? Arranging your data into tables at an early stage in the analysis may help you to identify significant patterns or groupings.

Arranging data for analysis

Jon firstly compiles a simple table recording the satisfaction levels of centre users (see Table 6.12).

It is a good idea to express results as both percentages and numbers. Giving only percentage scores might be misleading; for example, a study might show that 80 per cent of subjects in a study showed a drastic improvement when treated with a particular drug. However, if the total size of the study population was only 10 people (and 8 people showed an improvement as a result of treatment), the results would be suggestive but not conclusive. Further, larger scale surveys would be required in order to establish a causal relationship between treatment and improvement.

Jon starts to wonder about those people who rated the service as only fair to poor. When he produces a table to show the ethnicity of centre users against satisfaction levels, his new table gives cause for concern (see Table 6.13).

Table 6.12 Centre users: by level of satisfaction with service (N=50)

Rating	Number	Percentage
Excellent	1	2%
Good	25	50%
Average	15	30%
Fair	5	10%
Poor	4	8%
Total (N)	50	100%

Table 6.13 Centre users: by ethnicity and satisfaction levels (N=50)

Rating	White UK	Minority Ethnic (ME)	Total
Excellent	1 (2%)		1
Good	25 (50%)		25
Average	14 (28%)	1 (2%)	15
Fair	4 (8%)	1 (2%)	5
Poor	1 (2%)	3 (6%)	4
Total	45 (90%)	5 (10%)	50

(Note: using shading for alternate lines on a chart can help the reader to assimilate the data, especially when tables are very long.)

By introducing the additional variable of ethnicity, Jon's table now shows that people from minority ethnic (ME) communities attending the centre rate the service there, at best, as average. The majority of this group, four out of five people, rated the service as fair or poor. This finding is shown even more dramatically when the data set is expressed as a bar chart (see Figure 6.09).

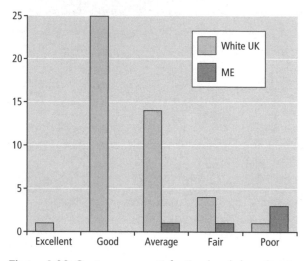

Figure 6.09 Centre users: satisfaction levels by ethnicity

This visual representation shows clearly that very few centre users are from minority ethnic communities. This has more impact than the numerical data set in Table 6.12. Secondly, it shows that centre users from White UK groups are much more satisfied with the centre than minority ethnic users. They are also in the majority, with very few centre users coming from ME groups.

Jon makes another analysis of centre users, this time by ethnicity and area of residence. This shows that all five of the parents from minority ethnic groups live in Snaresley, one of the areas shown to have a high number of lone-parent households but a low number of centre users. Snaresley also has a relatively high number of residents from minority ethnic groups, so Jon wonders whether the lone parents who live in Snaresley may find the centre unattractive because of something to do with the way in which the needs of people from minority ethnic communities are met (or not).

Jon knows that **correlation** does not necessarily imply causality (see also page 240). Nevertheless, he uses this analysis to justify the use of disproportionate random sampling when moving into the second phase of this study (in-depth interviews). Clearly, the five centre users from minority ethnic groups are not at all satisfied with the service offered at the centre. Jon is, therefore, perfectly justified in interviewing all of these subjects, even though they represent only 10 per cent of centre users. The interview information may reveal important information for managers and planners.

> **Correlation** – a link between two data sets, or two (or more) variables within a data set.

Pie charts can also be used to express data visually, as Figure 6.10 shows. Note that it is usually a good idea to give both numbers and percentages, as when expressing data in table form.

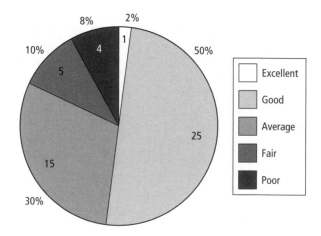

Figure 6.10 Centre users: satisfaction levels

Another way that Jon can show his data more visually is as a graph. He has collected information about travelling distances to the centre, which has a catchment area of about 3 miles in radius. Figure 6.11 shows how far centre users travel to reach the centre. The graph clearly shows that the majority of centre users (30 people) travel no further than 1 mile to get to the centre. Relatively few centre users live further than 2 miles away.

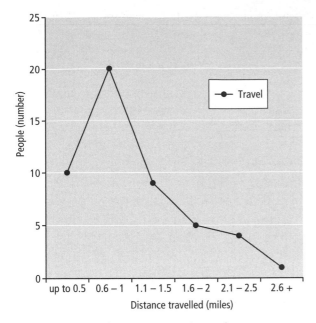

Figure 6.11 Travel to centre: numbers of centre users by miles travelled

Another good way to present quantitative information visually is by means of a pictograph. Similar to a bar chart, this uses a picture or symbol to represent the quantities or values being expressed in a data set. A pictograph using some of the data from Table 6.13 (Centre users: by ethnicity and satisfaction levels) is given in Figure 6.12.

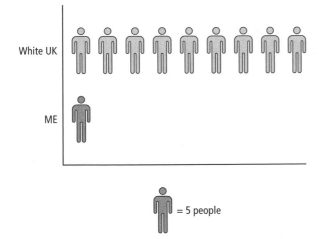

Figure 6.12 Pictograph of centre users by ethnicity

The way to make a pictograph is to:

- choose a symbol representing what you would like to show
- allocate a value to each symbol (for example, 10 people, 10 travel passes, etc.)
- plot a chart allocating the relevant number of symbols to each bar.

As far as Jon's study is concerned, using this method of showing the ethnicity of centre users really flags up the low take-up by people from minority ethnic groups.

Over to you

There are a number of other visual data presentation techniques, including histograms, Venn diagrams and sociograms. Find out about these additional methods of data presentation.

Further quantitative analysis: mean, median and mode

If meaningful inferences are to be made from quantitative data, there are a few mathematical concepts which can be helpful. These are the **mean**, the **median** and the **mode**.

> **Mean** – the average score.
> **Median** – the middle value of all the scores.
> **Mode** – the most frequently occurring score.

Jon has collected quantitative data on the number of sessions attended by each centre user. First of all, he expresses this as a table (see Table 6.14).

The centre holds two sessions per day, making a total of ten sessions per week. Because there are 50 regular centre users, this makes a possible 500 person/sessions weekly. Jon's table shows that one person is attending for eight sessions, but that most other people are attending for four sessions or less (five people attend four sessions; ten attend three sessions; and so on). This makes a total of 122 person/sessions per week.

The mean score from this data is very similar to what is referred to as the 'average' in arithmetic. Basically, if the total number of person/sessions (122) is divided by the total number of persons (50), this gives a mean score of 2.44. In other words, the average usage of the centre per person per week is 2.44 sessions.

However, in this case, the median and modal scores give a slightly more realistic figure. In both cases, the value here is two – as Table 6.14 shows, 30 centre users are attending for only two sessions. The reason for the discrepancy between the mean score and the median and modal scores is that the relatively high usage of the centre by just one user (8 sessions) has pushed up the score fractionally. However, in many surveys, the mean score may be the most useful. The small size of this sample and the clarity afforded by the table makes it desirable to use the median or modal scores as a truer indication of service use in this case.

Analysing qualitative data

Collecting stories

Jon has decided to conduct ten in-depth interviews using a mix of structured and unstructured data collection. This means he can quantify the responses to the more structured questions (for example, 'How many sessions a week do you attend the centre?') and show the answers in table or other visual form.

However, some of Jon's data is unstructured. He invites respondents to talk freely about their satisfaction level with the centre. By doing this, he discovers that some people for whom English is not a first language are having difficulties in relating both to staff and to other centre users. In order to conduct these interviews, Jon has had to use the services of a translator (for Albanian) and a signer who uses British Sign Language (to communicate with a deaf centre user).

Other respondents say they would like more flexible use of the centre to be an option, rather than having to commit to specified sessions.

Jon finishes up with ten sets of notes as a result of holding the in-depth interviews. Some of this data can be quantified (as explained above), but some of it requires a more flexible method of analysis. People express their views in their own way and in their own words, but it is possible to group responses into broadly similar categories.

Jon finds that a number of interviewees say they would like more flexible use of the centre

Table 6.14 Sessional use of day centre

Number of people	Number of sessions per person	Total person/sessions
1	8	8
5	4	20
10	3	30
30	2	60
4	1	4
50		122

to be an option, rather than having to commit to specified sessions. One person says that 'the opening times are not always convenient for me', whilst another says 'it would be nice to start at eleven and leave at two, instead of coming at nine and leaving at twelve'. Jon sees a pattern in these answers, and so he keeps a record of these on a chart that he prepares especially for this analysis. He ends up with statements from seven of the ten interviewees that are very similar. This is a significant finding, which he will put into his report as worthy of further investigation. It may be that another, short survey of all 50 centre users will show whether this is a general feeling, and perhaps give some pointers as to how opening times and centre use can be improved.

Jon's quantitative data has already established that although Snaresley has a high concentration of lone-parent households, the take-up from this area has been low (see page 136). Snaresley also has a high concentration of residents from minority ethnic groups, which led Jon to wonder if the centre is not catering sufficiently to meet the needs of people from such communities. The five in-depth interviews with centre users from ME groups reveal that service users for whom English is not a first language are clearly struggling to make good use of the centre. This group of users speak Albanian and Croatian. There are a host of issues to explore here, including the availability of translators, the use of other languages for signs and documentation, and the way in which the centre is advertised to speakers of other languages. If the centre were to attract more people from different cultural groups, centre users from other communities might begin to feel more comfortable having others from their own communities present. Jon will flag this up as another issue that requires urgent attention from managers and planners.

Interestingly, the ME centre users are from the new cultural groups entering the UK as a result of the expansion of the European Union, and not from those communities who have been resident in the UK for several generations (such as the Black and Asian populations defined in the Census). However, Jon needs to remember that correlation does not necessarily imply causality. The ME communities shown in the Census as living in Snaresley are, apparently, not using the centre at all. There may be cultural reasons for this, but it is certainly something worth investigating.

By allowing subjects the space and time to give their own views on services, the collection of qualitative data can reveal additional issues not covered elsewhere. Qualitative data collection is often vital at the pilot stage of a project, particularly large-scale studies. Establishing key issues at an early stage can avoid costly mistakes in the conduct of a large study. For example, Jon has shown that flexible times may be significant to centre users as a whole. Because this is only a small population (50 users in total) it is relatively easy to go back and get more data on this topic. However, if the survey population was much larger, perhaps over 1000 people, it would be a much more costly matter to redo the survey to collect this data. Researchers should always listen to their respondents, and piloting the project (even simply testing out the questionnaire) is always a good idea.

What does it all mean? Drawing conclusions from your data

How good is your data?

In research methodology, there are two concepts that relate to the quality of the data collected and, consequently, to the significance of the conclusions reached. These are reliability and validity (see page 234).

Aggregate – to aggregate data is to combine information collected at different times, and possibly from different sources.

For a small-scale research study, it should not usually be necessary to apply scientific tests of reliability or to spend a great deal of time on the measurement of validity. However, it will be important to demonstrate an awareness of the ways in which the reliability of data may be affected by the circumstances under which they were collected, and to build this into any conclusions or inferences made at the end of the project. It is also important to make sure that you focus on your objectives and design data collection tools to do the task in hand.

What does the data show?

A researcher should always be looking for patterns in the data collected, so it is advisable to query the data in as many ways as possible. Are there, for example, differences between men and women in the sample? Are there differences between people of different ages? Is there anything particularly significant about one group of people (for example, those who have been using a service for a long time or who have a particular disability)? The different categories that can be distinguished within data sets are referred to as **variables**.

Variable – something that can occur in different forms, i.e. it can vary in its characteristics.

A variable might be social class (in Census data), use of a particular drug (in medical research) or a type of mental health problem (in a piece of social research). The concern of researchers is often to establish whether one particular variable has a causal relationship to another. For example, they might be seeking to establish whether people of a certain social class or group tend to have fewer qualifications than people from a different group. Researchers may also be looking for variables that suggest further lines of enquiry. For example, people of a certain ethnic background might be under-represented in a particular group; researchers would want to find out why by designing further studies.

Correlation and causal inference

In some cases, researchers may say that the data allows them to establish a correlation between data sets, or between certain variables. If a pattern is distinguished, for example, a high proportion of people who smoke also experience early ageing of the skin, then researchers say there is a correlation to be made between these two variables. In some cases, the data may be strong enough for a **causal inference** to be made. In the Chief Medical Officer's Report from 2003, a causal inference has been made between smoking and facial ageing based on a relatively high number of separate studies. It is important to remember, however, that the correlation of two variables does not necessarily imply causality. Data has to be substantiated from a number of studies and the potential impact of other variables taken into account before a causal inference can be made.

In small-scale studies, conclusions will often be expressed in terms of inference or suggestion, particularly since the sample size is small.

Relatability and generalisation

Other key concepts in the expression of findings are relatability and generalisation.

Relatability
The extent to which the findings of the study of a specific population may be applicable to another, similar population sample (for example, two groups of smokers).

Generalisation
The extent to which the findings of a study may be generalised to a much wider population (for example, the smokers in a study and all smokers in the wider population).

Jon's findings are, in the main, specific to this population of centre users. He was not aiming to test out a specific hypothesis and, therefore, his findings will not necessarily have great applicability to other research. However, the following generalisations can be made:

● Jon's research has highlighted the dangers of not paying enough attention to the needs of minority groups when planning a service.
● Several centre users have said they would like more say in how the unit is run, which supports arguments for greater service-user empowerment (this is in line with much current national guidance on planning and service delivery).

● Findings on distances travelled to the centre, together with information about public transport use, may be of interest to the Borough's planning department when working on future local amenities.

As long as the results are used with caution, Jon's research may provide useful background information to other planning activity.

Presenting the findings

Presenting a written report

A very common way of presenting research findings is as a written report. There is a standard way of setting this out, which is described below. At the end of the analytical process, you will have created a number of tables and other visual ways of showing the data. For the final report, choose only the graphics that demonstrate the key findings of the study. If the findings are inconclusive, this is itself worth reporting.

Jon's study has revealed a number of interesting facts about current usage of the centre, together with some significant issues that deserve further investigation. His report will take all this into account. In writing up his results, he uses the structure set out in Table 6.15 (see page 242).

A professional research report will always begin with an abstract, which is a very short summary of the project, together with its key findings. The introduction sets out the aims and rationale of the study, and may also be the place to set out any interesting secondary research that has been used to inform the project. In the methodology section, an explanation of how the study was conducted should be given, including a description of how the population sample was chosen, how many people were in the study, how long it lasted and the data collection methods and tools used.

Actual specimens of data collection tools can be put into the appendix. The presentation and analysis sections of the report should be as

1. Abstract	Summary of study, with key findings
2. Introduction	Aims, rationale; may include relevant secondary research/background information
3. Methodology	Details of research methods and tools; sampling, sample size, etc.; process followed
4. Presentation of data	Select from tables, bar charts, diagrams, graphs, pie charts, pictographs, Venn diagrams and sociographs, as appropriate, to enhance presentation
5. Analysis of results	Any significant trends or relationship between variables is highlighted
6. Conclusion	Sets out possible causal inferences, relatability to other populations; inconclusive data also highlighted
7. Evaluation	Critical reflection on the study; strengths, weaknesses; how things might be done differently next time
8. Recommendations for future research	Lines of enquiry suggested by findings
Appendices	Specimen data collection tools; data from other sources, if relevant

Table 6.15 Research reports: key elements

succinct as possible. Quantitative data should always be expressed visually (for example, tables, bar charts) as well as in words.

The conclusion should make the findings and inferences clear. Often, a researcher will describe how the findings might be relatable to other similar situations, or if inferences may be made from this study to a wider population. There will usually be limited scope for this in a small-scale study.

It is essential to evaluate the study after it is finished. (Evaluation is considered in more detail on pages 244–246).

Finally, it might be possible to see how the study could be followed up. Suppose, for example, in a small study of a reminiscence session, eight out of ten people were found to have trouble getting to the venue. This is an important finding which would be worth following up with another piece of research. Jon's study showed that language issues were important for a small but significant group of centre users. It also showed that very few people from black or minority ethnic groups use the centre. He recommends that both these matters should be followed up.

Making an oral presentation about your research findings

Sometimes, a researcher may be required to set out his or her findings as part of an oral presentation. If you are in this position, you may find the following observations and checklist helpful.

There is a saying about giving a good talk. First of all you tell the audience what you are going to tell them (the introduction); then you tell them (the main body of your talk); then you tell them what you've just told them (the summary and conclusion at the end). In other words, the structure of a talk should be:

- TELL THEM what you are going to tell them
- TELL THEM
- TELL THEM what you've just told them.

This is a tried and tested approach used by public speakers, whether politicians, salespeople or entertainers. Good teachers and lecturers also use this structure. What is important about this system is that it uses the principle of repetition, which is also a central aspect of teaching and learning.

If you set out what your talk will be about in a clear and memorable introduction, you have created an expectation in your audience about what they will hear. The central body of your talk should then elaborate on these points, using only information or material that is relevant. A summary and conclusion will remind the audience about what they have just heard and make it more likely that they will remember the key aspects of the talk. People who are taking notes at a talk always appreciate a speaker who keeps to the point and follows a structure as laid out in the introduction.

The key points of a talk will be designed to achieve the aims and objectives that have already been decided. This is critical. There is no point is telling your audience to expect a talk on communicating with children and then digressing to include a mass of anecdotes about working with older people.

The same is true of any supplementary material that you decide to use. Visual material should enhance the points you are making. This might be carefully chosen photographs or projected images showing the points you are making in bullet-point form. It is a mistake to show too much printed or written material on an overhead – it will be too much for your audience to take in and can detract from what you are saying.

If you are using audio-visual aids such as a video, DVD or CD recording, make sure that you know how to use the equipment that will be available to you on the day. For a short talk, it is advisable to keep the use of such supplementary material to a minimum.

If there is too much material for the time available, but you feel it's really vital to tell the audience about certain things, handouts can be used to give out additional information. Handouts can also be used to reinforce the key points of the talk.

It is not a good idea to read out from the text of the written report. Some people use prompt cards, on which are written the main points. They then speak naturally when elaborating on these key items. Other people write out the key points onto a sheet of paper.

Table 6.16 Managing your material for an oral presentation: some tips

Structure your talk	<ul><li>Introduction</li><li>Body of talk</li><li>Summary/conclusion</li></ul>
Link your talk to your aims and objectives	Choose relevant material that supports your case
Visual aids	<ul><li>Should be clear and concise</li><li>Should enhance the talk, not detract from what you are saying</li></ul>
Audio-visual material	<ul><li>Keep to a minimum for a short talk</li><li>Make sure you can use the equipment</li></ul>
Aides-mémoires	Options include:<ul><li>reading from full text</li><li>prompt cards</li><li>notes on sheets of paper</li></ul>
Visual aids	<ul><li>Should be clear and concise</li><li>Use white space to effect (don't clutter your overheads with too many words)</li><li>Should enhance (not detract from) your talk</li></ul>
Supplementary material	You can use handouts to give extra material
Rehearse your talk	<ul><li>Always have at least one run-through before the actual event</li><li>Make sure you keep to time</li><li>Allocate time to each item</li></ul>

Evaluating a research project

Making an objective assessment

> **Evaluation**
> Evaluation is the process of looking back at something in order to review it and assess its worth, value or importance. This should be done critically and objectively. This means assessing the facts in a neutral, non-emotional way.

The following scenario illustrates how emotions can sometimes get in the way of objective thinking.

Keeping things in perspective

Rav has been assessing the effects of the introduction of a music therapy session in a day unit for older people. He collected data from 20 people, using self-completion questionnaires. He then interviewed some of the older people individually, using a semi-structured approach. Five of the six interviewees were very positive about the music therapy and appeared to enjoy talking to Rav. However, the sixth person, Mrs Da Silva, became angry and abusive during the interview. Her care manager had to intervene and the interview was terminated. Rav was very upset and began to feel that the whole project had been a bad idea.

1 Why is it important for Rav to sit back and evaluate what has happened objectively?

2 What reasons might there be for Mrs Da Silva's behaviour?

Once Rav recovered from the experience of having a difficult interview, he met with the care manager to evaluate the situation – not only the incident itself, but also the project as a whole. The care manager explained that Mrs Da Silva has painful arthritis, which sometimes makes her irritable. Furthermore, the day of the interview was the anniversary of her husband's death. Her behaviour was thus due to a combination of physical and emotional factors, and nothing at all to do with Rav's interviewing skills. Rav also realised, by discussing his work with his tutor, that he had collected plenty of meaningful information in the 20 self-completion questionnaires, which has given him sufficient quantitative data. The five semi-structured interviews have resulted in some good, anecdotal information, which will add a qualitative dimension to his conclusions.

Making an objective evaluation has helped Rav to overcome the negative feelings he experienced during and after the difficult interview, and also to appreciate the value of the rest of his work.

Questions to ask

Even if there have been no obvious incidents or upsets during the course of a research study, it is still important to be as critical as possible when reflecting on the project and its outcomes. The following checklists may be helpful when going through this process. It is also important to involve another person in the evaluative process. This might be your tutor or someone who supervised you during the data collection process. The following checklists might serve as a useful starting point for ordering your thoughts before meeting with whoever is going to help you with the evaluation.

Checklist: evaluating research methodology

- Were the aims and objectives of the project clear?
- Was the data reliable and valid?
- How representative was the target population?
- Was the sampling method appropriate?
- Were the data collection methods appropriate to the objectives?
- Did you observe ethical principles in choosing and applying data collection methods?
- How effective were the chosen data collection methods?

- Were the aims and objectives of the project met?
- Were there any unexpected outcomes of the research?

Checklist: evaluating the research process

- How thorough was the planning process?
- How thorough/useful was the secondary research?
- If you did a pilot study, how helpful was this?
- What can be learned from the process of implementing the research?
- How well did you observe ethical principles when implementing your research?
- How well were the principles of confidentiality and anonymity observed?
- Were there any unexpected events or surprises as a result of conducting the research?

Checklist: evaluating the research report

- Does the report contain all the necessary components?
- Are the conclusions clear?
- Is the language used in the report clear and concise?
- Do charts, diagrams and tables, etc., enhance the findings of the research?

In evaluating his research, Jon notes that he is glad he piloted the data collection form. Observations by people who tested it out for him revealed a number of ambiguous questions, and one or two helpful alternative questions were suggested. One question was deleted from the schedule as being irrelevant to Jon's objectives.

During the course of the in-depth interviews, one of the interviewees had become a little aggressive and, for a time, Jon's confidence was undermined. The manager had intervened at this point and it turned out that this particular centre user was worried about her other child, who had gone to school that morning despite having been sick in the night. It was decided to contact the school to check on the child's health, but Jon had remained upset for a while as he felt he should have checked out how this particular individual was feeling before they launched into the interview. The manager pointed out that Jon did respond appropriately as soon as he realised that something was not quite right. However, the incident has made Jon determined to be more sensitive when eliciting in-depth data from people. He also plans to ask his own manager for some further training on interviewing and interpersonal skills.

Jon's research: the outcomes

Jon's work has yielded a significant amount of valuable information for managers and planners. He has shown that not enough attention has been given to the needs of people from minority ethnic communities, and also to disabled and deaf people. Centre users have expressed a desire for more flexibility in the way services are offered. In terms of the purposes of research described at the start of this chapter, Jon has reviewed the impact of a new service and (to some extent) described the needs of a specific population (those people using the centre).

Jon's report is presented to managers and planners at a meeting of the Service Planning Committee, and Jon is invited to attend to answer questions. As a result, the planning department is asked to cost up proposals to provide translators at the centre and produce all of the centre's leaflets in Albanian and other languages. Further research is commissioned into how the needs of deaf people and those with disabilities can be met. The council is working on its Disability Equality Scheme (which has to be in place by the end of the year), and Jon's work has flagged up how easy it is to overlook the needs of disabled people.

Jon's tutor, the manager of the centre and Jon himself are all very pleased with this piece of work. By careful planning, thoughtful implementation, thorough analysis and clear presentation, Jon has produced a study that will make a significant contribution to service delivery. The people who took part in the study said how much they appreciated being consulted on these issues and having their views heard. The final report was made available at the centre (in several languages), which reassured centre users that the work was of genuine value and would actually make a difference to them on a day-to-day basis.

Perhaps your own research will have an impact in a similar way to Jon's research. In any case, developing research skills will provide you with a number of transferable tools and will enhance your performance as a professional working in the fields of health and social care.

Test yourself

1   Name four key purposes of research in health and social care.
2   What is epidemiology?
3   Explain the differences between:
    a) primary and secondary data
    b) qualitative and quantitative data.
4   Why is it important to set clear goals for a research project?
5   What is the meaning of the term 'population' with respect to research?
6   What is sampling?
7   Define what is meant by an 'open' question.
8   What instrument or tool might a researcher use when conducting a structured interview?
9   What is a longitudinal study?
10 Define the concept of bias in relation to research methodology.
11 Describe four principles of good practice when conducting research.
12 Why is it important to give numbers as well as percentages on a table of data?
13 In research terminology, what is 'reliability'?
14 Why does correlation not necessarily imply causality?

Further reading

References

- Bell, J. (1993) *Doing Your Research Project*. (2nd ed.) Buckingham: Open University Press
- Coles, A. and Cox, A. (2002) 'Does early treatment of multiple sclerosis prevent the progression of disability later on?', *Way Ahead*, 6 (1): 4–5
- Department of Health (2004), *On the state of the public health: Annual Report of the Chief Medical Officer 2003*, accessed via Department of Health website
- Gross, R. (2003) *Key Studies in Psychology*. (4th ed.) Abingdon: Hodder and Stoughton
- Halliday, S. (2001) 'Death and miasma in Victorian London: an obstinate belief', *British Medical Journal*, 323: 1469–71
- Harris, P. (1986) *Designing and Reporting Experiments*. Buckingham: Open University Press
- Milgram, S. (1963), 'Behavioural study of obedience', *Journal of Abnormal and Social Psychology*, 67: 371–8
- Snow, J. (1855) *On the Mode of Communication of Cholera*. London: John Churchill
- Wakefield, A.J. (*et al.*)(1998), 'Ileal-lymphoid-nodular hyperplasia, non-specific colitis and pervasive developmental disorder in children', *The Lancet*, 351: 637–41

Useful websites

The following websites can be accessed via the Heinemann website.
Go to www.heinemann.co.uk/hotlinks and enter the express code 4256P.

- Census Data (local)
- Cochrane Collaboration
- Department of Health
- Institute for Public Policy and Research (IPPR)
- NHS Gateway
- Joseph Rowntree Foundation
- Medical Research Council
- National Centre for Social Research
- National Institute for Health and Clinical Excellence (NICE)
- National Statistics Online
- Prince of Wales's Foundation for Integrated Health
- Research Council for Complementary Medicine
- Sociological Research Online
- Office of Public Sector Information (access to government publications)
- Valuing People
- What Doctors Don't Tell You (WDDTY)

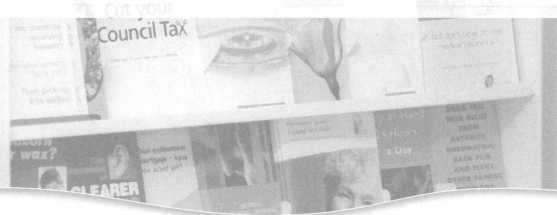

CHAPTER 7

Promoting good health and well-being

Key points

- There are many factors that can have a positive or negative effect on the health of individuals.
- Health means different things to different people.
- There have been a multitude of health initiatives from a variety of sources over the last 30 years.
- Health promotion can be approached in a variety of different ways.
- Health promotion priorities are identified following population studies.
- Health promotion involves initiatives from home to international organisations.
- Health promotion can create some ethical dilemmas.
- People still behave in an unhealthy way despite a wealth of information available to advise us how to keep healthy.

Introduction

Every human being is born with a potential life expectancy, but a wide range of factors can detrimentally affect this. Infants rely entirely on others to keep them safe and well. As children grow into young people, parents' and carers' opportunities to keep them safe and well diminish. Young people have to learn to make decisions about their lifestyle; these decisions can have far reaching consequences for their health in adulthood and old age. Some health promotion is beyond the scope of the individual and is addressed by the medical world under the influence of government policy.

In this chapter you will explore the many factors that can affect health and well-being, and the extent to which the individual can achieve the life expectancy potential with which he or she was born. You will also explore how health promoters can have a positive effect on the health of others.

Factors that affect health

There are a range of factors known to detrimentally affect health, and these are described in the following section.

Genetic influence

An individual's potential life expectancy at birth is dictated by genetic make-up. The Human Genome project, completed in 2003, identified specific genes responsible for the development of inherited conditions. However, this is not the whole picture. Some humans inherit an increased likelihood of developing certain conditions which it may be possible to avoid by taking certain medicines or adopting a particular lifestyle. Medical knowledge of these lifestyle changes is still in its infancy, and there is much to be discovered before concrete advice can be given to those identified to be susceptible. There are also many ethical issues surrounding the debate over whether scientists should be allowed to genetically test people to discover their potential profile of health and disease.

Over to you

Find out more about the Human Genome project, including the ethical debate about genetic testing, by going to www.heinemann.co.uk/hotlinks and entering the express code 4256P.

Screening for cancer genes

The Human Fertilisation and Embryology Authority announced in May 2006 that it will permit embryos to be screened for three genes that can cause an 80 per cent chance of breast or bowel cancer developing in adulthood.

Consider the three viewpoints below then discuss the ethical issues around genetic screening.

- My aunt and grandmother died of breast cancer when they were in their fifties. I am planning to start a family and want to have embryos screened before implantation to ensure they do not carry the gene BRCA1.
- A life insurance company has decided to ask all future female applicants to undertake a test for the BRCA1 and BRCA2 genes. If they test positive, the company will not insure them against developing breast cancer.
- I am a 43-year-old GP recovering from breast cancer. If my mother had known that I had the BRCA1 gene when she was pregnant, she may have had the pregnancy terminated.

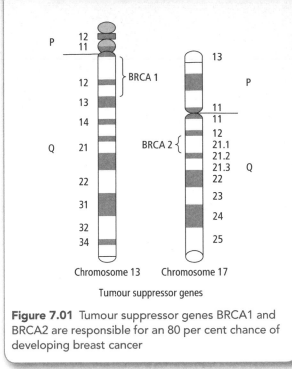

Figure 7.01 Tumour suppressor genes BRCA1 and BRCA2 are responsible for an 80 per cent chance of developing breast cancer

Socio-economic factors

There is a huge temptation to inextricably link social class with wealth, and whilst it is generally true that the middle classes are comfortably off, the upper classes are wealthy and the working classes are the least well off, social class is not really about wealth. It is more about attitude and behaviour. Indeed, the terms upper, middle and working classes have disappeared from use by researchers and government reports. Socio-economic grouping is determined by job status, as can be seen by looking at Figure 7.02. If a working-class family won the lottery, they would not automatically become upper class, and if a member of the aristocracy became bankrupt, he or she would not usually start behaving like a member of the working classes.

There is strong evidence that social class does have an influence on health, and this can largely be explained by looking at lifestyle. The behaviours that have the biggest detrimental effect on health are:

- smoking
- high alcohol consumption
- lack of exercise
- consumption of a high-fat and high-sugar diet.

These behaviours are more common among lower social classes (Naidoo & Wills, 2000).

Smoking

In 2003–04, 20 per cent of managerial and professional men smoked compared to 29 per cent of male intermediate workers and 36 per cent of male routine and manual workers (*Living in Britain*, 2002).

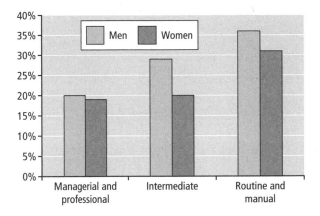

Figure 7.02 Prevalence of cigarette smoking among adults by sex and socio-economic group

> **Did you know?**
>
> *'Smoking has been identified as the single greatest cause of preventable illness and premature death in the UK... it is estimated that half the difference in survival to 70 years of age between social class I and V is due to higher smoking prevalence in class V.' (Wanless, 2004)*

Smoking causes a wide range of disorders, including lung cancer and heart disease. Less well-known conditions include **peripheral vascular disease**, which can lead to **gangrene** and ultimately leg amputation. Smoking can also increase the risk of cancer of the bladder, of which 37 per cent of deaths are attributable to smoking, and chronic obstructive lung disease, of which 84 per cent of deaths are blamed on smoking. You can find out more about smoking-related illness at the Action on Smoking and Health (ASH) website; to access this site, go to www.heinemann.co.uk/hotlinks and enter the express code 4256P.

> **Peripheral vascular disease** – narrowing of the blood vessels that carry blood to leg and arm muscles, which may cause pain when exercising.

Income

There is no doubt that those living in poverty have worse health than those who are better off. Much has been done over the years to attempt to redress the balance. The Department of Health ensures that people on low incomes have access to medical services through free prescriptions, dental care and optical care. **Income support** guarantees that those without an adequate income receive some financial assistance to enable them to afford basic essentials. Those unable to work through ill health or disability are similarly able to claim benefits. Despite this, statistics show that there is still a divide between the health of low-income individuals and that of the better off. This can be explained to some extent by considering how money is spent.

Income can also affect living conditions and working and living environments. Poor housing may be damp, for example, increasing the risk of respiratory disease. People on a low income are more likely to be working in manual jobs or to be unemployed. Those in manual jobs are more likely to develop work-related disorders due to inhaling dust or fumes or accidents at work. Those on a low income often live in inner city environments where pollution is greater and, again, this can cause or exacerbate respiratory disorders (see Figure 7.03).

Gender

The average life expectancy of men in the UK in 2002 was 76 years, and for women was 81 years. This can be explained by looking at differences in lifestyle between men and women as well as biological factors. In 2004–05, 26 per cent of men and 23 per cent women were cigarette smokers. Male smokers smoked on average 15 cigarettes a day, compared with 13 for women. Men are over three times more likely than women to die from road traffic accidents and suicide, and twice as likely to die from cancers of the mouth and throat. Women are more likely to die from blood disorders, behavioural disorders, Alzheimer's disease and strokes than men. (Source: National Statistics Online)

The gender difference in mortality due to road traffic accidents is explained partially by the fact that men drive more than women. A survey carried out in 2004 by the Scottish Executive found that 9 per cent of male drivers drove over 15,000 miles per year compared with 3 per cent of female drivers. In 2002, 56 per cent of men over 17 years of age drove daily, compared to 36 per cent women. (Source: Scottish Executive website)

Women are protected from heart disease by the hormone oestrogen until they reach the menopause, so tend to be a little older than men before signs of coronary heart disease start to appear.

Age

Unsurprisingly, the incidence of ill health increases with age. However, some older people are much fitter than others. This is generally related to genetic make-up, lifestyle and/or the nature of their job before retirement. The University of Texas carried out a seven-year research project on 1558 robust older people, which was published in the journal *Psychology and Aging* in 2004. It found that people with a positive mental attitude were less frail at the end of the seven years. There are links between positive mental health and good physical health, particularly in relation to reduced risk of heart disease.

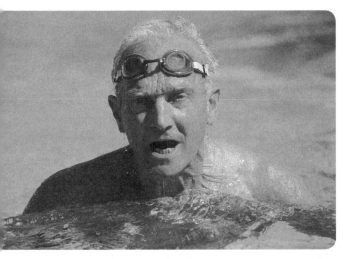

Good mental health and well-being are as important for older people as for any other age group

Over to you

Read the article on the BBC website entitled 'Positive Attitude Delays Aging' (available at http://news.bbc. co.uk/1/hi/health/3642356.stm). Consider how knowledge of this report might affect the way you work with elderly people. Try to think of ways you could maintain a positive attitude in older clients.

Older people are more susceptible to degenerative diseases, such as arthritis and dementia, much more likely to develop cancer, and the majority of people affected by heart disease, hypertension and strokes are over 65 years of age. (Source: National Statistics Online)

Culture

Some disease patterns can be seen to be more prevalent in particular cultural groups. Part of the reason for this is inheritance, and part is due to lifestyle, in particular diet. The British now eat more fast food than any other nationality in Western Europe. They also have the highest obesity rate. Obesity has been linked to heart disease, cancer, diabetes, arthritis, high blood pressure, infertility and strokes. (Schlosser, 2002)

People from minority ethnic groups have higher than average incidence of heart disease, strokes and diabetes. Sickle cell anaemia is a genetic disorder found in people of African Caribbean origin.

What do we mean by health?

People's ideas vary about what the word 'health' means, depending on their own situation. This will be influenced by the person's age, gender, ethnicity, and level and quality of education, as well as those ideas adopted from family members, whether the person has a disability and various additional factors.

Over to you

Ask some people you know, who have no training in health topics, to define the word 'health'. Ask a variety of people, including children, older people and those from different ethnic and socio-economic backgrounds to you. Discuss the different answers with other members of your group. Compare them to the ideas under Types of health on page 254.

Types of health

Physical health

Physical health refers to the mechanical functioning of the body. A person is physically healthy when the body systems are working properly and he or she does not need any medical treatment to achieve this.

Mental health

Mental health refers to a person's ability to cope with life in a positive way, and his or her having positive self-esteem.

Emotional health

Emotional health refers to a person's ability to respond in an appropriate way to situations. Consider, for example, a woman with post-natal depression. This can occur even if a woman has given birth to a healthy baby that was planned and the family is financially secure and stable. The depression is, therefore, an irrational reaction to what should be a happy event.

Social health

Social health is the ability to make and sustain relationships and to behave in a socially acceptable manner according to the person's cultural expectations. Social health relies on having good support and guidance from care givers, usually family. Some children find it difficult to behave in a socially acceptable way. This may be due to poor parenting in the early years and, despite the efforts of foster parents, etc., it can be very difficult to undo the harm of the early childhood years.

Models of health

'Model of health' is another term for a concept, definition, view or idea about what the word health means.

Lay model of health

The word 'lay' means non-professional. A lay model of health is an idea of what the word health might mean to a person who has no education or training in the field of health. For example:

- Young people without any chronic illness or disability may only think of themselves as healthy when they are free of pain, full of energy, and without any infections such as a cold or influenza.
- People with physical disabilities who use a wheelchair might always have some pain or stiffness. They might consider themselves healthy if they are well enough to go to school or college or to participate in sport. Many people with disabilities cope very well, are independent, are able to hold down a full-time job, and are reliable and productive employees; because of this they consider themselves to be healthy.

Both these 'lay concepts' of health are views held by people without professional expertise in health.

Some people would define health as 'not being ill'. This is a negative definition – that is, it says what health is not rather than what it is.

Many researchers have examined the topic of concepts of health related to a variety of socio-economic factors. Some of their findings are shown in Table 7.01.

Medical model of health

Once people start to train in a health-related occupation, their ideas about health evolve. Healthcare workers understand health as something that can be demonstrated through the results of tests and examinations. This tends to be related to physical health and, to an extent, mental health. They learn the normal range for

Socio-economic group	Concept of health
Older people	Inner strength; ability to cope
Young people	Fitness, energy, strength
Middle-class people	Enjoying life; being fit and active
Working-class people	Able to get through the day; not being ill
Men	Being fit
Women	Able to carry out everyday tasks

Table 7.01 Concepts of health by socio-economic group

healthy pulse, blood pressure and haemoglobin levels, and the signs of ill health.

Plenty of non-medically trained people also understand health in more technical terms; for example, many people are aware of an acceptable range for blood pressure.

Cultural model of health

People of Western origin tend to think of health and illness more in physical terms. In the UK, most of the population would attend their general practitioner if they were feeling ill and many would expect a prescription to restore them to health.

In eastern cultures, it is not unusual for people to seek treatment from acupuncture. Acupuncture focuses on improving the overall well-being of the person rather than the isolated treatment of specific symptoms. According to Chinese philosophy, health is dependent on the body's motivating energy – known as Qi – moving in a smooth and balanced way through a series of meridians (channels) beneath the skin.

Over to you

Find out more about acupuncture by visiting the website of the British Acupuncture Council. You can access this site by going to www.heinemann.co.uk/hotlinks and entering the express code 4256P.

Holistic model of health

Some people see health as incorporating a whole range of issues, from physical well-being to social ability, emotional stability and inner peace. There is much to be said for this approach, since a fully functioning body will not make you feel healthy if you are affected by depression or acute anxiety. Indeed, mental illness may manifest as physical symptoms, such as palpitations, tightness of the chest and breathlessness, all of which could also be symptoms of several physical illnesses. A person who is unable to make and/or maintain friendships may experience low self-esteem, feel rejected and become very introvert, so here, too, it would be difficult to describe the individual as healthy.

Did you know?

The World Health Organisation in 1946 defined health in the preamble to its constitution as, 'a state of complete physical, mental and social well-being and not merely the absence of disease or infirmity.' (See also Chapter 3, page 67.)

Health promotion

Health can be promoted when people are fully fit, have a permanent disability or are chronically sick. Health promoters aim to enable people to be as well as possible.

Types of health promotion

Health promotion can be primary, secondary or tertiary. Table 7.02 lists twenty different health promotion strategies.

Primary health promotion
Primary health promotion means preventing ill health occurring at all.

Secondary health promotion
Secondary health promotion involves detecting illness in early stages through screening or medical examination, and giving treatment to correct any abnormality.

Tertiary health promotion
Tertiary health promotion involves preventing an existing condition from worsening.

Table 7.02 Twenty health promotion strategies

Initiative	Primary (✓)	Secondary (✓)	Tertiary (✓)
1. Diabetic clinic			
2. Counselling sessions			
3. Food hygiene training			
4. Filling teeth			
5. Guthrie test (screening for PKU)			
6. Childhood immunisation			
7. Five-a-day initiative			
8. Eye tests			
9. Water and sewage treatment			
10. Bullying strategies in school			
11. Fluoride toothpaste			
12. Teaching parents to check for head lice			
13. Antenatal care			
14. Child health surveillance			
15. Asthma clinic			
16. Free gym membership for employees			
17. Cholesterol tests			
18. Breast screening			
19. **Statins**			
20. Safety in the sun			

Statins – a relatively new group of drugs used to lower blood cholesterol levels, thus reducing the risk of heart attack.

The development of modern approaches to health promotion

It wasn't until the 19th century that it was realised that the health of the population could be improved by public health measures. In the early days, public health was improved by the provision of clean water and the construction of sewers. The government passed several pieces of legislation aimed at improving the health of the population, resulting in improvements in housing, and the establishment of the Ministry of Health. The NHS was founded in 1948, ensuring that the whole population had access to medical care, free at the point of delivery. This was followed by routine childhood immunisation which began in 1960. These measures were responsible for a substantial increase in the life expectancy of the British population. However, the 1980s saw a real development in the academic study of health promotion. This section examines the way in which inequalities in health were identified, and the development of present-day strategies to further improve the health of the British population.

'Health for All' by the year 2000

The Alma-Ata Declaration was adopted at the International Conference on Primary Health Care in 1978. It stated:

> *... that health, which is a complete physical, mental and social well-being, and not merely the absence of disease or infirmity, is a fundamental human right and that the attainment of the highest possible level of health is a most important world-wide social goal whose realisation requires the action of many other social and economic sectors in addition to the health sector.*

The declaration challenged governments, organisations and the whole world community to ensure, by the year 2000, a level of health that would permit all peoples to lead a socially and economically productive life. The focus from an international perspective was to redress the balance between developing and developed countries. 28 years later, however, this imbalance is still true.

1 Why do you think that developing countries still have much lower life expectancy than developed countries?

2 What are the differences in disease patterns between developing and developed countries?

Approaches to health promotion in the UK

The Working Group on Inequalities in Health was set up in 1977, under the chairmanship of Sir Douglas Black, to investigate the relationship between health and social class. In 1980, the Black Report was published. It identified patterns of inequalities of health across Britain and made recommendations for health improvement. By 1987, GPs were given financial incentives to hit targets for various health promotion activities, such as immunisation. In 1988 the Acheson Report was published, which again highlighted health inequalities in the UK.

The Health of the Nation

The Black and Acheson reports kick-started an initiative in the UK to improve the health of the population, entitled 'The Health of the Nation'.

The main areas of concern identified were:

- cancer
- coronary heart disease and stroke
- HIV and sexual health
- accidents
- suicide.

The initiative was launched in 1992 by setting out measurable targets to improve these specific areas. Using numerical data, the incidence of ill-health was then compared over a specific period. For example, one target for coronary heart disease was 'to reduce death rates in those aged under 65 years by 40 per cent by 2000, and in those aged 65–74 years by 30 per cent by the year 2000'. The target for stroke was 'to reduce death rate for stroke in those aged 65–74 years by 40 per cent by 2000'.

By 1996, the proportions of those under 65 years dying of coronary heart disease had fallen by just 10.7 per cent, and those aged 65–74 years by just 7.7 per cent. Other targets were also significantly missed. However, good progress was being made towards 11 of the 27 targets; some progress was being made on a further 6 targets; but for some targets, it was too soon to assess progress. (Source: National Audit Office)

Our Healthier Nation

Our Healthier Nation was launched in 1999 to replace the original targets with more realistic ones. The new target for coronary heart disease was 'to reduce the death rate from heart disease and stroke and related illnesses amongst people under 65 years by at least a further third by 2010 from a baseline at 1996'. In other words, the government had effectively given itself another 10 years to achieve the original targets.

The areas of focus were reduced to four: cancer, coronary heart disease and stroke, accidents and mental illness. The initiative was to be carried out by investing money in:

- smoking cessation programmes
- NHS Direct
- Healthy Living Centres
- the instigation of Health Action Zones for

areas identified as having significant health issues within their population.

These initiatives form the basis of health promotion strategies in the UK.

Initiatives linked to Our Healthier Nation

Smoking cessation programmes

These programmes are locally run and have different names. People can refer themselves by telephone or the Internet. Help is provided on a one-to-one or group-work basis. They provide free or reduced cost Nicotine Replacement Therapy, and specialist help for pregnant women and non-English-speaking clients. They also train other professionals, such as school nurses, occupational health nurses and youth workers, to enable them to give support to smokers trying to quit.

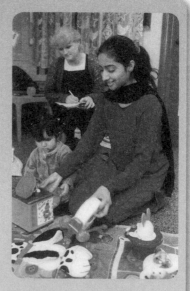

Stephanie

I am 23 years old and work as a nursery assistant at a Day Nursery in Dover, Kent. I started smoking when I was 17 years old, when I started college. Most of the girls in my group smoked. They went outside for a cigarette between every lesson. I did not want to feel left out, so when someone offered me a cigarette, I took it. Although I didn't enjoy the first few cigarettes, I enjoyed being part of the crowd. Before long, I was also smoking two or three cigarettes before college and the same on the way home. My Dad saw me smoking as I came down the road one day.

He didn't seem that bothered, so I started smoking at home as well. By the time I left college, I was smoking 20 cigarettes a day. I started to notice a cough developing, but didn't take it seriously until one day I developed breathlessness and chest pains. I was at work at the time and the first aider called an ambulance. I was admitted to hospital. The doctor said the symptoms were almost certainly due to my smoking habits. My grandparents were both heavy smokers. My grandmother died of lung cancer at the age of 59, and my grandfather died of emphysema aged 63. It was then that I realised that if I did not give up smoking, I was running a huge risk of following them to an early grave.

When I got home from hospital I immediately called the NHS Smoking Helpline, and was referred to the local NHS Stop Smoking Service. I made an appointment for a one-to-one session with a practice nurse, who coached me through the giving-up process. She gave me advice on how to quit and some Nicotine Replacement Therapy patches. The nurse, Mel, was brilliant and really spent time with me. She talked through why and when I had been smoking, and helped me to think of a way to stop. I was going out in my breaks to have a cigarette, usually on my own, as my colleagues at work are mainly non-smokers. So that bit was easy. The difficult part was going out with friends in the evening. Mel suggested we went to the cinema or ten-pin bowling instead of the pub. She made me realise that if I changed my habits away from the normal routine, I wouldn't miss cigarettes as much. And she was right! I have not had a cigarette now for six months. I feel so much fitter, and haven't put on any weight at all. I am also £30 a week better off. I am saving it up and intend to go on holiday with what I've saved.

1 Why do some non-smokers feel that the only way they will be accepted into a social group of smokers is to smoke as well?

2 Find out if anyone in your group has found themselves in this situation and managed to remain a non-smoker. Discuss the experience with this person.

NHS Direct

The NHS Direct telephone service was set up to give people access 24 hours a day to health advisers. Although the majority of calls are about medical problems, the service also provides information on a wide range of health topics. It is also linked to a website where people can access information themselves to determine whether to seek professional medical help. This was, in part, an attempt to empower individuals to take more control over their own health and thus relieve the NHS from unnecessary consultations. However, the number of visits to the GP has not decreased significantly, despite good use of NHS Direct.

Over to you

Use the NHS Direct website (to access the site, go to www.heinemann.co.uk/hotlinks and enter the express code 4256P) to investigate a health promotion topic of interest to you. Think about your own health behaviour and the area you think you need to improve on. Make yourself a health improvement plan and see if you can stick to it for a week. At the end of the week, evaluate how feasible it would be to make the changes permanently.

Healthy Living Centres

There are 350 Healthy Living Centres nationwide that target the most disadvantaged sectors of the population. The centres have been funded from the National Lottery's Big Lottery Fund and will receive funding for up to five years. The Healthy Living Centres initiative is intended to complement the 'Our Healthier Nation' targets by offering projects in local areas specifically aimed at making progress towards achieving the targets. The centres are about initiatives, partnerships and networks rather than about specific buildings, so you cannot necessarily visit a Healthy Living Centre. They are intended to offer additional provision to services already existent in an area.

Healthy Living Centres offer a wide range of services to people of all different ages and backgrounds. The centres offer innovative and holistic approaches to healthy living, including:

- exercise groups for older people
- cafés serving healthy foods
- drug and alcohol awareness programmes
- stress counselling
- smoking cessation
- community allotments, which enable people to grow their own vegetables.

The centres are encouraged to monitor the health of their users in order to be able to evaluate the impact centres are having on the health of the local population. This will also ensure that the Big Lottery Fund is being spent effectively.

Healthy Living Centre, Blackburn

The Blackburn Healthy Living Centre initiative has encouraged members of the predominantly Asian community to participate in sporting activities such as swimming and aerobics. One of the most innovative projects is a walking group. Social walking is an alien concept to much of the Asian community, and some organisations who lead guided walks have received criticism for failing to attract people from minority ethnic groups. The incidence of coronary heart disease, strokes and high blood pressure in people of Asian origin is high, and walking is known to improve cardiac health. The walking group initially catered for men, most of whom had been referred by their GP. Following a family walk, women started to attend as well. The first walks were to local beauty spots, and now different grades of walks are offered. Some of the walkers have gone on to become walk leaders.

They have been encouraged to join other groups, such as the Ramblers Association, but the majority prefer to walk with their peers, who speak the same language.

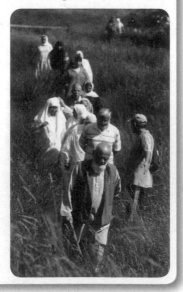

Blackburn Healthy Living Centre's walking group

Over to you

Your school nurse has become very concerned at the numbers of children who are participating in binge drinking sessions. She has decided that the school can no longer ignore this behaviour, as letters home seem to have had no impact whatsoever. The school nurse comes to your health and social care lesson to say that she wants you to help her devise a project to tackle the problem. She will then put in a bid to the local Healthy Living Centre, to try to get funding for the project.

Developing the project

As a group, devise a strategy to attract fellow pupils away from binge drinking sessions and encourage them to use their time better. Divide yourselves into the following sub-groups:

- Group 1 – write a justified proposal to present with the bid, explaining what you are hoping to do and how this will reduce binge drinking. Try to incorporate some reference to theory about how to change behaviour (see also Chapter 4, pages 144–148).
- Group 2 – create materials to promote the scheme to other pupils, thinking carefully about the design and language used and making it suitable for the target audience.
- Group 3 – work out the costing of the scheme. This would include marketing materials, the cost of any activities, and staffing.
- Group 4 – devise a tool, such as a questionnaire, to monitor the effectiveness of the project. This would be used to give feedback to the Healthy Living Centre six months into the scheme.

Evaluation

1 What difficulties did you encounter in carrying out this project?
2 How difficult was it to design the project using actual theory rather than your own ideas?
3 How did you tackle the costing?
4 Try out the monitoring tool, devised by Group 4, to establish how easy it would be to produce a report suitable to send to the Healthy Living Centre. Would you be able to give concrete evidence about the success or failure of the project?

Health Action Zones

There are 26 Health Action Zones (HAZ) in England targeting the most deprived areas in the country. The HAZ focuses on four main areas of action:

- improving health and reducing health inequalities
- improving access to services
- ensuring that local people have a voice in decision making about health
- better integration of social and health care services that will meet the needs of the most vulnerable families and young people.

(NHS: The Improvement Network website)

Special projects are set up and initiatives are specifically designed to meet the needs of the area, such as drop-in centres for young people to give advice about contraception and sexual health. The aim of such projects is to reduce teenage conceptions and sexually transmitted infections in the local area. This is done by offering contraception and sexual health services for young people aged 12–25 years, as well as a drop-in facility offering advice.

Charlene

I am 14 years old. I had been drinking cider in the park with friends one evening and chatting to Rob, who I'd been attracted to for some time. When he walked me home I realised my Mum was out, so I invited Rob in. We ended up having unprotected sex. The next morning, I realised what an idiot I'd been because I was worried I might be pregnant. Fortunately, a few weeks earlier a peer educator from a project based at my local health centre had come to my school and talked to my tutor group in PSE. She had mentioned the 'morning after' pill. I decided that I wanted to take this, because if I waited for my next period and then found out that I was pregnant, that would be really awful.

I went to the health centre after school, but the office was closed although a nurse was there. I was told go into the city, but couldn't think of a valid

reason to tell my Mum why I would not be at home when she returned from work. Luckily, the nurse was able to issue emergency contraception to me there and then. I told the nurse that there was no way I could have taken this action were it not for the project.

(Source: Adapted from Nottingham Health Action Zone (HAZ) final evaluation report for KISS – Knowledge and Information about Sexual Health and Sexuality. Dara Coppel, 2002)

Target setting

Target setting for GPs has become a common strategy to increase uptake of health promotion strategies. In addition to childhood immunisations, target setting now includes initiatives such as cervical smear tests and the prescription of statins.

GPs are paid on a *per capita* (average per person) basis. For some initiatives, the practice receives a lower rate per person if the practice fails to hit the target, for example, the target for childhood immunisation is 90 per cent. This is an incentive for GPs to make a greater effort to encourage parents to bring children in. Thus, whereas years ago, parents would be expected to remember to bring children to the clinic for vaccination, today reminders are sent out and repeated if parents fail to present their children for vaccination. The health visitor's role is to give further encouragement. A similar system is in place to encourage women to attend for cervical smear tests.

Health Improvement Programmes

Health Improvement Programmes were instigated in 1999. They are rolling three-year local frameworks which bring together local health authorities, primary care trusts, health professionals such as dentists and pharmacists, local authorities and others. The participants work together to improve the health of the local population, tackle health inequalities and improve local services. The programmes identify the most important health needs of the local population and develop strategies to meet these needs. This also involves developing new services where insufficient services exist to meet local needs.

Health Protection Agency

The Health Protection Agency (HPA) was created in April 2003 to provide better protection against infectious diseases and other dangers to health, including chemical hazards, poisons and radiation. The functions of the HPA are as follows:

● The HPA aims to identify and respond to health hazards and emergencies in the UK through the Centre for Emergency Preparedness and Response. To this end, the HPA runs training courses for practitioners and co-ordinates exercises to monitor the country's ability to cope in a major health emergency situation.

● The HPA anticipates and prepares for emerging and future threats such as avian influenza (should it mutate into a form easily transmitted between humans). The agency identifies the severity of the risk of new diseases emerging, and develops strategies to minimise the impact on those living and working in the UK.

● The agency alerts and advises the public and government on health protection through the distribution of explanatory leaflets and by using the media to bring issues to the notice of the general public.

● The HPA provides specialist health protection services, such as genito-urinary medicine (GUM) clinics.

● The HPA supports others in their health protection roles through offering training courses.

(Source: Health Protection Agency website)

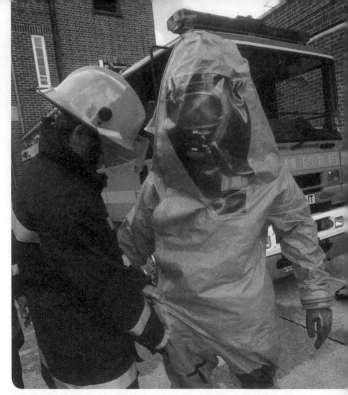

Part of the HPA's work is training emergency staff to cope in a major health emergency situation

The aim of the HPA is to protect the health of the population, prevent harm and prepare for threats to health and well-being. About 2700 people work for the Health Protection Agency including:

● specialists in communicable disease control, who tackle outbreaks of infectious diseases and prevent the spread of disease through vaccination and other measures

● public health specialists

● infection control nurses

● emergency planning advisers

● microbiologists, who study the organisms that cause infectious diseases

● epidemiologists, who monitor the spread of disease

● toxicologists, who study the effects of chemicals and poisons on the body

● laboratory scientists and technicians

● information specialists, who organise information and make it accessible to other members of staff

● information technologists, who input data onto computers to assist with analysis of information.

Other health promotion initiatives in the UK

Initiatives in schools

The School Health Service aims to promote the health of school-age children through prevention of ill health, early detection of illness and developmental delay, and by maximising the health of children with chronic health problems. The service was created to prevent children falling behind with their education for health reasons. This is achieved through a programme of routine medical checks at regular intervals through a child's school career, which make sure that children are growing and developing within the normal range. This includes routine checks on eyesight and hearing. Any problems detected can be referred to the appropriate specialist services. The School Health Service also continues the immunisation programme started before children attend school. School nurses provide health promotion within the national curriculum, delivering sessions to whole classes, small groups and individuals as appropriate. The School Health Service also employs paediatricians, who are doctors specialising in child health.

The School Fruit and Vegetable Scheme is part of the 5-a-day campaign to increase consumption of fresh fruit and vegetables. All children aged 4–6 years are entitled to a free piece of fruit each day.

Health centres

Although most people associate health centres with ill health, there is also a range of health promotion services available.

Well-person checks

Well-person checks are available to anyone who feels they need one. These are nurse-led clinics in which individuals are able to discuss their lifestyle and the risks associated with it. In addition, the individual's general health can be assessed by a series of tests to check for diabetes, raised blood cholesterol and weight/height ratio.

Health checks are available on an annual basis to monitor the health of over 75 year olds, particularly those who have not visited their GP for more than 12 months. They offer advice on maintaining health, and routine checks are made, such as blood pressure measurements.

Antenatal care

Antenatal care is offered to all pregnant women and is designed to keep both mother and baby well. Women are offered advice about such issues as diet and smoking cessation, which is designed to prevent complications as the pregnancy progresses. Routine examinations and investigations detect any abnormalities as early as possible and enable treatment to be given quickly or plans to be made to provide care that will minimise the risks of harm to mother or child. This might include identifying that the baby is lying in an unusual position and planning a caesarean delivery to safeguard the baby.

Child health surveillance

Child health surveillance is carried out by a health visitor and general practitioner. Babies are monitored for growth and weight gain, as well as the age at which they reach developmental milestones in their physical, intellectual, language, social and emotional development. It is vital that developmental delay is detected as early as possible to minimise the effect on the child's overall development. In conjunction with this, parents are invited to bring their babies for immunisation, to prevent a wide range of childhood illnesses, some of which can lead to disability in some children.

Age of child	Immunisations offered
Birth (only in infants at risk)	• Tuberculosis
2 months	• '5-in-1': Diphtheria; Pertussis (Whooping Cough); Tetanus; Polio; Haemophilus Influenzae type B (Hib) • Pneumococcal conjugate vaccine (PCV)
3 months	• '5-in-1': Diphtheria; Pertussis (Whooping Cough); Tetanus; Polio; Haemophilus Influenzae type B (Hib) • Meningitis C (meningococcal group C)
4 months	• '5-in-1': Diphtheria; Pertussis (Whooping Cough); Tetanus; Polio; Haemophilus Influenzae type B (Hib) • Meningitis C (meningococcal group C) • Pneumococcal conjugate vaccine (PCV)
12 months (approx)	• Meningitis C (meningococcal group C) • Haemophilus Influenzae type B (Hib)
Around 13 months (approx)	• Measles, Mumps and Rubella (MMR) • Pneumococcal conjugate vaccine (PCV)
Pre-school (between 3 years 4 months and 5 years)	• Diphtheria; Pertussis (Whooping Cough); Tetanus; Polio • Measles, Mumps and Rubella (MMR)
13 to 18 years old	• Diphtheria; Tetanus; Polio (given by school nurse)

(Source: NHS Immunisation Information website, 2006)

Table 7.03 Routine immunisation schedule for children in the UK

Over to you

Investigate the complications associated with the childhood diseases included in the routine immunisation schedule in the UK (Table 7.03).

Travel advice clinics

Travel advice clinics are another example of primary prevention, as immunisations given before travel overseas should prevent a range of very serious illnesses prevalent particularly in tropical countries.

Over to you

Choose a country that you might like to visit for an exotic holiday and find out what immunisations you would need. Do they have any side effects or contra-indications? What are the signs and symptoms of the diseases you would be at risk of contracting? Would you still want to go ahead with your holiday plans?

Occupational health

Since the Health and Safety at Work Act 1974 (see Chapter 5 page 193), employers have had to take responsibility for the welfare of their employees. There is no requirement for staff in the UK to have access to occupational health staff, although many workplaces do offer such facilities. Employers are, however, obliged to provide a safe working environment, which not only means that staff should be protected as far as possible from the risk of accidents but also that risk assessments should be carried out to ascertain if the workplace increases employees' risks of developing particular diseases.

The health risks of welding

Welders have an increased risk of cancers of the lung, larynx (voice box) and urinary tract, caused by inhaling welding smoke, which can contain cadmium, nickel, beryllium, chromium and arsenic. Welders may also develop retinal damage, cataracts, chronic respiratory problems, heart disease, stomach disorders, kidney damage, hearing loss and poor sperm quality. Clearly there are a lot of hazards, but the risks can be reduced, for example, by ensuring good ventilation, wearing helmets and ear defenders, and using techniques that minimise the amount of fumes, smoke and noise produced. In addition:

- the air quality should be monitored
- welders should receive annual medical checks specifically designed to test for the conditions described above
- welders should be thoroughly trained to ensure they know how to minimise the risks associated with their work.

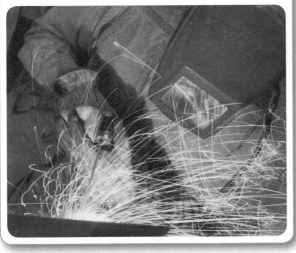

Over to you

Think of a job that appears very hazardous or choose from the following list:

- *coal miners*
- *nurses*
- *IT workers*
- *radiographers.*

Find out what hazards these workers face and what measures should be taken to reduce the risks to health and safety.

Reducing the risks of MRSA

The Health and Safety at Work Act 1974 requires employees to take responsibility for their own health and that of colleagues, visitors and those in their care. The spread of MRSA is dependent upon staff adopting very strict hygiene procedures. Consider the perspectives below:

- I am a nurse working on a busy ward. As far as I am concerned, none of the patients on the ward has MRSA. I am simply doing the observations of temperature, pulse and blood pressure.
- I have recently been discharged from hospital and have subsequently discovered that I contracted MRSA during my stay. My wound is taking a long time to heal and I have to take some very strong antibiotics. The ward was very busy, and I know that although the nurses looked after me very well, they did not always wash their hands between patients.

1 How would you feel if you were the patient that has contracted MRSA?

2 How would you feel if you were the nurse and a patient asked you if you had washed your hands?

International health promotion initiatives

World Health Organisation

The World Health Organisation (WHO), established in 1948, is an agency of the United Nations. It is governed by 192 member states through the World Health Assembly, whose task it is to approve the WHO programme and budget. WHO's key objective is, 'the attainment by all peoples of the highest possible level of health'. Programmes in 2006 include:

- the Intersun Programme, which aims to raise awareness of the risks associated with exposure to UV radiation
- the Diabetes Programme, which aims to develop international standards for diabetes treatment and contribute towards research into prevention of diabetes.

WHO's Three-Year Programme (TYP) aims to strengthen the organisation's capacity to support member states in preparing for and responding to crises, such as the South Asian Earthquake and the Central African Republic crisis (where two-thirds of the population live on less than $1 a day). In these situations, the WHO assesses health priorities, co-ordinates health stakeholders, ensures gaps are identified and filled, and supports local capacity to provide services.

Save the Children

Save the Children is an example of a voluntary organisation that promotes health on an international scale. One example of the work of Save the Children is the Saving Newborn Lives programme, which aims to reduce the horrendous infant mortality rate in developing countries. Every year, four million babies die worldwide in the first month of life. Three million of these lives could be saved by low technology solutions such as a providing a hygienic environment for delivering infants, immunising pregnant women against tetanus, and breastfeeding rather than bottle feeding.

Health behaviour theory

Why do people not follow health advice?

It is an interesting anomaly that, despite a wealth of advice about how we should behave to keep ourselves healthy, many people ignore some, most or all of the advice about healthy lifestyles.

The above is a substantial list of advice, which many people find overwhelming and too restrictive. Some people simply do not have this amount of control over their lives. Those who believe in an 'external locus of control' (see Chapter 4, page 140) consider that their health is controlled by things outside of their body, such as luck, God, people more powerful than themselves. Those who take responsibility for their own health tend to have an 'internal locus of control' (see Chapter 4, page 140). Such people recognise the positive influence they can have on their life; they know that if they behave in an unhealthy way, they must accept responsibility when something goes wrong.

Ignoring health advice

About 65,000 people are diagnosed with skin cancer in the UK each year. In 2003, Cancer Research UK published a survey which showed that 75 per cent of people questioned are concerned that exposure to the sun can cause skin cancer. However, only 6 per cent of those questioned avoid the midday sun, less than 5 per cent wear hats, sunglasses and T-shirts, and less than 40 per cent use high-factor sunscreen. According to the same survey, 70 per cent of people think suntans make them look healthier and more attractive. (Source: Cancer Research UK) This may be true in the short term, but one of the long-term effects of substantial exposure to the sun is premature ageing.

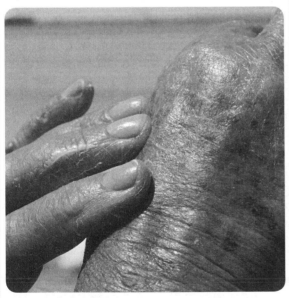

Many people risk premature ageing of the skin through sunbathing and the use of sunbeds

1 Why do you think people still sun-bathe without adequate sun protection, especially when there are so many products on the market to give skin a tanned appearance?

2 What do you think would make people change this behaviour?

Essential elements for change

To successfully persuade a person to change his or her behaviour, he or she must want to do so. In addition, he or she must:

- be currently worried about the potential effects of his or her lifestyle on personal health
- feel that the benefits of changing outweigh the consequences of not doing so
- be in a position to carry out the change, including having control over that aspect of lifestyle
- have the support of friends and family.

Essential element	Reason to change
Current fears about lifestyle	Risk higher than I realised; over 1 in 1000 people in the UK develop skin cancer annually.
Benefits of changing	Reduced risk of skin cancer and, therefore, having to endure operation(s), unpleasant treatment and possible early death. Won't have such wrinkled skin when I am older.
Consequences of not changing	Won't look tanned and healthy in summer. Possibly less self-confidence.
Ability to change	If I find really good fake tan. This, and the high factor sun cream, will be expensive, but if I can afford it I will do it.
Support needed	People to admire my fake tan. Family and friends not complaining if I want to keep out of the sun between 11am and 3pm.

Table 7.04 Desired health behaviour: always use sunscreen

Running a health promotion campaign

Health promotion campaigns are devised following identification of a need to change health behaviour to reduce incidence of ill health. The Department of Health uses data sources such as the Office of Population Census and Surveys to identify current patterns of disease in the UK. Where there are obvious differences between incidences in one population group to another, the potential for health improvement is noted. Research determines exact causes of certain diseases, and this information can be used to produce advice to enable people to reduce their risks. One such example is the research carried out in the 1950s by Sir Richard Doll, which linked cigarette smoking to the development of lung cancer. More recently, passive smoking has been proven to increase the risk of cot death and asthma. This has enabled health promoters to target families with young children, to educate them of the risks they pose.

There are a variety of methods used to promote health; some of these are listed in Table 7.05. Methods are chosen according to a variety of factors, including budget and resources available, appropriateness for target group and perceived effectiveness.

Methods	Examples
Medical intervention	Immunisation; mammography
Educational	Parentcraft classes; sun safety
Shock tactics	Drink-drive advertisements; warnings on cigarette packets
Cultural change	Healthy work initiatives; free fruit for schools; media pressure on food industry
Client-centred	Smoking cessation; contraception
Environmental control	Pollution control; water treatment
Legislation	Health and Safety at Work Act 1974; Control of Substances Hazardous to Health Regulations 2002

Table 7.05 Methods used to promote health

Medical intervention

Medical intervention tends to be an effective way to prevent disease. It takes responsibility away from the individual. People generally trust the method, as strategies have been developed scientifically, with extensive trials to prove effectiveness.

One example of medical intervention is mammography. Mammography is a low-dose x-ray of the breast, which can detect tumours that cannot be detected through self-examination. All women in the UK aged 50–70 years are offered three-yearly mammograms. Women who have two or more close female relatives who have had breast cancer will be able to attend from a younger age.

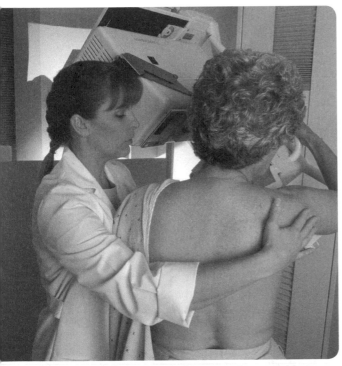

Mammography is a medical intervention available to women aged 50–70 years in the UK

Did you know?

Further information on the NHS Breast Screening Programme can be found on the NHS Cancer Screening Programmes website. To access the site, go to www.heinemann.co.uk/hotlinks and enter the express code 4256P.

Educational method

This involves giving factual information that allows individuals to make an informed choice about health behaviour. One example of the educational method is parentcraft classes. These teach prospective parents how to safely care for a new baby. They are not intended to impose values. For example, both breastfeeding and bottle-feeding are discussed, and the advantages and disadvantages of both methods are explained. Although it is known that breastfeeding has more advantages for the baby than bottle-feeding, some mothers are unable to breastfeed due to insufficient milk supply or illness after a difficult delivery, for example. Others do not like the idea of breastfeeding. Whatever the reason for opting for bottle-feeding, mothers must not be made to feel guilty because bottle-fed babies can still grow up to be healthy and happy.

Shock tactics

Presenting individuals with the potential consequences of their behaviour can be enough to frighten some people into changing their lifestyle. For example, television and radio adverts about drink-driving use horrific sounds or sights to emphasise the dangers of driving whilst under the influence of alcohol. The adverts are particularly aimed at young adults. Shock tactics are also used as health warnings on cigarette packets (see Chapter 4, page 159). However, this does not seem to have had a dramatic effect on reducing cigarette smoking. Indeed, there is no real evidence that shock tactics work.

Reflection

Based on your reading of the essential elements for change earlier in this chapter (page 267), can you think of any reasons why shock tactics might be an ineffective method of changing behaviour?

Social change

When traditional behaviour of a society is proven to be unhealthy, a cultural change has to be achieved to improve health.

One example of a cultural change regarding working practice in the UK, is that ear defenders should be worn by anyone who is exposed to loud noise in their job. Workers are sometimes initially reluctant to wear ear protection, considering it contrary to their 'macho' image. However, the Health and Safety at Work Act 1974 requires employers to provide, and employees to use, safety equipment. If employers rigorously enforce the wearing of ear defenders, it becomes the norm, so workers do not feel embarrassed.

Client-centred

Some health promotion is best tackled on a one-to-one basis with individuals. Contraception, for example, is a very personal issue and can be quite complex. There is a wide variety of methods to choose from, each with advantages and disadvantages. As each person is different, one-to-one sessions are the most effective way of ensuring that people get the best product to meet their individual needs and, just as importantly, know how to use the contraception properly to avoid conception and sexually transmitted infections.

Environmental control

Reduction in disease incidence has been achieved more by improvements in environmental conditions than by any other initiative.

Contaminated water

Contaminated water still causes millions of unnecessary deaths in developing countries today. According to the World Health Organisation, in 2000, 1.1 billion people worldwide did not have access to clean water. The WHO also estimated that, every year, 4 billion cases of diarrhoea and millions of other cases of illness are caused by unclean water consumption. The latter can include diseases caused by washing in infected water and diseases spread by insects that breed near water. Some parasites enter the body through the skin. Schistosoma larvae, for example, enter humans through unbroken skin, and migrate through the lungs to reach the liver. After 45 days they are mature. Males and females pair off, and the male transports the pair to a blood vessel, where they can live for years. They produce many eggs each day, which break from the blood vessel into the human bladder, and if excreted in a river, hatch into larvae and then penetrate a particular type of snail. Once inside the snail the larvae asexually reproduce thousands more larvae, which leave the snail and enter the water, and the cycle is complete. About 40 per cent of people infected with schistosomiasis live asymptomatically for years, but 50 per cent do have symptoms and 20 per cent have severe symptoms. The serious symptoms include blood in the urine (haematuria) and impaired physical and intellectual development.

In the UK, very strict controls ensure that tap water is safe to drink and waste water is safely carried away via sewers to be made clean enough to discharge into rivers or the sea. There are also strict controls over air pollution, refuse removal and industrial waste.

Legislation

The Health and Safety at Work Act 1974 and the many regulations that have since been incorporated into that legislation, ensure that workers are protected from risks to their health and safety in the working environment. Employers are obliged to provide training and protective equipment as well as ensuring that thorough and regular maintenance of equipment is carried out. Employees must attend training and use equipment supplied according to instructions. This also protects individuals using the service and members of the public. It affords protection from harmful substances and practices, and has resulted in a significant fall in industrial disease.

The Manual Handling Regulations 1992 cover moving and handling training, which focuses on avoiding lifting whenever possible. There are many aids available to assist care workers in transferring individuals unable to do so independently (see also Chapter 5, page 195). These regulations have significantly reduced the incidence of back injury in the health and social care sector.

Health promotion materials

Health promotion materials are designed with their intended audience in mind. Language, vocabulary and style need to be appropriate to the target age and gender. TV and radio adverts can be used to dramatic effect, with shocking images to remind listeners and viewers of the potential consequences of irresponsible behaviour. Leaflets can be widely distributed by making them available in public places such as libraries, pharmacies, health centres and schools.

The Internet has become a very useful tool to access health promotion advice. It is particularly useful when information on sensitive issues is required. However, there is also the danger that some people will look at descriptions of conditions and become convinced that they are seriously ill (when signs and symptoms are similar). This can cause unnecessary worry and visits to the GP.

Ethical issues in health promotion

Although health promotion aims to improve well-being, there are also ethical issues to consider.

It is not the place of health professionals to make value judgements on the way others choose to live, particularly if their behaviour does not cause harm to others. When considering particular health promotion initiatives to determine the ethical issues they raise, there are questions that can be used as a tool.

Ethical issues surrounding the rubella vaccine

GPs are currently under a lot of pressure to achieve a 95 per cent plus uptake of measles, mumps and rubella (MMR) immunisation. Until 1988, rubella vaccination was given to teenage girls at approximately 13 years of age. This was to ensure that they were immune to rubella before conceiving a child, as maternal rubella can have devastating effects on the developing embryo. (Congenital rubella syndrome is characterised by poor vision or blindness, congenital heart disease, loss of hearing, enlarged liver and learning disability.) The vast majority of teenage girls prior to 1988 would have had rubella as a young child, and consequently be immune, thus not requiring the immunisation. So, one ethical issue is that of giving unnecessary immunisations, rather than doing a blood test for rubella immunity and only immunising those girls who had not developed immunity naturally.

Since 1988, the MMR immunisation has been given to both girls and boys at about 15 months of age. Rubella is usually a fairly mild infection, so immunising boys is not generally necessary for their own protection. The main reason that boys and girls are immunised is to reduce the amount of rubella in the community, thus reducing the chance of an infectious child coming into contact with a non-immune pregnant woman. Therefore, this is an example of a health promotion measure given to one person to protect another, rather than to protect the actual person receiving the vaccine.

Another ethical issue could also be linked to this practice. Clearly, it is sensible to prevent as many babies as possible from being damaged by this condition. However, one reason for spending money immunising boys could be to save the cost to the country of providing care services for a child with congenital rubella syndrome.

Think of a health promotion campaign. Use the questions below to determine whether there are any ethical issues associated with that campaign.

- *Is the health promoter going to financially benefit from people following their advice?*
- *Does the campaign exaggerate the degree of risk of the activity you are trying to discourage?*
- *Is there advice for people who want to continue the unhealthy lifestyle but reduce the risks?*
- *Is the information given in language appropriate for the target group?*
- *Is the advice suitable for all, or should there be different advice for people from different religious, ethnic or other groups?*
- *Are there mixed messages? Does the advice keep changing?*
- *Is the information up to date with the most recent research and advice?*
- *Is the advice unbiased?*
- *Is the method 100 per cent reliable? If not, is the failure rate stated?*
- *Are potential side-effects of interventions clearly stated?*
- *Are people pressurised into conforming or made guilty for not doing so?*
- *Is the advice for the benefit of the person or for the wider community?*
- *Is the government committed to the initiative or worried about loss of revenue from taxation?*
- *Will savings be made in the long term if people follow the advice? Could this be the motive behind the campaign?*
- *Are there political motives – does the government want to be seen to be 'doing something'?*
- *Is it possible to prove that one particular campaign is more effective than other methods?*
- *Is personal responsibility taken away from individuals, or should it be?*
- *Should personal responsibility be given to individuals?*
- *Is the campaign aimed at protecting someone else, rather than the individual?*
- *Is there too much temptation around to allow people to easily follow the advice? Why is that temptation there? Could it be removed?*

Reflection

Life expectancy has risen from 49 years for women and 45 years for men in 1901 to 81 years and 76 years respectively in 2005.

- *The number of children dying from measles across the world has fallen by 40 per cent between 1999 and 2003. Successful vaccination programmes have led to the fall.*
- *Death rates from cardiovascular disease have been falling since the 1970s. In the last decade, the death rate for those under 75 years has fallen by 38 per cent, and for those under 65 years by 44 per cent.*

However, it is predicted by some that life expectancy rates in the UK will soon start to fall, and that it will become more common for some parents to outlive their children.

- *Since 1971, the incidence of cancer has risen by around 20 per cent in men and 30 per cent in women.*
- *Mortality rates for deaths related to alcohol consumption have been rising in England and Wales for many years, but this rise has been especially marked over recent years.*

1 Do you think that we have reached the limit on extending life expectancy?

2 Do you think the science fiction image of people living for centuries could ever become a reality?

Give reasons for your answers.

1 What are the main factors that determine longevity?

2 Apart from lung cancer, what diseases are far more prevalent in smokers?

3 What can affect a person's perception of what is meant by the word 'health'?

4 What is the difference between primary, secondary and tertiary health promotion?

5 In what ways has health been promoted by government policy and legislation?

6 What measures do individuals have to take to maximise their health?

References and further reading

- Acheson, D. (1998) *Independent Inquiry into Inequalities in Health*. London: HMSO
- Blaxter, M. (1990) *Health and Lifestyles*. London: Tavistock/Routledge
- Calnan, M. (1987) *Health and Illness*. London: Tavistock
- Coppel, D. (2002) *Final Evaluation Report for KISS – Knowledge and Information about Sexual Health and Sexuality*. Nottingham Health Action Zone
- Croghan, E. (2005) 'Supporting adolescents through behaviour change'. *Nursing Standard*, 19, 34; 50–53
- Hippisley-Cox, J., Fielding, K. and Pringle, M. (1998) 'Depression as a risk factor for ischaemic heart disease in men: population based case control study'. *British Medical Journal* 316: 1714–9
- Naidoo, J. and Wills, J. (2000) *Health Promotion: Foundations for Practice*. (2nd ed.) London: Baillière Tindall
- National Audit Office Press Office. *Health of the Nation: A Progress Report*. 14 August 1996
- Schlosser, E. (2002) *Fast Food Nation*. London: Penguin
- Von Ah, D., Ebert, S., Ngamvitroj, A., Park, N. and Kang, D.H. (2004) 'Predictors of health behaviours in college students'. *Journal of Advanced Nursing*, 48, 5; 463–74
- Walker, A. *et al.* (2002) *Living in Britain*. London: TSO
- Wanless, D. (2004) *Securing Good Health for the Whole Population*. London: TSO
- Williams, R. G. A. (1983) 'Concepts of Health: an analysis of lay logic'. *Sociology* 17: 183–205
- World Health Organisation 1946 Constitution. WHO, Geneva

Useful websites

The following websites can be accessed via the Heinemann website.
Go to www.heinemann.co.uk/hotlinks and enter the express code 4256P.

- British Acupuncture Council
- American Federation of State, County and Municipal Employees
- Action on Smoking and Health
- BBC
- BUPA
- Cancer Research UK
- NHS Cancer Screening Programmes
- Blackburn North Healthy Living Centre
- British Heart Foundation Statistics Website

- Health Protection Agency
- NHS Immunisation Information
- The Science Museum: Making the Modern World
- National Audit Office
- NHS Direct Online
- Big Lottery Fund
- Your Right to Health (debates healthcare in the United States)
- Wellcome Trust Sanger Institute (genome research)
- Schistosomiasis Control Initiative
- Scottish Executive
- Spartacus Educational
- National Statistics Online
- NHS Improvement Network (East Midlands)
- United Nations Children's Fund (UNICEF)
- World Health Organisation

Appendix 1: Physical, intellectual, emotional and social development

The following pages are intended to collate the key points of physical, intellectual, emotional and social development. You will find them useful for essay construction, revision points for external assessment and as a memory aid for class participation. To complement the diagrams on pages 278–285, several It's my story and Scenario features are included with associated questions.

Physical development

Laura

I went to my GP's surgery one afternoon feeling rather foolish because I didn't feel there was really anything wrong with me. The weather had been extremely hot, I couldn't sleep at night, I was sweating uncontrollably and consequently was extremely irritable and short-tempered, both at home and at work. I had a complaint against me at work for being unacceptably rude to a colleague when she asked for some clarification, and my partner was getting very fed-up with my attitude. I knew that my teenage children were keeping out of my way and although I felt awful, I couldn't help it. My GP examined me and took a detailed medical history after which she said that I was menopausal. I told her that I was only 44 years old! She told me that it can happen as early as that in some women. She prescribed some medication to help me and we agreed that I would return in three month's time.

1. What is meant by the term 'menopause'?
2. Explain the physiological process responsible for the menopause.
3. What are the signs and symptoms of the menopause?
4. What does the menopause mean for a woman's fertility?

Tracey

Some people will tell you that I have always been flighty. Certainly, I didn't attend school very much after I was 14. My mam ran a busy market stall as a way of keeping our home going and I was more interested in making money by helping her out. I married my boyfriend as soon as I could because I was expecting. After we were married, we lived with my mam and my four brothers and sisters. I was stunned when I had twins. They weren't identical: a boy and a girl and as different as chalk and cheese. That was when I wished that I had learned more at school. They fascinated me and I watched them constantly. Sara was the active one, crawling, walking and riding her little tricycle; trying to skip long before John. Even as they grew older, she continued to run about and play games while John put great concentration into doing little things, like trying to draw and do up his buttons and laces on his trainers. We said that John was the studious one while Sara was more like me.

1. What is the technical term for skills such as crawling and walking?
2. What is the technical term for skills such as drawing and fastening buttons?
3. Which of these skills uses large muscle groups?
4. Which skill is more precise and complex?
5. Which of the two skills develop first?
6. Explain why it takes longer to develop the later skills.

Intellectual development

Developing numeracy skills

Tony is 14 years old and has specific needs. He is often described as a 'slow learner'. He learned to count and get a grasp of addition and subtraction after a struggle. He is now able to multiply and divide simple numbers by using his fingers, but larger numbers are still beyond him. Anything he cannot identify with real objects is too difficult and he loses interest.

Using Piaget's theory of cognitive development as a guide, explain (as far as numeracy is concerned):

1 the stages of cognitive development that Tony has passed through
2 the stage he has reached at the age of 14
3 the stage he has yet to achieve as an adolescent
4 the cognitive development of an adult.

Leon

My mum told me that I was very slow to talk, and it has seemed to be so all my life. I have never been very good at expressing my feelings or starting conversations. At school, reports always seemed to comment somewhere about my lack of language. I hated class discussions as I could never think of anything to say. Other children laughed at me and thought I was stupid. I was not very good at putting words down on paper either. I'm 28 now and I have felt a failure all my life. I still live with my mum and dad and work as a builder's labourer, basically carrying things around the site.

1. Outline the stages of language development in infants and children.
2. Explain the links between communication skills and social, emotional and intellectual development.

Emotional development

Rasheed

I was at school with Leon (see Leon's story) and tried to befriend him when others laughed at him. He seemed to be wary of me because I was good at sport, popular with the girls and keen to learn. After school, I went to college to study health and social care and graduated as a psychiatric nurse last year. I realise that Leon has a negative self-concept and it has been that way since his teenage years. I met Leon again last week and invited him round for supper with my partner. He made a feeble excuse and said his mum would be expecting him home and off he went. I saw him across the street yesterday and he avoided me.

1. Explain the term 'self-concept'.
2. Describe some of the characteristics shown by a person who is said to have a negative self-concept.
3. How would you describe Rasheed's self-concept? How do you justify your answer?
4. Suggest one realistic way in which Leon's self-concept might be improved.

A growing pain!

Christine's son Adam is 16 years old and impossible to live with. His bedroom is always a mess and he knows that his mother is very house-proud. Last week he wrote some graffiti on his bedroom walls and there are posters of his favourite pop groups and football team stuck everywhere. One moment Adam is cheerful and fairly optimistic, the next he is depressed and saying that he is going to fail all his exams. He treats his family home like a hotel, coming in in the early hours after being with his friends and raiding the fridge. He has had several girlfriends but doesn't stay with any of them for very long. Every time Christine tries to scold him, he shouts back at her and then sulks for days. He won't discuss any problems with either Christine or his father. Christine is fed up with him.

1 What life stage is Christine's son passing through?
2 Discuss the idea that many of Christine's complaints can be attributed to this life stage.
3 Explain why you think Christine cannot get Adam to confide in her or her husband.
4 What pressures can impact on those passing through this life stage?

Social development

Roger

I that know my son is passing through adolescence in a fairly typical way, just like I did I suppose (see the Scenario on page 276). My wife Christine believes he is deliberately trying to be difficult and she chooses not to listen to me because she cannot remember being a trial to her parents. Socialisation is an important part of growing up in today's society. I know these problems will pass, but it's difficult to live with an unhappy wife and a moody son, believe me! Some days, I want to go and live on a mountain top.

1. Explain the term `socialisation'.
2. Primary socialisation occurs in early childhood. Explain the process of primary socialisation.
3. Secondary socialisation occurs in adolescence. Using Christine and Roger's son Adam as an example, explain secondary socialisation.

Adam

I was a pain to my parents when I was a teenager, but I knew I had to establish some freedom to go out with my mates. After I passed my exams and graduated from university with a business degree, I got a good job in a bank advising business clients and moved up rapidly to be a manager of large accounts. I am always being told that my communication skills are very good and this helps me tremendously when dealing with clients. I am happily married with two small children, a nice home in the suburbs and a fantastic social life. My parents are very proud of me and visit regularly.

1. Do you think Adam has well-developed social skills? How do you justify your answer?
2. Discuss the factors which have led to his successful social development using the diagram of social development on pages 284–5 to assist you.

LATER ADULTHOOD (65+ years)

Skin elasticity reduced
Bone density reduced
Senses deteriorate (taste, smell, hearing, sight)
Mobility reduces; stiffer joints
Balance impaired, particularly turning round
Blood pressure rises
Body systems less efficient leading to health problems
Constipation as muscles decline
Anaemia as food less well absorbed

MIDDLE ADULTHOOD (46–65 years)

Long-sightedness develops (presbyopia)
Skin elasticity starts to decline
Weight gain around trunk in some people as activity declines

Females:
Onset of menopause
Fertility declines and stops
Menstruation stops
Night sweats
Hot flushes
Irritability

Males:
Male menopause? – controversial

EARLY ADULTHOOD (18–45 years)

Completion of growth and muscle development
Selecting a partner
Sexual activity with partner(s)
Childbirth and rearing of children
Physical activity at peak
Home management
Starting work/career
Male hair thins

INFANCY (0–2 years)

Primitive reflexes, e.g. milestones of development = norms = average age for significant stages.

Gross motor skills:
Head control
Limb control
Back control
Sitting
Crawling
Walking
Running
Jumping

Fine motor skills:
Pincer grasp
Hand to hand
Holding spoon
Holding crayon

Physical changes:
Testes descend into scrotum
Growth of head and brain
Growth of trunk and limbs
Increase in weight and height

PHYSICAL DEVELOPMENT

CHILDHOOD (2–8 years)

Developing physical skills for activities/games
Fine tuning co-ordination of gross and fine motor skills

Gross motor skills:
Climbing stairs
Control of bladder and bowel
  movements
Riding scooter, bicycle
Climbing frames, swings
Hopping, skipping
Kicking a ball

Fine motor skills:
Tying shoelaces
Handling buttons
Using scissors
Writing
Drawing
Painting
Making necklaces of
  beads, daisies

ADOLESCENCE (9–18 years)

Growth spurt; muscular development; body hair; acne; tonsils/adenoids shrink.

Females:
Breasts grow
Ovulation
Menstruation
Growth of ovaries, uterus and vagina
Hips widen, altering body shape and gait
Deposition of fat changes shape
Voice less shrill

Males:
Voice breaks
Growth of penis and testes
Chest hair
Facial hair
Sperm production
Gland secretion
Shoulders widen
Increased strength

Cognitive Skills

Early infancy – responses mainly due to physical stimuli: hunger, temperature, discomfort, pain.

Infancy and childhood – Piaget described four stages, as follows:
- Sensori-motor (0–2 years) – learning through using senses and muscles.
- Pre-operations (2–7 years) – children do not always understand meaning and are unable to imagine perceptions of others, viz. pre-logical. Egocentric – focussed on the way they see things.
- Concrete operations (7–11 years) – logical thinking (problem-solving) provided that the issues are 'down to earth' and not abstract. Fact collection common.
- Formal operations (11 years+) – logical thinking beyond reality, using imagination.

Adulthood
Adults can reason through problems and construct hypotheses (probabilities from known facts) leading to reasoned investigations.
Adults continue to develop mental skills to cope with uncertainties, inconsistencies and contradictions.
Able to make judgements and to think flexibly.
Develop memory skills more effectively than in adolescence.

Later adulthood
Up to middle 70s, changes are small and often unnoticeable.
Late 70s onwards, generally some decline and reduction in speed at working out problems.
However, experience may lead to better judgements and decisions. Loss of memory may become more noticeable.

Dementia

Not a natural part of ageing, however, 1 per cent of adults over 60 years develop dementia and the rate doubles every 5 years. Symptoms include:
- difficulty with communication, expressing thoughts and understanding
- more difficulty in controlling emotions
- loss of memory
- problems with daily living
- difficulty with recognising people, places and things
- being unaware of where you are
- not knowing what is going on around you.

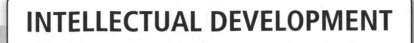

INTELLECTUAL DEVELOPMENT

How 'thinking' or cognitive skills and language are built and maintained

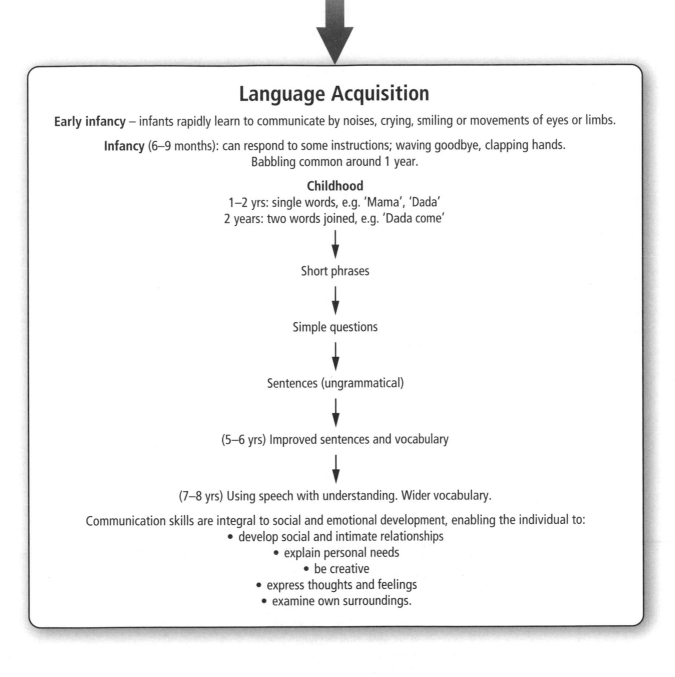

Language Acquisition

Early infancy – infants rapidly learn to communicate by noises, crying, smiling or movements of eyes or limbs.

Infancy (6–9 months): can respond to some instructions; waving goodbye, clapping hands. Babbling common around 1 year.

Childhood
1–2 yrs: single words, e.g. 'Mama', 'Dada'
2 years: two words joined, e.g. 'Dada come'

Short phrases

Simple questions

Sentences (ungrammatical)

(5–6 yrs) Improved sentences and vocabulary

(7–8 yrs) Using speech with understanding. Wider vocabulary.

Communication skills are integral to social and emotional development, enabling the individual to:
- develop social and intimate relationships
- explain personal needs
- be creative
- express thoughts and feelings
- examine own surroundings.

ADULTHOOD

Success and fulfilment of potential in working life and sexual life generally leads to an enhanced self concept. Responsibilities of having a partner, home and children present different perspectives according to circumstance. Self-concept may change in later adulthood.

Self-concept said to be a combination of self-esteem and self-image (and ideal self).
Self-esteem: how you feel/value/perceive yourself.
Self-image: how you see yourself as a person (not how you look).

Self-concept is a learned idea that you have of yourself as distinct from other people. Your self-concept may change as a result of life stages or life events, and may be positive or negative.

Positive self-concept:
Self-confident
Keen to accept new challenges
Motivated to do things
Happy in life
Likely to achieve or be successful
Plan ahead for future
Mix confidently with others
Not afraid to meet new people
Communicates successfully
Able to form intimate relationships
Happy with work and love
Clear thinking
Can work problems through
Accepts responsibility

Negative self-concept:
Lacks self confidence
Timid in approach
New challenges likely to fail, so doesn't try
Lack of motivation
Bumbles along through life
Settles for less than best
Thinks of today, not tomorrow
Reluctant to mix with others
Reluctant to meet new people
Has difficulty with intimate relationships
Confused thinking
Lets problems build up
Not particularly happy with life; may make excuses/blame others
May result in aggression, conflict, tension
Shuns responsibility

Merges into…

ADOLESCENCE

Knowledge of what makes you feel good/happy
Comparison of self with others
Rapid mood swings ('touchy')
Friends become main emotional support
Often idealistic or fanatical, e.g. about environment, politics, sport
Can be rebellious, angry
Low self-esteem, negative self-image and low self-confidence are common
Sometimes depressed

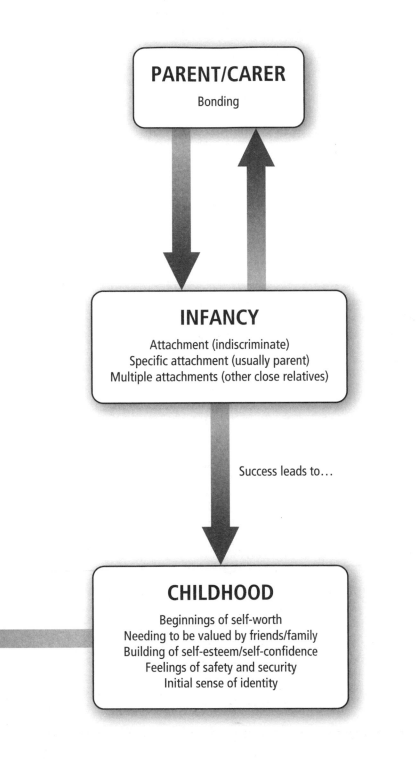

EMOTIONAL DEVELOPMENT

How individuals develop a sense of self/identity and develop feelings towards others

PARENT/CARER

Bonding

INFANCY

Attachment (indiscriminate)
Specific attachment (usually parent)
Multiple attachments (other close relatives)

Success leads to…

CHILDHOOD

Beginnings of self-worth
Needing to be valued by friends/family
Building of self-esteem/self-confidence
Feelings of safety and security
Initial sense of identity

Builds…

RELIGIOUS AND CULTURAL BELIEFS

CHILDHOOD

Primary socialisation takes place in early childhood. Acquisition of language, norms and values of the culture and society to which the child belongs.

'Socialisation is the process whereby the helpless infant gradually becomes a self-aware, knowledgeable person, skilled in the ways of the culture into which he or she is born.' (Giddens, 1997) Socialisation involves learning the social norms of your culture.

Secondary socialisation takes place in late childhood and adolescence. Acquisition of norms, values and behaviour of group membership to which the young individual belongs.

ADOLESCENCE

SOCIAL CLASS

Registrar-General's socio-economic ranking of groups of people based on occupation, wealth and status.

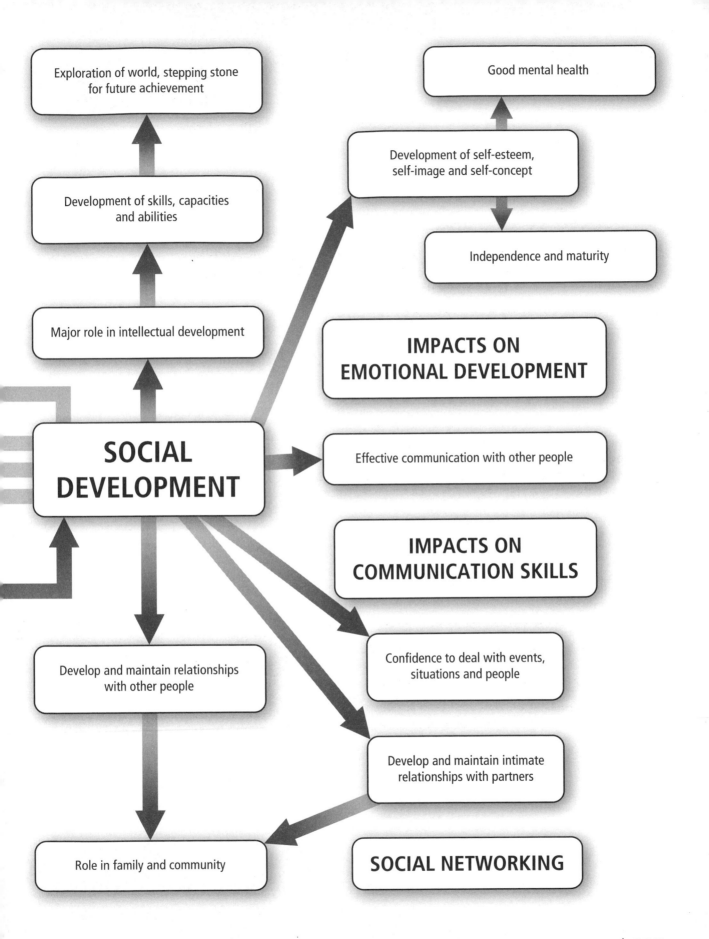

Exploration of world, stepping stone for future achievement

Development of skills, capacities and abilities

Major role in intellectual development

Good mental health

Development of self-esteem, self-image and self-concept

Independence and maturity

IMPACTS ON EMOTIONAL DEVELOPMENT

SOCIAL DEVELOPMENT

Effective communication with other people

IMPACTS ON COMMUNICATION SKILLS

Confidence to deal with events, situations and people

Develop and maintain relationships with other people

Develop and maintain intimate relationships with partners

Role in family and community

SOCIAL NETWORKING

Appendix 2: Study skills

Introduction

Studying should be an exhilarating and rewarding experience in itself, not just a means to an end. Of course, it's great when the qualification has been achieved. This may be the key to a better or different career, promotion or entrance to university. These are all wonderful outcomes to the study process.

However, some people regard study as a 'necessary evil' that has to be endured in order to achieve the goal. If you are one of these people, the aim of this section is to persuade you that this need not be the case – that you can positively enjoy your time as a student and perhaps experience the personal transformation that often results from taking an extended course of study. If you are already hooked and can't wait for the next course to begin, then that's great. Perhaps you will find a few helpful tips in this section that will make your studies even more enjoyable.

Study: a multi-skilled activity

Successful study is a multi-skilled experience. It includes self-awareness and good planning, reading and note-taking skills, expertise with words and numbers, and the ability to construct and sustain logical trains of thought. You will enhance your ability to perform well by knowing your own strengths and weaknesses with respect to this range of abilities. Once you have this awareness, you can play to your strengths whilst working on the areas that need development.

This range of abilities can be expressed visually in terms of a spider's web. Have a look at Figure A1 then use it to make a preliminary assessment of your current levels of expertise.

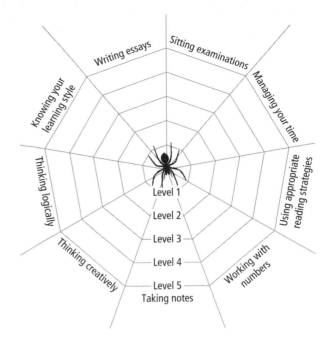

Figure A1 A 'spider's web' approach to study

Over to you

Take a pencil and block in segments of the web for each subject. Start at the centre of the web. If you are very confident about a specific set of skills, then block in four or five segments. If you are less confident, block in only one, two or three segments. The resulting web will give you a visual analysis of how you rate your study skills at this stage.

This appendix considers each of these topics in turn, as follows:

1 Getting organised – managing your time; knowing your learning style.
2 Using your brain – logical thinking; creative thinking; working with numbers.
3 Reading and writing – using appropriate reading strategies; note taking; writing essays.
4 Sitting examinations.

However, as space is very limited, there is room for only a few ideas under each heading. There is a list of supplementary reading at the end of this section.

Getting organised for study

Managing your time

How good are you at managing your time?

Use Table A1 to analyse how you currently spend your time. Be brutally honest.

Table A1 Time management chart

	Monday	Tuesday	Wednesday	Thursday	Friday	Saturday	Sunday
Morning							
Afternoon							
Evening							

Does your chart show that you could make better use of your time? Could you prioritise what you do? Do you need extra help with certain things? For example, if you have childcare responsibilities, could you use additional support to help you free up more time? Are some activities moveable – perhaps they could be better done at another time? If you are about to start a course of study, when might your study time be best scheduled? If you are already studying, could you benefit from being more systematic in your time management? However, you should always schedule in some rest and recreation. There is no point in burning yourself out by week eight of a thirty-week course.

1 *Use Table A2 to further analyse how you spend time.*

Table A2 Time management analysis

Time	Task	Notes
9am		
10am		
11am		
12 noon		
1pm		
2pm		
3pm		
4pm		

2 *Change the hours on the grid for evening tasks.*

Do you put things off? Are there a lot of distractions whilst you work? Perhaps you need a dedicated, quiet place to study. Do you have trouble concentrating or settling to the task in hand? In some cases, a 'pacing and reward' system can be helpful. Do you work better at certain times of day? If so, then rescheduling other tasks might be the answer. Whatever the issues are for you, it is important to devise a strategy to maximise your efficiency.

Time management: some tips

- Have a dedicated study space.
- Set clear boundaries (both in time and space) and ask whoever you live with to respect these.
- Establish your own framework for your working day.
- Manage your own personal 'time wasters'.
- Have a good filing system (to minimise time spent looking for relevant items).

- Set goals for tasks, both large and small (for example, finish reading a certain chapter, write an essay, etc.).
- Prioritise on a daily basis.
- Be flexible.
- Use travelling time wisely.
- Never underestimate what can be done in fifteen minutes.
- Schedule time off.
- Pace yourself to avoid fatigue (rest five minutes in each hour, etc.).
- Have a reward system for tasks achieved.
- Use techniques such as visualisation to focus on what needs to be done.

Knowing your learning style

The consultants Peter Honey and Alan Mumford have devised a very clear analysis of learning styles, which has proved a useful starting point for self-awareness for many students. A much simplified and adapted version is given in Table A3 below.

ACTIVIST	REFLECTOR
Learns best from: • new learning activities • short experiential activities like role play, simulated situations • no constraints on learning (e.g. no imposed format or structure) • being the focus of attention (e.g. leading a discussion) • difficult tasks • working with others (e.g. groupwork, team-based problem-solving) • 'having a go'.	Learns best from: • watching, thinking • listening, observing (e.g. day centre groupwork; film, video) • thinking before taking action (e.g. preparing in advance) • doing detailed research • doing thoroughly thought-through analyses and reports • exchanging views with others in a safe, structured environment • minimal pressure/deadlines to achieve targets.
THEORIST	PRAGMATIST
Learns best from: • material presented as part of a system, model or theory • time to explore connections between ideas, events, situations • chance to question/investigate methodology, assumptions, logic behind something • being intellectually stretched • structured situations with clear aims • material that emphasises logic and rationality • generalising from making an analysis • material containing interesting ideas/concepts (even if not directly relevant to the task in hand) • taking part in complex activities or projects.	Learns best from: • clear links between the topic and its application at work • techniques that have practical applications (e.g. speed reading) • trying out techniques with feedback from a credible expert • observing a clear model to copy (e.g. a specimen report; a film of a manual handling technique) • techniques applicable to own job • immediate opportunity to apply what has been learned • high 'validity' in learning activity (e.g. case studies based on real people) • concentrating on practical tasks (e.g. planning for a project).

Table A3 What kind of learner are you? (Adapted from Peter Honey and Alan Mumford, *The Manual of Learning Styles*, 2nd edition, 1986)

Self-awareness is a considerable strength. It is important to recognise how you like to learn, because you will then be able to capitalise on your strengths and work on your weaknesses. None of these styles is any better or worse than the others. For example, if your preferred style is activist, you may be an asset in a groupwork situation, giving a strong lead and injecting energy into the activity.

Using your brain

Thinking logically

Academic work is based upon the application of logical thinking. This is not to say that creative and imaginative thought does not play a role in study (see below); however, to succeed academically it is vital to master and apply a logical approach.

Some key aspects of logical thinking are:

- identify the issues/questions clearly
- question everything
- consider all the options (including advantages and disadvantages)
- be objective
- look for evidence
- look for similar examples from elsewhere
- be precise throughout the thinking process.

It is essential to define the question you are seeking to answer, together with associated issues. Often, you will be given an essay title as a starting point, but sometimes you will have to generate the questions for yourself whilst you are working. Useful questions might be:

- What evidence is there to support this theory?
- Have I seen something similar elsewhere?

- Is this argument subjective?
- Is this writer trying to manipulate scanty material to support a case?

The important thing is to question everything you read, and even to question your own assumptions and statements. In this way, you will be driven to explore many options.

Alison is in the first year of a degree in social work. She has an essay to write. The task is to review a number of theories on child development, then to apply one of them to a specific individual (she is doing a placement in a day unit for parents with small children).

- *What steps should Alison take to research and write her essay?*

Alison needs to:

- identify and read about those theories which are relevant
- identify a child to study
- take notes about each theory (the evidence used, its application), testing out how it might be applicable to the chosen child
- keep a 'work in progress' log, linking the theoretical reading to the child's observed behaviour.

Thinking creatively

Creative thinking also has a role to play in the academic process. Use of the imagination and visualisation techniques can be very powerful tools, often resulting in insights and connections that can radically enhance the logical process. The use of meditation and relaxation to enhance cognitive processes is now accepted. Music is also used, both to improve 'active' learning work (such as essay writing, active thinking) and to deepen the more 'passive' activities such as listening to a recorded voice or memorising material (see below).

The writers Edward de Bono and Tony Buzan (among others) have written extensively about thinking processes and how the brain works. They both encourage imaginative and unusual thinking (usually performed by the right-hand side of the brain) to enhance and complement logical thinking (usually performed by the left-hand side of the brain).

Making connections

Alison has a look at *Make the Most of Your Mind* (1988) by Tony Buzan and decides to try one of the exercises. She finds what she considers to be an unusual exercise. Forty items such as potato, shoe and pigeon are listed. The task is to think of ways in which 'paper clip' can be associated with each item.

Alison has problems with this, as she is a very structured thinker. She associates paper clips principally with their use in the office, although she has occasionally straightened one out and used it to unblock or clean something, such as the nozzle on a washing-up bottle. When she looks at the possible associations that might be made between paper clips and the forty items on the list, she realises how rigid her thinking can be.

The suggested connections include extending the paper clip and piercing the potato, then putting it in the oven. The paper clip will act as a transmitter of heat so that the potato will cook more efficiently. The clip could be used as an emergency shoelace or for cleaning the ridges on the sole. Finally, the clip could be used to attach an identity tag or a message to the pigeon's leg. The value of such a thought process lies in the ability to think 'outside the box'. Making unusual connections can enhance the logical thought process. If you can connect a paper clip with a potato, you will certainly be able to connect aspects of theories on child development to specific children.

Buzan encourages people to make uncensored connections around problems or issues that need to be worked on. This could include your essay questions. If you write the essay question in the middle of the page, and then start to generate ideas around it, no matter how far-fetched these may seem at the time, you are sure to come up with some stimulating and interesting connections. Buzan called this method 'mind mapping', and you can also use it for note taking (see below, and also Buzan and Buzan 1995 for a detailed account of this method).

Working with numbers

In order to apply logical thought processes to the material you study, it will sometimes be necessary to analyse numerical data. Chapter 6 (page 293) contains some advice on interpreting data, including devising tables, bar charts, graphs and pie charts. You will need to be able to decide what a set of figures actually proves (or otherwise). It will be important to ask whether a run of figures represents a significant trend (for example, annual temperatures that represent a trend towards global warming) or whether a recurring variable is significant (for example, the people using a particular service tend to be from a particular ethic group).

You do not need to be a mathematical genius, but simply need to have a questioning approach to any numerical data that is presented as part of an argument. A creative approach to the use of numbers can also be found in the work of Tony Buzan (1988).

Reading and writing

Using appropriate reading strategies

If you develop a strategy for approaching your reading list, you will put yourself in control of the material.

Reading: a strategy

- Identify the key issues/questions that you need to find out about.
- Skim books or articles to determine their relevance.
- Scan books/articles to identify relevant sections.
- Read relevant material in depth.
- Check back to your starting analysis: did you find out what you wanted to know?

Reading with purpose

Consider how Alison approaches her own reading list in tackling the essay on theories of child development.

Alison has a general booklist that was issued at the start of this module on working with children. She uses it to plan her reading and research for the essay on child development theories. She gets hold of three of the books, skimming them to see whether they will be of any use. She skims the contents lists and the summaries at the start of each chapter. One book contains nothing of relevance, and she rejects it for the purposes of the current essay. However, her skimming process has shown that the other two books are worthy of further attention.

She then scans the relevant chapters of each book, looking for items and references that will be of help. As a result, she decides that she needs to read all of the relevant chapters in depth, taking notes as she goes along.

Note that Alison has been selective in her reading and takes notes as she works. In the next section, you will consider some alternative ways of recording both the material and your thoughts.

Note taking

Taking notes from written material

Figure A2 Index card

Why take notes?

Note taking will enable you to:

- identify books/articles and their content
- summarise the gist of a book/article
- record the content/argument of a book/article in detail.

In the scenario above, Alison rejected one of the books she skimmed because it was not relevant to the essay. However, she feels that it may be useful at a later date, so she records the full publication details on an index card, together with a line summarising the contents (see Figure A2).

> **Did you know?**
>
> *There are several different conventions for recording the details of publications. However, you must record author, title, publisher and place of publication. For articles, page references must also be given. All these pieces of information will be vital if you need to find the work again or make a reference to it in your own written work.*
>
> *The following two examples show how typed references might be made.*
>
> - Smith, J. (2002) *Child's Play: Ideas for developmental activity in the early years.* London: Maxton's Publishing
> - Jones, S. (2005) 'Boys versus Girls: gender differences in an early years centre', *Journal of Education and Development* 97, 212–23

Smith, J. (2002) Child's Play: Ideas for developmental activity in the early years. London: Maxton's Publishing

Over to you

What differences are there between recording a book and recording an article? What system does your college/university use?

For recording details in greater depth, there are a range of options. The method you use depends to some extent on your preferred learning style. If you like the usual structure of working from left to right and top to bottom of the page, then the linear form of note taking may be for you. (This is, of course, the convention for written English; people who use other languages such as Arabic may prefer a different format.) On the other hand, if you respond well to visual stimuli and are not constrained by the 'normal' page layout, then pattern notes or mind maps may be your preference. All three are described below.

Linear notes

In this case, Alison has typed her notes using the publisher's convention of italicising the title of a work. She has used bold font for her own benefit, for the title and also for chapter headings. She uses white space around the chapter descriptions to help her when skimming her notes at a later date. She has also added the library shelf-reference to save time should she need to refer to it again. Linear notes (indeed all notes) can be enhanced by using highlighters, different fonts and careful use of upper- and lower-case letters.

Pattern notes

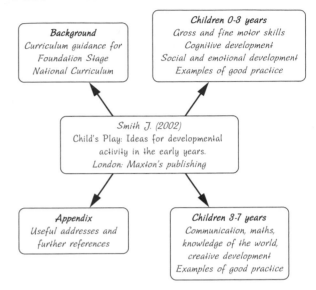

Figure A4 Pattern notes

This version records exactly the same information as the linear notes but simply rearranges it to give a more visual impression. Some people prefer this style, finding it more memorable, and both quicker and easier to read.

Figure A3 Linear notes

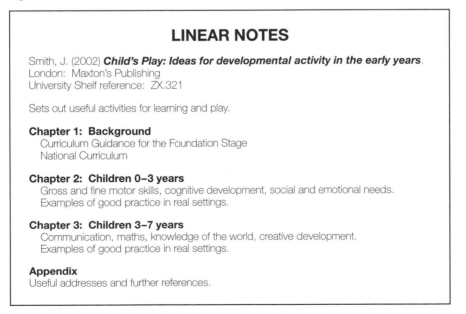

LINEAR NOTES

Smith, J. (2002) ***Child's Play: Ideas for developmental activity in the early years***. London: Maxton's Publishing
University Shelf reference: ZX.321

Sets out useful activities for learning and play.

Chapter 1: Background
Curriculum Guidance for the Foundation Stage
National Curriculum

Chapter 2: Children 0–3 years
Gross and fine motor skills, cognitive development, social and emotional needs.
Examples of good practice in real settings.

Chapter 3: Children 3–7 years
Communication, maths, knowledge of the world, creative development.
Examples of good practice in real settings.

Appendix
Useful addresses and further references.

Mind mapping

Finally, a less structured approach to note taking is the mind mapping technique, which has been most thoroughly described and explored by Tony Buzan (Buzan and Buzan, 1995). This is a very flexible and associative technique that allows the note-taker freedom to reassemble information and ideas in a meaningful way.

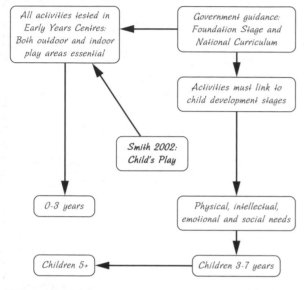

Figure A5 Mind map

Did you know?

The important thing is to find a note-taking method that suits you. None of these methods is any better or worse than another.

Taking notes from lectures

As with reading, it is a good idea to have a strategy for taking notes from lectures. Some tips for getting the best from lectures are:

- try to prepare in advance – be aware of the issues and have some questions ready
- devise your own shorthand system (see below)
- tape-record the lecture (ask permission first)
- pair up with a colleague to compare notes afterwards
- ask the lecturer for handouts or summaries.

Using shorthand

You can also devise your own shorthand system. Should you do this, you may find the following advice useful:

- Keep to the same acronyms for words and expressions you use frequently (for example, SW = social worker, SU = service user, etc.).
- Devise your own abbreviations and contracted forms for common words (for example, w = with; yr = your; nxt = next; man = manager, etc.).
- Use symbols/numbers/single letters as word substitutes (for example, + = and; 4 = for; R = are, etc.).

Taking notes from audio-visual media

Note taking from TV programmes, videos or DVDs can be difficult, as it is hard to watch the images whilst writing at the same time. Using a combination of the above options, however, can aid the process. There is also the added advantage of being able to play back the programme or film to check on misunderstood or missed items.

When taking notes from audio-visual media, remember to:

- prepare in advance (as for lectures)
- use your own shorthand system
- compare notes with a colleague
- play back to check your understanding.

Writing essays

There are some excellent books to consult on this subject. Of particular value is the very readable work by Good and South (1988) and the Open University Good Study Guides by Chambers and Northedge (1997) and Northedge (1990).

Key points on essay writing

Academic essays usually require you to be able to do four tasks, as follows:

1 describe or explain something (for example, the main features of a theory, a case study, etc.)

2 present an argument (for example, the view that global warming has almost reached the point of being irreversible)

3 evaluate two or more theories or viewpoints (for example, the case for and against providing complementary and alternative therapies on the NHS)

4 reflect on experience (this is especially important for students in the health and social care fields).

When you are working towards a particular piece of work, always bear in mind the title, being clear about what you have been asked to do. Essay questions will often include instructions such as *analyse*, *critically evaluate*, *explain*, *outline*, *state* or *summarise*. These are vital clues to the approach you are expected to take in your essay.

Essay writing – the process

The process of essay writing includes the following stages:

- jot down your main points
- organise these into a structure (see below)
- as you work, consider all possible viewpoints and options (it is fine to change your mind as you go along)
- make a first draft
- edit (cutting and adding as appropriate)
- get someone else to read it
- write the final version.

Remember, changing your mind is great – it shows that you are really thinking about the work.

A simple but useful essay structure would be:

- introduction
- paragraph 1
- paragraph 2
- conclusion.

Use the introduction to summarise what you plan to say, giving the tutor a clear idea as to the gist of your response to the question. Keep to one topic per paragraph. Use the conclusion to reiterate your argument (briefly).

A logical essay structure

Alison's essay asks her to review and critically evaluate several theories on child development, applying one of these to a specific child. Her essay structure might be:

- *Introduction*: This essay will review Theories (X) and (Y), and then apply Theory (X) to child (Z).
- *Paragraph 1*: Theory (X): whose theory it is and where/when it was set out. Key features of this theory. Evidence to support this theory; its weaknesses.
- *Paragraph 2*: Theory (Y): whose theory it is and where/when it was set out. Key features of this theory. Evidence to support this theory; its weaknesses.
- *Paragraph 3*: Anonymised description of Child (Z): age, characteristic behaviours and developmental issues.
- *Paragraph 4*: How Theory (X) is relevant to Child (Z)'s development. Ways in which it doesn't apply.
- *Conclusion*: Although in a few respects, Theory (X) does not apply to Child (Z), there are enough points of correspondence to suggest that this is a useful theory for understanding Child (Z)'s behaviour and development.

Alison has done everything the essay question has asked. She concludes that Theory (X) is useful for understanding Child (Z), but has anticipated criticism by pointing out ways in which this theory doesn't apply.

Now Alison has to express her argument clearly. Besides sticking to the structure and the rule of one idea/topic per paragraph, Alison is careful to use plenty of 'signpost' words to give her tutor clear guidelines as to where her argument is going.

'Signposting' in essays

Use words and expressions such as:

- firstly
- on the other hand
- conversely
- nevertheless
- in conclusion
- as has just been explained
- an alternative viewpoint is
- Theory (Y) will now be considered.

Your college or university may have guidelines on essay writing and style. Some colleges require a formal style, whilst others allow more intimacy and informality.

Over to you

Consider the following sentences.

A. Observation of the principle of confidentiality is mandatory when working directly with service users.

B. Professionals must observe the principle of confidentiality when working with service users.

C. As professionals, we must make sure that information about service users is kept confidential.

- *Which of these styles do you think is most suitable for writing an academic essay and why?*

Sentence A is the most formal and 'distant' of the three styles, and is the style usually preferred for university or college essays. Sentence C is rather informal and seeks to create a close link between writer and reader (note the use of 'we). This style might be suitable for writing guidelines or giving a talk. Sentence B is a blend of the two styles, and is also likely to be suitable for an essay.

The style you choose for your essay will depend on your college guidelines, your tutor's preference and your own expertise. It's a good idea to experiment with sentence structures, expressing the same idea in different ways to see what effect you get. Enjoy being creative and you may surprise yourself. If you have command of language and can use it in different ways to suit the context (whether written or spoken), your expertise as a communicator is greatly enhanced.

Sitting examinations

Andrew Northedge (1990) has described sitting an exam as a performance, comparable to playing a piano sonata or taking the lead role in a play. Musicians and actors prepare and rehearse exhaustively, working towards giving a superb performance at the end of this process of hard work and preparation.

Thinking about exams in this way is very helpful: it serves as a reminder that the exam is not just a one-off event for which you must make a last-minute effort. Rather, the exam is the natural culmination of a series of carefully planned tasks; if the tasks are carried out thoroughly during the course of a year (or more), then the performance is more likely to go smoothly. The exams, just like the essay, can be thought of as a process rather than a product.

This means that you need to start planning your exam strategy almost as soon as the course begins. This doesn't mean that you need to wind yourself up into a state of excessive anxiety months before you sit your exam. Rather, you should have the exam and its requirements in mind throughout your studies, keeping notes that will be useful during revision, putting aside copies of articles or books that will help, chatting to colleagues or to people who have already done this particular exam, and then carefully planning the time leading up to the exam so that revision is incorporated naturally into your schedule and there are no unfortunate clashes of commitment.

Some tips for devising an overall exam strategy are:

- know what's expected of you in each exam (study the exam requirements)
- don't leave revision to the last minute (see below)
- create notes that anticipate revision needs
- do test questions in exam conditions
- visit the exam room in advance: familiarity can give added confidence
- take advice from your tutor
- work out ways to control your anxiety

- keep things in perspective
- use a mentor to support you through the exam period (preferably someone who also has exam experience)
- avoid negative or over-anxious people during the exam period.

Revision: some ideas

- Make sure you've covered all compulsory topics.
- Be selective with optional topics (see below).
- Work towards the exam throughout the course.
- Make course notes with revision in mind.
- Use both active and passive learning strategies (see below).
- Have a revision timetable.
- Work with (positive) friends to share revision sessions.

The concept of active and passive learning requires a little explanation. Active learning is not the same thing as Honey and Mumford's 'Activist' learning style (see page 287). Rather, active learning involves performing tasks in which the learner is actively doing something concrete, for example, essay writing, making notes, making a video, creating a mind map, etc. Passive learning, on the other hand, requires the learner to be in a more receptive frame of mind, as when listening to a lecture, watching a video or meditating on a topic, for example. Of course, there is indeed something happening when a student is involved in passive learning – the brain is working continuously to process ideas, and it is possible to be engaged in a 'passive' task and to suddenly be galvanised into action as a result of making a significant connection of ideas. By and large, however, the broad distinction between active and passive learning techniques holds good as a working concept.

Active revision strategies

- Create and use memory devices (for example, rhymes, mnemonics).
- Edit information down to essential points.

- Create visual aids (e.g. index cards with pattern notes).
- Record your own voice to play back to yourself (facts, ideas, etc.; see scenario below).
- Use fast-paced music to enhance your creativity and boost your levels of brain activity.
- Complete old exam papers in exam conditions.
- Work with a group of friends to revise specific topics.

To balance your active strategies, passive techniques are desirable as they offer contrasting forms of occupation. This can be refreshing, allowing you to relax and learn at the same time, thus minimising the risk of exhaustion or burnout.

Passive revision strategies

- Listen to revision tapes (either your own voice, or commercially prepared).
- Listen to slow-paced music to aid receptivity whilst reflecting on a topic
- Watch videos and DVDs, etc. without making notes.
- Visualise your exam performance (a successful one!).
- Meditate to clear the mind.

Music can be very effective in boosting brain activity, and is useful for both active and passive learning techniques. Ostrander and Schroeder (1995) describe in detail the effect that music has on the brain, and how it can be used to speed up cognitive and creative processes, or to enhance retention and memory.

Music can also be used to enhance concentration whilst engaged in the active tasks of writing essays or reading, although it is essential to use this technique scientifically, applying the principles described by Ostrander and Schroeder. Playing your favourite *Black Sabbath* album whilst reading about Bowlby's theory of attachment is unlikely to be helpful. There is more on using music for a range of tasks in Campbell (1997).

The writer and thinker Tony Buzan has produced a vast range of books on aspects of the mind, learning and memory, and the items listed in the references at the end of this section are strongly recommended if you are looking for some ideas to liven up your learning in general and revision in particular.

Finally, a few tips for sitting the examination itself are given below.

Sitting an exam: some advice

- Get a good rest the night before (midnight-oil burning will not help at this stage).
- Arrive at the venue in good time.
- Use relaxation techniques in the half hour leading up to the exam (for example, deep breathing, visualisation).
- Read the paper carefully.
- Always comply with instructions.
- Choose optional questions that play to your strengths.
- Allocate time to each question.
- Read each question carefully.
- Plan each answer and stick to what is asked.

- Keep to a layout that enhances your answers (for example, use of white space, paragraphs, underlining, etc.).
- Write clearly and simply.
- Stay focused on the task.
- Ignore what everyone else is doing: your performance alone is important.

As with revision, a good performance on examination day comes down to planning, and staying calm and focused. Don't be put off by what other people are doing (either just before or during the exam itself). Everyone has his or her own methods (for example, going through pattern notes on index cards in the last fifteen minutes, or walking up and down reciting lists) – stick to what works for you. Similarly, don't be concerned by others' performance during the exam – that person who seems to have written reams after only 45 minutes may not have devoted enough time to proper planning. Or he or she may simply be a very quick writer. Either way, it doesn't matter. Your technique is the only one that matters. If you have prepared adequately and know how you are going to tackle the questions, you are invincible.

References and further reading

- Buzan, A. (1988) *Make the Most of Your Mind*. London: Pan Books
- Buzan, A. (1989) *Use Your Memory*. (Revised ed.) London: BBC Books
- Buzan, A. (2000) *The Speed Reading Book*. (Revised ed.) London: BBC Books
- Buzan, A. and Buzan, B. (1995) *The Mind Map Book*. London: BBC Books
- Campbell, D. (1997) *The Mozart Effect*. London: Hodder & Stroughton
- Chambers, E. and Northedge, A. (1997) *The Arts Good Study Guide*. Milton Keynes: The Open University
- Good, M. and South, C. (1988) *In the Know: 8 Keys to Successful Learning*. London: BBC Books
- Honey, P. and Mumford, A. (1986) *The Manual of Learning Styles*. (2nd ed.) Maidenhead: Available from the authors
- Northedge, A. (1990) *The Good Study Guide*. Milton Keynes: The Open University
- Ostrander, S., Schroeder, L. and Ostrander, N. (1994) *Super-learning 2000*. London: Souvenir Press

GLOSSARY

Acute   illness which flares up suddenly and is not long-lasting

Adrenaline   a hormone produced by the adrenal glands which boosts the heart and breathing rates and increases the strength of the heartbeat

Advocate   someone who speaks on behalf of another person

Aggregate   to aggregate data is to combine information collected at different times, and possibly from different sources

Allele   half a gene. Each gene, responsible for a characteristic, consists of two alleles, one from each parent. The alleles may be similar or different, dominant or recessive. Dominant alleles always show in the individual when present; a recessive allele will only show when both alleles are recessive

Amoeba   a single-celled microscopic animal living in water which moves by changing shape by flowing

Angiogram   an X-ray photograph of blood vessels, taken after injecting the vessels with a substance opaque to the rays

Antigen   a substance that causes the immune system to produce antibodies against it. Antigens are proteins (or sometimes carbohydrates) inserted into the surface coats of pathogens

Antigenic   types of inherited protein markers existing on the surface of an individual's body cells; blood cells are usually used as these are easy to obtain

Asbestos   fireproof material. Inhalation of asbestos fibres can lead to lung cancer and lung disease

Audit   a quality check (usually involving a detailed examination of an organisation's systems, structures and processes)

Auto-immune disease   disease in which the individual develops antibodies against his or her own tissues

Autonomic nervous system   consists of sympathetic and parasympathetic branches serving internal organs and glands. There is no conscious control over this system

Benign   any condition which, untreated or with symptomatic therapy, will not become life-threatening. The term is used particularly in relation to tumours

Bias   distortion of the results of a piece of research, due to the undue influence of a specific factor

Biopsy   examination of cells, tissue or fluid which has been surgically removed, in order to form a diagnosis

Bolus   masticated ball of food ready for swallowing

Bundle of His   a strand of conducting tissue that bridges the fibrous ring between the atria and ventricles

Causal inference   a strong suggestion that one particular variable has a specified effect upon another

Chromosome   long, thread-like structure located in the cell nucleus made of two parallel strands, which plays an important role in cell division. Genes are located on chromosomes

Chronic   illness which is deep-seated and long-lasting

Citation   the act of making reference to another piece of research

Cognitive   aspects of mental activity that involve the manipulation of material in an abstract way. This includes thinking, memory, perception and problem solving

Coronary heart disease   a number of illnesses that are a consequence of narrowing or blocking of the coronary arteries which supply blood to the heart muscle; they include angina, arteriosclerosis and myocardial infarction (heart attack)

Corpus luteum   a yellowish body in the ovary formed from the follicle cells after the ovum has been released. The corpus luteum secretes several hormones including progesterone

Correlation   a link between two data sets, or two (or more) variables within a data set

Covert   hidden; concealed

Demographic variable   aspects of the population surveyed; for example, age, gender, ethnicity, social class, level of education, type of occupation, level of wealth etc.

Demography   the large-scale study of populations

Dermatitis   inflammation of the dermis, the outer layer of the skin, caused by contact with an external substance

Dialect   words and pronunciation of words that is specific to a geographical community

Discourse analysis   a research technique in which speech or conversation is recorded and then analysed to determine how someone uses and structures language

Discriminate to treat a person differently (unfairly) because of prejudices (bias) about his or her sex, race, religion etc.

Emulsify the mixing of two liquids which do not readily make a smooth mixture, such that one is dispersed within the other as tiny droplets, e.g. water and oil

Enzyme biological catalyst promoting the rate of chemical change. Catalyst molecules are themselves unchanged at the end of a reaction and can be used over and over again

Epidemiology the study of the geographical incidence of disease in order to demonstrate potential causes (and cures)

Epithelium (or epithelial tissue) lining tissues which exist on external and internal surfaces of organs, blood vessels and body cavities

Ethnicity the customs of a particular cultural or racial group

Fibrillation uncoordinated contraction of muscle fibres in the heart

Gamete sexual reproductive cell; it cannot develop further unless united with a gamete of the opposite sex. The male gamete is a spermatozoon (sperm); the female gamete is an ovum (egg)

Gangrene the death of body tissue caused by a loss of blood flow, especially in the legs and feet. Gangrenous tissue turns black and smells offensive

Gender indicating differences in biological sex, i.e. whether a person is male, female, transgender etc.

Gene a unit of inheritance responsible for passing on specific characteristics from parents to offspring through constituent alleles. Chemically, alleles and genes are composed of deoxyribonucleic acid, or DNA

Gestation the period of development from conception to birth; a technical term for the duration of a pregnancy

Goblet cells mucus-producing cells

Gonads organs which are also sex glands; they produce gametes and hormones. They are the ovaries in females and the testes in males

Harassment to continually distress, annoy, pester or trouble another person

Homeostasis the processes by which the body maintains a constant internal physiological environment

Hormones chemicals secreted by the endocrine system which have both behavioural and physiological functions

Income support financial help given by the government to people aged between 16 to 60 years old who live on a low income or who have no income

Interpersonal between two people

Ionise to be converted into ions. An ion is an electrically-charged particle, having either a positive or negative charge

Jargon terminology that people in a specific social or occupational speech community use

Joint place where two or more bones meet

Language register the degree of formality or informality of language

Longitudinal study a research study that lasts for a significant period of time, allowing the impact of a number of variables to be taken into account

Malignant the term describes a clinical course that progresses rapidly to death

Mean the average score

Median the middle value of all the scores

Meditation suspending the stream of thoughts that normally occupy the mind to induce mental calmness and physical relaxation

Micro-organisms life forms seen only under a microscope. They include bacteria, viruses, fungi and parasites

Mode the most frequently occurring score

Negative feedback mechanism occurs when the increased output of a substance stimulates a change which in turn inhibits the increasing output and thereby re-establishes the norm

Nerve impulse an electro-chemical burst of activity, often known as an action potential

Neurones nerve cells

Neurotransmitter a chemical that is released by a neurone and taken up by another neurone

Noradrenaline a hormone secreted by the adrenal muscle as part of the 'fight or flight' response. It is also a neurotransmitter in the nervous system and affects parts of the brain where attention and impulsivity are controlled

Nucleus a membrane-bound structure that contains the cell's genetic information and controls the cell's growth, function and reproduction

Open question a question that cannot be answered with 'yes' or 'no'; it requires a response to be made in the person's own words

Osmosis the movement of water molecules from a high concentration to a low concentration through a partially permeable membrane. The partially permeable membrane is usually the cell membrane of single-layered epithelial cells

Output areas the small local divisions within which Census data is counted

Overt   open to view; not concealed

Pacemaker   artificial device for controlling the heart rate

Paraphrase   to express something a person had said in your own words

Pathogen   any disease-causing micro-organism, virus, bacterium or fungus

Peripheral vascular disease   narrowing of the blood vessels that carry blood to leg and arm muscles, which may cause pain when exercising

pH   a measure of Hydrogen ions. A scale of the measure of acidity or alkalinity of a substance which ranges from 1 (strongly acidic) to 14 (strongly alkaline), with pH 7 representing neutral (neither acidic nor alkaline)

Phagocytosis   process by which leucocytes change shape and engulf foreign material

Placebo   something that looks like a medical intervention, but which is in fact inactive

Plasma   a yellowish fluid that is the liquid part of blood; it is mainly water in which various substances are carried

Pleura   membranes covering the lungs and inner chest wall

Puberty   time of life when the secondary sexual characteristics develop and the capability for sexual reproduction becomes possible, usually between the ages of 10 and 17 years

Purkinje fibres   modified muscle fibres forming the conduction tissue of the heart

Race   group of people of common descent and with a common set of characteristics

Respondent   a person who takes part in a survey and who responds to the questions (either by self-completion of a questionnaire or during interview)

Role model   a person who is admired for any reason and whose behaviour may be imitated by others

Serotonin   a neurotransmitter found in the brain that affects mood and appetite. It is also thought to influence physical co-ordination, body temperature and sleep, and to play a role in the mechanism of migraine headaches

Sexuality   a person's sexual orientation, i.e. heterosexual, homosexual, bisexual

Slang   informal words and phrases that are not found in standard dictionaries but are used within specific social groups and communities

Statins   a relatively new group of drugs used to lower blood cholesterol levels, thus reducing the risk of heart attack

Stereotype   a fixed way of thinking involving generalisations and expectations about an issue or group of people

Steroid   substance from a lipid/fat base using cholesterol as a source

Substrate   the substance or substances on which an enzyme acts

Umbilical cord   long, 'rope-like' structure containing umbilical blood vessels which connects the foetus to the placenta

Variable   something that can occur in different forms, i.e. it can vary in its characteristics

Visualisation   concentrating on or imagining something very strongly as a visual image. A visualisation technique is often used to treat disease by inducing relaxation in the individual

Zygote   formed during fertilisation, when the nuclei of the ovum and sperm fuse; the start of a new human life

INDEX

A

abuse 38, 51–2
accidents, reporting 183–4
acid-base balance 68
action research 228
active listening 10, 18
acupuncture 255
acute, defined 74
addictions 158–9
  alcohol 160
  smoking 159–60
adrenaline 73, 118
advocacy 55–6
affirmative action 58
age and health 253
aggregate, data 240
aggression, dealing with 170–2
alcohol
  addiction to 160
  and heart disease 86
alimentary canal, structure and
  function of 91–6
allergies, treating 204–5
Alma-Ata Declaration 257
amino acids 96
analysing research data 234
  drawing conclusions 239–41
  qualitative data 238–9
  quantitative data 235–8
anaphylactic shock 205
antenatal care 263
anti-discriminatory practice
  actively promoting 59–60
  effects of personal beliefs and
    values 60–2
  national initiatives 52–9
anti-diuretic hormone (ADH) 112,
  118
anti-harassment 58
antigenic, defined 116
anxiety reduction 156–8
appendix 94
arteries 79–80
arthritis 123
asthma 74, 160

first aid for 202
attributional style 139–40
audits, quality checks 57
auto-immune disease 123
autonomic nervous system 83–4,
  127, 128–9

B

bacteria 187
barriers to communication 7–9
behavioural changes needed for
  healthy lifestyle 143–8, 266–7
beliefs 37, 60–1
benign conditions 148
bias in data collection 223, 231
biofeedback 157–8
birth process 105–6
bites and stings, treating 204
bleeding, first aid for 201
blood cells 80–2
blood circulation 77–8
blood pressure 84, 84–5
blood transport of oxygen 72–3
blood vessels 79–80
body language 4–6
bomb scares 172–3
breastfeeding 269
breathing 68–71
  checking for 199
  control of 73
bronchial asthma 74
bronchitis 74–5
bullying 50–1, 58, 59–60
burns, first aid for 201–2

C

caecum 94
cancer screening 250–1, 269
capillaries 79–80
cardiac cycle 82–4
cardiac muscle 78, 120, 121
cardiac output 83
cardio-pulmonary resuscitation
  (CPR) 198–9
cardiovascular system

arteries and veins 79–80
  blood cells 80–2
  cardiac cycle 82–4
  disorders of 84–9
  heart, functions of 74–9
care homes 41–2
Care Standards Act (2000) 53
care values 18–20, 44–5, 60
'caring presence' 14
caring relationships 13–14
case studies 228–9
causal inference 240–1
cell respiration 73
census data 209–10
charters, health 54
child health surveillance 263–4
Children Act (1989 and 2004) 53
choices, taking account of 50, 52
chromosomes 100
chronic pain 148–9
cleaning
  of equipment 189
  hand washing 188
  of spillages 189–90
closed questions 216
Cochrane Collaboration 227
codes of practice 18–19, 44–5
  professional conduct 54–5
  residential care 54
colonoscopy 99
communication barriers, overcoming
  7–9, 49
communication skills 45–6
  barriers to effective 7–9
  for developing understanding
    10–12
  non-verbal 4–7
  providing emotional
    support 13–16
  SOLER principles 12–13
  verbal 3–4
community cohesion 43–4
community hazards 169
complaints procedures 57
confidentiality 44–5, 58–9

learning styles 289–90

legislation

anti-discriminatory 52–3

codes of practice 54–5

equality and rights 55–6

health and safety 190–7

organisational policies 56–9

promoting health 270–1

leucocytes 81–2

life-saving procedures 198–200

life expectancy 272

lifestyle

adopting healthy 143–6

lifestyles

and heart disease 86, 89

lifting techniques 193–5

listening skills 10–11, 18

locus of control 140–3

logical thinking 290

lone workers, protecting 170–2

longitudinal studies 227

luteinising hormone (LH) 102, 103, 118

M

macro- and micro nutrients 91

male reproductive system 101–2

malignant, definition of 148

mammography 269

Manual Handling Operations Regulations (1992) 193–5, 271

Maslow, Abraham, hierarchy of needs 16

mean/median/mode 237–8

mechanical digestion 91–2

medical interventions, health promotion 269

medical model of health 254–5

meditation 151

menstrual cycle 102–3

mental health, definition of 254

Mental Health Act (1983) 52

Mental Health Order (1986) 52

metabolism 68

micro-organisms 186

migraine headaches, reducing with biofeedback 157

mind mapping 294

MMR controversy 228

models of health 254–5

Moon, Jennifer, levels of reflection 24–5

mouth-to-mouth resuscitation 199

movement 121–2, 127–8

MRSA (methicillin resistant Staphylococcus aureus) 265

Multidimensional Health Locus of Control Scale 141–2

multiple sclerosis (MS) 129–30, 227

muscle tone 120

musculo-skeletal system

disorders of 122–4

movement 121–2

muscle types 120–1

protective function 122

support functions 120

myocardial infarction 86

N

National Census 209–10

National Institute for Health and Clinical Excellence (NICE) 227

negative reinforcement 145

nephrons 110–11

nervous system

autonomic 128–9

disorders of 129–30

functions of 126–7

neurones 125–6

somatic 127–8

neurones 73

structure and function of 125–6

neurotransmitters 161

NHS Direct 259

NICE (National Institute for Health and Clinical Excellence) 227

non-judgemental attitude, importance of 17

non-verbal communication 4–7

noradrenaline 161

note taking 292–4

Nursing and Residential Care Homes Regulations (1984/2002) 53

nursing care settings 42–3

nutrients in the bloodstream 91, 96

O

obesity 148, 253

observation, research method 225–6, 230

occupational health 264–5

oestrogen 103, 118

older people

factors affecting health 253

safety needs of 181

one-to-one health promotion 270

operant conditioning 145–6

operations, providing information to deal with 153–4

opportunities see equal opportunities

opportunity sampling 218

organisational policies 56–9

osmosis 81

osteoarthritis 123

osteoporosis 123

Our Healthier Nation, UK initiatives 258

Health Action Zones 261

Health Improvement Programmes 261–2

Health Protection Agency 262

Healthy Living Centres 259–60

NHS direct 259

smoking cessation programmes 258–9

target setting for GPs 261

overt discrimination 34

P

pacemakers 88

pain

perception of 149–50

physiological responses to 150–1

psychological explanations 151

types of 148–9

panic attacks 162

parasites 187

parasympathetic nervous system 83, 128–9

Parkinson's disease 129

peer pressure and smoking 159

people with disabilities, working safely with 182–3

peptic ulcers 97–8

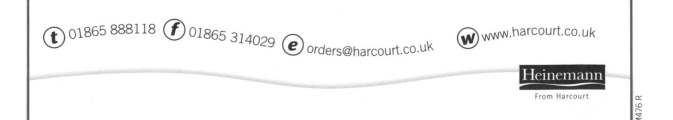